UCLA Symposia on Molecular and Cellular Biology, New Series

Series Editor, C. Fred Fox

RECENT TITLES

Volume 108
Acute Lymphoblastic Leukemia, Robert Peter Gale and Dieter Hoelzer, *Editors*

Volume 109
Frontiers of NMR in Molecular Biology, David Live, Ian M. Armitage, and Dinshaw J. Patel, *Editors*

Volume 110
Protein and Pharmaceutical Engineering, Charles S. Craik, Robert J. Fletterick, C. Robert Matthews, and James A. Wells, *Editors*

Volume 111
Glycobiology, Ernest G. Jaworski and Joseph R. Welply, *Editors*

Volume 112
New Directions in Biological Control: Alternatives for Suppressing Agricultural Pests and Diseases, Ralph R. Baker and Peter E. Dunn, *Editors*

Volume 113
Immunogenicity, Charles A. Janeway, Jr., Jonathan Sprent, and Eli Sercarz, *Editors*

Volume 114
Genetic Mechanisms in Carcinogenesis and Tumor Progression, Curtis Harris and Lance A. Liotta, *Editors*

Volume 115
Growth Regulation of Cancer II, Marc E. Lippman and Robert B. Dickson, *Editors*

Volume 116
Transgenic Models in Medicine and Agriculture, Robert B. Church, *Editor*

Volume 117
Early Embryo Development and Paracrine Relationships, Susan Heyner and Lynn M. Wiley, *Editors*

Volume 118
Cellular and Molecular Biology of Normal and Abnormal Erythroid Membranes, Carl M. Cohen and Jiri Palek, *Editors*

Volume 119
Human Retroviruses, Jerome E. Groopman, Irvin S.Y. Chen, Myron Essex, and Robin A. Weiss, *Editors*

Volume 120
Hematopoiesis, David W. Golde and Steven C. Clark, *Editors*

Volume 121
Defense Molecules, John J. Marchalonis and Carol L. Reinisch, *Editors*

Volume 122
Molecular Evolution, Michael T. Clegg and Stephen J. O'Brien, *Editors*

Volume 123
Molecular Biology of Aging, Caleb E. Finch and Thomas E. Johnson, *Editors*

Volume 124
Papillomaviruses, Peter M. Howley and Thomas R. Broker, *Editors*

Volume 125
Developmental Biology, Eric H. Davidson, Joan V. Ruderman, and James W. Posakony, *Editors*

Volume 126
Biotechnology and Human Genetic Predisposition to Disease, Charles R. Cantor, C. Thomas Caskey, Leroy E. Hood, Daphne Kamely, and Gilbert S. Omenn, *Editors*

Volume 127
Molecular Mechanisms in DNA Replication and Recombination, Charles C. Richardson and I. Robert Lehman, *Editors*

Volume 128
Nucleic Acid Methylation, Gary A. Clawson, Dawn B. Willis, Arthur Weissbach, and Peter A. Jones, *Editors*

Volume 129
Plant Gene Transfer, Christopher J. Lamb and Roger N. Beachy, *Editors*

Volume 130
Parasites: Molecular Biology, Drug and Vaccine Design, Nina M. Agabian and Anthony Cerami, *Editors*

Volume 131
Molecular Biology of the Cardiovascular System, Robert Roberts and Joseph F. Sambrook, *Editors*

Volume 132
Obesity: Towards a Molecular Approach, George A. Bray, Daniel Ricquier, and Bruce M. Spiegelman, *Editors*

Volume 133
Structural and Organizational Aspects of Metabolic Regulation, Paul A. Srere, Mary Ellen Jones, and Christopher K. Mathews, *Editors*

Please contact the publisher for information about previous titles in this series.

UCLA Symposia Board

Cellular and Molecular Biology of Normal and Abnormal Erythroid Membranes

Cellular and Molecular Biology of Normal and Abnormal Erythroid Membranes

Proceedings of a UCLA Colloquium
Held at Taos, New Mexico
February 3–10, 1989

Editors

Carl M. Cohen

Cellular and Molecular Biology
St. Elizabeth's Hospital
Boston, Massachusetts

Jiri Palek

Biomedical Research
St. Elizabeth's Hospital
Boston, Massachusetts

Wiley-Liss, New York

The publication of this volume was facilitated by the authors and editors who submitted the text in a form suitable for direct reproduction without subsequent editing or proofreading by the publisher.

Library of Congress Cataloging-in-Publication Data

UCLA Colloquium "Cellular and Molecular Biology of Normal and Abnormal
   Erythroid Membranes" (1989 : Taos, N.M.)
     Cellular and molecular biology of normal and abnormal erythroid
   membranes : proceedings of a UCLA Colloquium held at Taos, New
   Mexico, February 3-10, 1989 / editors, Carl M. Cohen, Jiri Palek.
        p.   cm. -- (UCLA symposia on molecular and cellular biology ;
   new ser., v. 118)
     "The 1989 UCLA Colloquium "Cellular and Molecular Biology of
   Normal and Abnormal Erythroid Membranes""--Pref.
     Includes bibliographical references.
     ISBN 0-471-56750-7
     1. Erythrocyte membranes--Congresses.   2. Membrane proteins-
   -Congresses.   3. Molecular biology--Congresses.   4. Erythrocyte
   disorders--Congresses.   I. Cohen, Carl M.   II. Palek, Jiri.
   III. University of California, Los Angeles.   IV. Title.
     [DNLM: 1. Erythrocyte Membrane--pathology--congresses.
   2. Erythrocyte Membrane--ultrastructure--congresses.   3. Malaria-
   -pathology--congresses.   4. Membrane Proteins--congresses.
   5. Molecular Biology--congresses.   W3 U17N new ser. v. 118 / WH 150
   U17 1989c]
   QP96.U25   1989
   612.1'11--dc20
   DNLM/DLC
   for Library of Congress   89-70632
                                                                        CIP

Contents

Contributors.   xi
Preface
    Carl M. Cohen and Jiri Palek.   xvii

**I. BIOCHEMISTRY AND MOLECULAR BIOLOGY OF ERYTHROID
MEMBRANE PROTEINS**

Reversible Association of Spectrin With Brain Membrane Proteins and
Implications of a Dynamic Spectrin-Based Membrane Skeleton
    Joseph P. Steiner and Vann Bennett.   1
Localization of the Ankyrin Binding Site on the Cytoplasmic Domain of
Human Erythroid Band 3
    Kevin A. Davies, Samuel E. Lux, and Harvey F. Lodish.   27
Membrane Skeletal Protein 4.1 of Human Erythroid and Non-Erythroid
Cells is Composed of Multiple Isoforms With Novel Sizes, Functions,
and Tissue-Specific Expression
    Tang K. Tang, Zhi Qin, Thomas Leto, Vincent T. Marchesi, and Edward
    J. Benz, Jr.   43
Protein 4.1 mRNA Structure in Normal and Abnormal Erythroid
Membranes
    John G. Conboy.   61
The Erythrocyte Rh Polypeptides
    Peter Agre, Barbara L. Smith, Ali M. Saboori, Bradley M. Denker, and
    Marcel P. de Vetten.   75

II. REGULATION AND DEVELOPMENT OF ERYTHROID MEMBRANES

Phosphorylation-Mediated Associations of the Red Cell Membrane
Skeleton
    Carl M. Cohen, Bipasha GuptaRoy, and Richard Fennell.   89
Multiple Kinases Phosphorylate Spectrin
    Sheenah M. Mische and Jon S. Morrow.   113
Modulation of Erythropoietin Receptor Expression on Erythropoietin
Responsive and Unresponsive Cell Lines
    Virginia C. Broudy, Nancy Lin, Betty Nakamoto, and Thalia
    Papayannopoulou.   131

The Biogenesis of Membrane Skeleton in Mammalian Red Cells
Manjit Hanspal, Jatinder S. Hanspal, and Jiri Palek.   145

Transport of Phosphatidylserine Across Erythrocyte Membranes
Jerome Connor and Alan J. Schroit.   161

III. MOLECULAR BIOLOGY AND GENETICS OF ERYTHROID
MEMBRANE ABNORMALITIES

Molecular Anatomy of Erythrocyte Membrane Skeleton in Health and
Disease
Shih-Chun Liu, Laura H. Derick, and Jiri Palek.   171

Consequences of Structural Abnormalities on the Mechanical Properties
of Red Blood Cell Membrane
Richard E. Waugh and Sally L. Marchesi.   185

Use of the Polymerase Chain Reaction for the Detection and
Characterization of Mutations Causing Hereditary Elliptocytosis
K.E. Sahr, M. Garbarz, D. Dhermy, M.C. Lecomte, P. Boivin, P. Agre,
K. Laughinghouse, A. Scarpa, T. Coetzer, J. Palek, S.L. Marchesi, and
B.G. Forget.   201

Molecular Heterogeneity of α Spectrin Mutants in Hereditary
Elliptocytosis/Pyropoikilocytosis
Theresa Coetzer, Jack Lawler, Josef Prchal, Ken Sahr, Bernard Forget,
and Jiri Palek.   211

The Diversity of Hereditary Elliptocytosis in North Africa: Protein
Aspects and Molecular Genetics
L. Morlé, A.-F. Roux, F. Morlé, N. Alloisio, B. Pothier, K.E. Sahr,
B.G. Forget, J. Godet, and J. Delaunay.   223

Clinical Expression of Spectrin αI Variants
P. Boivin, M.C. Lecomte, M. Garbarz, C. Féo, O. Bournier, I. Devaux,
C. Galand, H. Gautero, and D. Dhermy.   235

IV. MOLECULAR AND CELLULAR EFFECTS ON THE ERYTHROCYTE
MEMBRANE OF MALARIAL PARASITE INVASION

A New Cytoadherence Property of Plasmodium falciparum-Infected
Erythrocytes: Rosetting With Uninfected Erythrocytes
Shiroma M. Handunnetti, Aileen D. Gilladoga, and Russell J. Howard. .   249

Discrete Sites of Permeation Induced in the Human Red Cell Membrane
by Malaria Parasites
Z. Ioav Cabantchik, Josefine Silfen, and Hava Glickstein.   267

A Modified Band 3 Protein, Expressed on the Surface of Erythrocytes
Infected With a Knobby Line Plasmodium falciparum (Human Malaria),
is Involved in Cytoadherence
I.W. Sherman and E. Winograd.   283

Invasion of Erythrocytes Deficient in Glycophorin C (β, β_1, and γ) by
Plasmodium falciparum **Malaria Parasites**
    T.J. Hadley, F.W. Klotz, D.J. Anstee, J.D. Haynes, and L.H. Miller. . . .   **301**

A Malaria Phosphatidylinositol-Specific Phospholipase C: A Possible
Role in Merozoite Maturation and Erythrocyte Invasion
    Catherine Braun Breton, Gordon Langsley, Jean-Christophe Barale, and
    Luis H. Pereira da Silva. **315**

Index. **333**

Contributors

Peter Agre, Departments of Medicine and Cell Biology/Anatomy, Johns Hopkins University School of Medicine, Baltimore, MD 21205 **[75, 201]**

N. Alloisio, CNRS URA 1171, Faculté de Médecine Grange-Blanche, 69373 Lyon Cedex 08, France **[223]**

D.J. Anstee, Division of Hematology/ Oncology, University of Louisville School of Medicine, Louisville, KY 40292; present address: Southwestern Regional Blood Transfusion Centre, Bristol BS105ND, England **[301]**

Jean-Christophe Barale, Department of Experimental Parasitology, Institut Pasteur, 75015 Paris, France **[315]**

Vann Bennett, Howard Hughes Medical Institute and the Department of Biochemistry, Duke University Medical Center, Durham, NC 27710 **[1]**

Edward J. Benz, Jr., Departments of Internal Medicine and Human Genetics, Yale University School of Medicine, New Haven, CT 06510 **[43]**

P. Boivin, INSERM U. 160, Hôpital Beaujon, 92118 Clichy Cedex, France **[201, 235]**

Odile Bournier, INSERM U. 160, Hôpital Beaujon, 92118 Clichy Cedex, France **[235]**

Catherine Braun Breton, Department of Experimental Parasitology, Institut Pasteur, 75015 Paris, France **[315]**

Virginia C. Broudy, Department of Medicine, Division of Hematology, University of Washington, Seattle, WA 98195 **[131]**

Z. Ioav Cabantchik, Department of Biological Chemistry, Institute of Life Sciences, Hebrew University, Jerusalem, Israel 91904 **[267]**

Theresa Coetzer, Department of Biomedical Research, St. Elizabeth's Hospital of Boston, Boston, MA 02135; present address: Department of Hematology, South African Institute for Medical Research, Johannesburg, South Africa 2000 **[201, 211]**

Carl M. Cohen, Department of Biomedical Research, St. Elizabeth's Hospital of Boston, Boston, MA 02135 **[89]**

John G. Conboy, Cancer Research Institute, University of California, San Francisco, San Francisco, CA 94143 **[61]**

The numbers in brackets are the opening page numbers of the contributors' articles.

Jerome Connor, Department of Cell Biology, The University of Texas M.D. Anderson Cancer Center, Houston, TX 77030 [161]

Luis H. Pereira da Silva, Department of Experimental Parasitology, Institut Pasteur, 75015 Paris, France [315]

Kevin A. Davies, Whitehead Institute for Biomedical Research, Cambridge, MA 02142 [27]

J. Delaunay, CNRS URA 1171, Faculté de Médecine Grange-Blanche, 69373 Lyon Cedex 08, France [223]

Bradley M. Denker, Departments of Medicine and Cell Biology/Anatomy, Johns Hopkins University School of Medicine, Baltimore, MD 21205; present address: Departments of Medicine and Nephrology, Brigham and Women's Hospital, Harvard Medical School, Boston, MA 02115 [75]

Laura H. Derick, Department of Biomedical Research, St. Elizabeth's Hospital of Boston, Boston, MA 02135 [171]

Isabelle Devaux, INSERM U. 160, Hôpital Beaujon, 92118 Clichy Cedex, France [235]

Marcel P. de Vetten, Departments of Medicine and Cell Biology/Anatomy, Johns Hopkins University School of Medicine, Baltimore, MD 21205; present address: Erasmus University School of Medicine, 3011 ML Rotterdam, The Netherlands [75]

Didier Dhermy, INSERM U. 160, Hôpital Beaujon, 92118 Clichy Cedex, France [201, 235]

Richard Fennell, Department of Biomedical Research, St. Elizabeth's Hospital of Boston, Boston, MA 02135 [89]

Claude Féo, INSERM U. 160, Hôpital du Kremlin Bicetre, 94275 Le Kremlin Bicetre Cedex, France [235]

B.G. Forget, Department of Medicine, Yale University School of Medicine, New Haven, CT 06510 [201, 211, 223]

C. Galand, INSERM U. 160, Hôpital Beaujon, 92118 Clichy Cedex, France [235]

Michel Garbarz, INSERN U. 160, Hôpital Beaujon, 92118 Clichy Cedex, France [201, 235]

Huguette Gautero, INSERM U. 160, Hôpital Beaujon, 92118 Clichy Cedex, France [235]

Aileen D. Gilladoga, Laboratory for Infectious Diseases, DNAX Research Institute, Palo Alto, CA 94304-1104 [249]

Hava Glickstein, Department of Biological Chemistry, Institute of Life Sciences, Hebrew University, Jerusalem, Israel 91904 [267]

J. Godet, CNRS UMR 4, Université Claude-Bernard Lyon-I, 69622 Villeurbanne Cedex, France [223]

Bipasha Gupta Roy, Department of Biomedical Research, St. Elizabeth's Hospital of Boston, Boston, MA 02135 [89]

T.J. Hadley, Division of Hematology, University of Louisville School of Medicine, Louisville, KY 40292 [301]

Shiroma M. Handunnetti, Laboratory for Infectious Diseases, DNAX Research Institute, Palo Alto, CA 94304-1104 **[249]**

Jatinder S. Hanspal, Department of Biomedical Research, St. Elizabeth's Hospital of Boston, Boston, MA 02135 **[145]**

Manjit Hanspal, Department of Biomedical Research, St. Elizabeth's Hospital of Boston, Boston, MA 02135 **[145]**

J.D. Haynes, Division of Hematology/Oncology, University of Louisville School of Medicine, Louisville, KY 40292; present address: Division of Communicable Disease and Immunology, Walter Reed Army Institute of Research, Washington, DC 20307 **[301]**

Russell J. Howard, Laboratory for Infectious Diseases, DNAX Research Institute, Palo Alto, CA 94304-1104 **[249]**

F.W. Klotz, Division of Hematology/Oncology, University of Louisville School of Medicine, Louisville, KY 40292; present address: Division of Communicable Disease and Immunology, Walter Reed Army Institute of Research, Washington, DC 20307 **[301]**

Gordon Langsley, Department of Experimental Parasitology, Institut Pasteur, 75015 Paris, France **[315]**

K. Laughinghouse, Department of Medicine, Yale University School of Medicine, New Haven, CT 06510 **[201]**

John Lawler, Department of Biomedical Research, St. Elizabeth's Hospital of Boston, Boston, MA 02135; present address: Department of Pathology, Brigham & Women's Hospital, Boston, MA 02115 **[211]**

Marie-Christine Lecomte, INSERM U. 160, Hôpital Beaujon, 92118 Clichy Cedex, France **[201, 235]**

Thomas Leto, Department of Pathology, Yale University School of Medicine, New Haven, CT 06510; present address: National Institute of Allergy and Infectious Diseases, National Institutes of Health, Bethesda, MD 20892 **[43]**

Nancy Lin, Department of Medicine, Division of Hematology, University of Washington, Seattle, WA 98195 **[131]**

Shih-Chun Liu, Department of Biomedical Research, St. Elizabeth's Hospital of Boston, Boston, MA 02135 **[171]**

Harvey F. Lodish, Whitehead Institute for Biomedical Research, Cambridge, MA 02139 and the Department of Biology, Massachusetts Institute of Technology, Cambridge, MA 02139 **[27]**

Samuel E. Lux, Department of Pediatrics, The Children's Hospital, Harvard Medical School, Boston, MA 02115 **[27]**

Sally L. Marchesi, Department of Pathology, Yale University School of Medicine, New Haven, CT 06510 **[185, 201]**

Vincent T. Marchesi, Department of Pathology, Yale University School of Medicine, New Haven, CT 06510 **[43]**

L.H. Miller, Division of Hematology/ Oncology, University of Louisville School of Medicine, Louisville, KY 40292; present address: Laboratory for Parasitic Diseases, National Institute of Allergy and Infectious Diseases, National Institutes of Health, Bethesda, MD 20205 [301]

Sheenah M. Mische, Laboratory of Pathology, Yale University School of Medicine, New Haven, CT 06510 [113]

F. Morlé, CNRS UMR 4, Université Claude-Bernard Lyon-I, 69622 Villeurbanne Cedex, France [223]

L. Morlé, CNRS URA 1171, Faculté de Médecine Grange-Blanche, 69373 Lyon Cedex 08, France [223]

Jon S. Morrow, Laboratory of Pathology, Yale University School of Medicine, New Haven, CT 06510 [113]

Betty Nakamoto, Department of Medicine, Division of Hematology, University of Washington, Seattle, WA 98195 [131]

Jiri Palek, Department of Biomedical Research, St. Elizabeth's Hospital of Boston, Boston, MA 02135 [145, 171, 201, 211]

Thalia Papayannopoulou, Department of Medicine, Division of Hematology, University of Washington, Seattle, WA 98195 [131]

B. Pothier, CNRS URA 1171, Faculté de Médecine Grange-Blanche, 69373 Lyon Cedex 08, France [223]

Josef Prchal, Division of Hematology/ Oncology, University of Alabama at Birmingham, Birmingham, AL 35294 [211]

Zhi Qin, Department of Pathology, Yale University School of Medicine, New Haven, CT 06510 [43]

A.-F. Roux, CNRS URA 1171, Faculté de Médecine Grange-Blanche, 69373 Lyon Cedex 08, France and CNRS UMR 4, Université Claude-Bernard Lyon-I Villeurbanne Cedex, France [223]

Ali M. Saboori, Departments of Medicine and Cell Biology/Anatomy, Johns Hopkins University School of Medicine, Baltimore, MD 21205; present address: Department of Environmental Health Sciences, Johns Hopkins University School of Hygiene, Baltimore, MD 21205 [75]

Ken Sahr, Department of Medicine, Yale University School of Medicine, New Haven, CT 06510; present address: Department of Biomedical Research, St. Elizabeth's Hospital of Boston, Boston, MA 02135 [201, 211, 223]

A. Scarpa, Department of Medicine, Yale University School of Medicine, New Haven, CT 06510 [201]

Alan J. Schroit, Department of Cell Biology, The University of Texas M.D. Anderson Cancer Center, Houston, TX 77030 [161]

I.W. Sherman, Department of Biology, University of California, Riverside, Riverside, CA 92521 [283]

Josefine Silfen, Department of Biological Chemistry, Institute of Life Sciences, Hebrew University, Jerusalem, Israel 91904 [267]

Barbara L. Smith, Departments of Medicine and Cell Biology/Anatomy, Johns Hopkins University School of Medicine, Baltimore, MD 21205 **[75]**

Joseph P. Steiner, Howard Hughes Medical Institute and the Department of Biochemistry, Duke University Medical Center, Durham, NC 27710 **[1]**

Tang K. Tang, Departments of Internal Medicine and Human Genetics, Yale University School of Medicine, New Haven, CT 06510; present address: Institute of Biomedical Sciences, Academia Sinica, Taipei 11529, Taiwan **[43]**

Richard E. Waugh, Department of Biophysics, University of Rochester, School of Medicine and Dentistry, Rochester, NY 14642 **[185]**

E. Winograd, Department of Biology, University of California, Riverside, Riverside, CA 92521 **[283]**

Preface

The 1989 UCLA Colloquium **Cellular and Molecular Biology of Normal and Abnormal Erythroid Membranes** was held during a truly impressive snowstorm in early February 1989 in Taos, New Mexico. Equally impressive, however, was the quality and quantity of new and exciting work that was presented at the meeting. One of the principal goals of the meeting was to bring together (1) basic scientists working on the cellular and molecular biology of erythroid membranes and (2) clinical researchers studying inherited hemolytic anemias, malaria, and other diseases affecting erythroid cells. From this point of view the meeting was clearly a great success, as attested by the contents of this volume and by the lengthy and vigorous discussions that took place each evening around the poster boards at the Kachina Lodge.

Considerable new information about ankyrins was presented, giving new insights into the primary structure and association of this protein in both erythroid and non-erythroid cells. Similarly, new chapters in the unfolding saga of erythroid and non-erythroid band 4.1 isoforms were presented. The above findings make it clear that the expression of these protein isoforms is both tissue-specific and developmentally regulated and that understanding the factors that regulate their expression will be a major challenge in the near future.

Studies of regulatory aspects of skeletal organization focused on spectrin and band 4.1 phosphorylation. These studies emphasized that skeletal protein phosphorylation plays a critical role in regulating the associations of skeletal proteins and that a new functional role can be assigned to spectrin phosphorylation. Regulation at a more fundamental level was addressed by several speakers dealings with the biogenesis of the membrane skeleton of both normal and abnormal red cells and the structure and expression of the erythropoietin receptor in erythroid precursor cells. The identification and structure of the receptor now offers new opportunities to study the specifics of the erythropoietin-dependent signal transduction pathway.

Studies of the ultrastructure of erythrocyte membrane skeletons with a variety of molecular defects and the analysis of defective cells using micropipet techniques emphasized the diversity of skeletal abnormalities available as experiments of nature.

Furthermore, a considerable amount of new information has been presented on the characterization of various skeletal protein mutations, in terms of their functional and clinical heterogeneity as well as the nature of the underlying defect both at the protein primary structure and the cDNA levels.

Finally, a session on malaria focused on some of the exciting advances being made in the study of this still-devastating disease. New information on how malaria-infected red cells adhere to endothelial cells was presented, and a possible relationship to a modification in band 3 was suggested. Several presentations highlighted parasite-induced alterations in the red cell membrane including permeability changes and lipid alterations. This session and the other sessions on skeletal defects gave many conference participants a glimpse of the tremendous impact that basic studies of erythroid membranes and membrane skeletons is likely to have in the near future on the diagnosis and treatment of diseases affecting erythroid cells.

The organizers would like to thank all those who attended the meeting for making it a memorable and stimulating occasion. Sponsorship for this meeting was provided by the Director's Sponsor Fund established by E.I. du Pont de Nemours & Co., Inc.; Hoffmann-La Roche, Inc.; Immunex Corporation; Monsanto Corporation; Schering Corporation; and the Upjohn Company. We also thank the staff of the UCLA Symposia for handling the meeting logistics and dealing with the myriad of details that inevitably arise.

Carl M. Cohen
Jiri Palek

Cellular and Molecular Biology of Normal
and Abnormal Erythroid Membranes, pages 1–26
© 1990 Alan R. Liss, Inc.

REVERSIBLE ASSOCIATION OF SPECTRIN WITH BRAIN MEMBRANE
PROTEINS AND IMPLICATIONS OF A DYNAMIC SPECTRIN-BASED
MEMBRANE SKELETON

Joseph P. Steiner and Vann Bennett

Howard Hughes Medical Institute and the Department of
Biochemisty, Duke University Medical Center,
Durham, NC 27710

ABSTRACT

Brain spectrin reassociates in in vitro binding assays
with protease sensitive sites in highly extracted brain
membranes quantitatively depleted of spectrin and ankyrin.
Spectrin binds with high affinity (K_D=3-10nM) to these
membrane sites, with a capacity (at least 50 pmol/mg
membrane protein) approximating the amount of spectrin in
brain. Brain membranes also contain high affinity binding
sites for erythrocyte spectrin, but with 4-fold lower
binding capacity than brain spectrin. The beta subunit of
brain spectrin contains the major ankyrin-independent
binding activity of brain spectrin. Erythrocyte spectrin,
and most likely brain spectrin as well, contain distinct
binding domains for ankyrin and brain membrane protein
sites, since the active M_r=72,000 spectrin-binding fragment
of erythrocyte ankyrin failed to compete for binding of
spectrin to brain membrane proteins. Some of the spectrin
binding-proteins associate with both isoforms of spectrin,
while some sites associate preferentially with either
erythrocyte spectrin or brain spectrin. A small number of
spectrin-binding sites (10,000-15,000 copies/cell) exists in
erythrocyte membranes, where brain spectrin binds to these
sites better than erythrocyte spectrin. Direct and
ankyrin-mediated linkages of spectrin are differentially
regulated by physiological concentrations of
calcium/calmodulin, where calmodulin has no effect on
spectrin-ankyrin interactions but blocks binding of brain
spectrin to ankyrin-depleted synaptosomal membranes.
Inhibition is due to a receptor-mediated process, and not

proteolysis, since the effect of calcium/calmodulin is
reversed by the calmodulin antagonist trifluoperazine and by
chelation of calcium with NaEGTA. The target of calmodulin
is most likely the spectrin attachment protein(s) rather
than spectrin itself. Direct linkage of spectrin to the
plasma membrane subject to calcium-dependent inhibition by
calmodulin has implications for membrane skeleton biogenesis
and assembly, targeting of spectrin isoforms to specialized
regions of cells, and regional, site-directed
disassembly/reassembly of a nonerythroid spectrin-based
membrane skeleton.

INTRODUCTION

Brain spectrin is a major structural protein in neural
tissues and is structurally and functionally similar to
erythrocyte spectrin. Both brain and erythrocyte spectrins
share common antigenic sites, contain a distinctive flexible
rod-like morphology (1-5), a similar association of alpha
and beta subunit heterodimers into tetramers, strikingly
conserved 106-amino acid repeats throughout the length of
individual spectrin subunits (6-8), and localization to the
membrane fractions in erythrocytes and nervous tissue,
respectively (9-11). Erythrocyte spectrin is the major
component of a two-dimensional network of proteins, referred
to as the spectrin-based membrane skeleton, which has been
visualized by electron microscopy (12-14) as a repeating
hexagonal array of proteins that lines the cytoplasmic
surface of the erythrocyte plasma membrane. This protein
meshwork provides mechanical support and is responsible for
cell shape and the elastic properties of the red cell plasma
membrane (15-18). Spectrin is attached to the plasma
membrane via high affinity interaction with ankyrin (19),
which is in turn linked to the transmembrane
bicarbonate/chloride transporter called band 3 (20). In
addition, erythrocyte spectrin also is linked to the plasma
membrane along with actin protofilaments by accessory
membrane proteins such as protein 4.1 (21,22).
A neural spectrin-based membrane skeleton most likely
exists and contains protein components similar in structure
and function to erythrocyte skeletal proteins spectrin,
ankyrin, protein 4.1 and adducin. Based on the erythrocyte
membrane skeleton model, one linkage of brain spectrin to
membranes is likely to be provided by brain ankyrin which
binds with high affinity to brain spectrin (23,24) and also

associates with high affinity with binding sites in brain membranes (25), one of which is the voltage-dependent sodium channel (26). However, brain spectrin is also likely to fulfill additional roles and interact with proteins not found in mammalian red cells. Recently, an alternative method of attaching spectrin to the plasma membrane was determined, where spectrin interacts directly with membrane proteins contained on highly stripped brain membranes depleted of spectrin and ankyrin (27). In addition, direct association of spectrin with synaptosomal membrane protein(s) was competitively inhibited by calmodulin in a calcium dependent manner (28). The purpose of this paper is to review these ankyrin-independent linkages of spectrin directly to brain membrane proteins and the regulation of these interactions by calcium/calmodulin. The implications of this alternative method for spectrin-membrane attachment with respect to membrane skeleton assembly, targeting of spectrin isoforms to specialized regions of cells, and site directed disassembly/reassembly of the spectrin-based membrane skeleton will be discussed.

METHODS

Procedures were performed as described (27,28).

RESULTS

Brain Spectrin Binds with High Affinity to Ankyrin-Independent Protein Sites in Stripped Brain Membranes.

Spectrin, purified from bovine brain, was demonstrated to bind specifically to bovine brain membranes depleted of spectrin, ankyrin, and other peripheral membrane proteins by alkaline pH extraction (Fig. 1). These in vitro binding interactions occurred optimally at physiological ionic strength and pH conditions (50 mM NaCl and pH 6.8-6.9) and are thus likely to be biologically relevant. Binding of spectrin to the stripped brain membranes requires a protein, since predigestion of membrane proteins with alpha-chymotrypsin destroyed specific spectrin-membrane interactions. Although this result indicates that the ankyrin-independent membrane binding site for brain spectrin involves a protein, membrane lipids may still participate in the interaction.

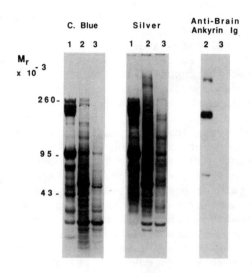

FIGURE 1. Sodium hydroxide-extracted brain membranes
are completely stripped of ankyrin and peripheral membrane
proteins. Demyelinated bovine brain membranes (1 mg/ml)
were extracted with 0.1 N NaOH and electrophoresed
on SDS-polyacrylamide gels and either stained with Coomassie
Blue, Silver Stain (Bio-Rad) reagent, or electrophoretically
transferred to nitrocellulose paper followed by
immunoblotting with anti-brain ankyrin Ig. Panel A,
Coomassie Blue-stained pig erythrocyte ghosts (lane 1),
demyelinated bovine brain membranes (lane 2), and
NaOH-extracted brain membranes (lane 3). Panel B contains a
silver-stained profile of samples contained in panel A.
Panel C shows anti-brain ankyrin immunoreactivity in lanes 2
and 3.

In order to quantitate spectrin-membrane protein
interactions, Scatchard analysis of binding as a function of
spectrin concentration (Fig. 2) revealed a curvilinear
binding isotherm, suggesting that either brain spectrin is
binding to at least two distinct classes of noninteracting
sites, or that binding occurs with negative cooperativity to
one class of proteins. Assuming multiple classes of
receptor proteins, a high affinity portion of the curve has

a K_D of approximately 3-4 nM and a capacity ranging from 25 to 45 pmol/mg NaOH-extracted membrane protein. This capacity for spectrin binding corresponds to a maximum of approximately 25 pmol/mg total demyelinated membrane protein, which is comparable to the amount of spectrin tetramer in brain (30 pmol/mg). Binding of spectrin also occurs to a lower affinity class of sites (K_D=30-50 nM) of indeterminate capacity (at least 50 pmol/mg membrane protein) in brain membranes. Alternatively, brain spectrin may associate with negative cooperativity with a single class of interacting sites. These nonlinear Scatchard plots of spectrin binding are very complex, and further interpretation of the data is not possible since: (a) brain spectrin consists of a mixture of two isoforms, each of which may bind differently to its own receptor, and (b) both subunits of brain spectrin may independently participate in binding interactions.

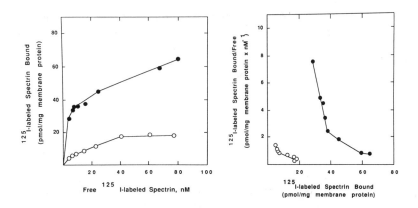

FIGURE 2. Binding of increasing concentration of brain (•) and erythrocyte (o) spectrin to brain membranes. Binding of ^{125}I-Bolton-Hunter-labeled brain spectrin (9.8 nM, 1.4×10^5 cpm/ug) and ^{125}I-Bolton-Hunter-labeled erythrocyte spectrin tetramer (9.9 nM, 1.8×10^5 cpm/ug) to

sodium hydroxide-extracted brain membranes was measured in
the presence of increasing concentrations of unlabeled brain
and erythrocyte spectrin tetramers, respectively. Values
for nonspecific binding using heat-treated (67°C, 15 min for
brain spectrin, 58°C for 15 min for red blood cell spectrin
tetramer) ^{125}I-labeled spectrins were subtracted. The
specific activity of the ^{125}I-labeled spectrins was
calculated at each data point of unlabeled spectrin
displacement, and the data was transformed into saturation
binding isotherms (A) and into Scatchard plots (B), where
B/F=N/K-B/K and B is pmol of spectrin bound/mg of membrane
protein, F is the concentration of unbound spectrin (nM), N
is the number of binding sites, pmol/mg membrane protein,
and K is the dissociation constant (Scatchard, 1949).

It was not possible to directly compare the
ankyrin-dependent and ankyrin-independent contributions of
spectrin-membrane binding, since methods are not available
for complete removal of spectrin without extraction of
ankyrin. There are at least 50 pmol/mg total membrane
protein of ankyrin-independent spectrin-binding sites (Fig.
2), while ankyrin is present in brain membranes at 100
pmol/mg membrane protein (24). The capacities of both
ankyrin and ankyrin-independent spectrin binding sites are
in excess of the amount of spectrin in brain membranes (30
pmol/mg membrane protein), suggesting that attachment of
spectrin to brain membranes may occur physiologically
utilizing either or both types of linkage.

Role of Brain Spectrin Alpha and Beta Subunits in Brain
Membrane Interactions.

The alpha and beta subunits of bovine brain spectrin
were purified as described (29) and compared with total
brain spectrin in ability to displace binding of
radiolabeled spectrin to brain membranes The major binding
activity is confined to the purified beta subunit, which
displaced 50% of binding at 18 nM unlabeled subunits
compared to 12 nM for total brain spectrin. Brain spectrin
alpha subunit also inhibited binding of brain spectrin, but
at 7-fold lower potency (about 110 nM required for 50%
inhibition). These results suggested that the beta subunit
contains the major binding activity, and alpha subunit a
minor activity, both of which together may cooperatively

form the complete reactive binding domain. Alternatively, the beta subunit may contain the binding domain for a higher affinity (K_D=3-4 nM) class of sites, and the alpha subunit may preferentially bind to a lower affinity class of binding sites indicated by the curvilinear Scatchard plot (Fig. 2).

Brain and Erythrocyte Spectrin Bind to Distinct
Ankyrin-Independent Sites in Brain Membranes.

Brain contains an isoform of spectrin with a beta subunit closely related to the beta subunit of erythrocyte spectrin that is localized in different regions of neurons from the major brain isoform of spectrin (30). It was therefore of interest to measure binding of erythrocyte spectrin to brain membranes. Human erythrocyte spectrin exhibited a nonlinear Scatchard plot similar to that observed for brain spectrin, although the capacity of binding sites was reduced 4-fold compared to brain spectrin (Fig. 2). The curvilinear Scatchard plots for human erythrocyte spectrin could be due to multiple spectrin-binding proteins or an interacting class of binding proteins, as similarly described above for brain spectrin. This data demonstrated that both brain and erythrocyte forms of spectrin can associate specifically to at least one class of ankyrin-independent binding sites in brain membranes with increased binding capacity for brain spectrin.

To determine if brain and erythrocyte spectrin are binding to the same classes of brain membrane proteins, both unlabeled erythrocyte and brain spectrin were tested for the ability to compete for membrane binding of labeled brain and erythrocyte spectrins. While unlabeled brain spectrin inhibited greater than 90% of binding of labeled brain spectrin and unlabeled erythrocyte spectrin inhibited the binding of labeled erythrocyte spectrin in a similar manner, both erythrocyte spectrin and brain spectrin partially inhibited membrane binding by the other spectrin isoform at 5 to 10 fold lower potency. These crossover inhibition binding studies suggested that spectrin in brain interacts with three types of sites, sites that bind preferentially to either brain spectrin or erythroid-like spectrin, and site(s) that interact with both isoforms of spectrin. A potential complication is that brain spectrin contains both fodrin and an erythrocyte-like form of spectrin, and these isoforms may account for some of the crossover inhibitory activity of the brain spectrin.

Brain and erythrocyte spectrin could associate with ankyrin-independent sites in brain membranes by two possible mechanisms: (a) Spectrin may interact at its ankyrin-binding site with proteins possessing conformational homology to ankyrin or (b) Spectrin may associate with brain membranes at site(s) distinct from the ankyrin-binding site. The $M_r=72,000$ spectrin binding fragment of erythrocyte ankyrin inhibits spectrin-ankyrin associations (31) and provides a tool to evaluate possible inhibition of spectrin-ankyrin interactions. While the $M_r=72,000$ ankyrin fragment inhibited greater than 90% of the binding of erythrocyte spectrin to ankyrin-containing erythrocyte vesicles, the ankyrin fragment was ineffective at competing for binding of either labeled erythrocyte or brain spectrin to stripped brain membranes. Therefore, erythrocyte spectrin and most likely brain spectrin, associates with a brain membrane protein at a domain on the beta subunit of spectrin distinct from the ankyrin-binding domain.

Ankyrin-Independent Site(s) for Brain Spectrin in Erythrocyte Membranes.

Removal of ankyrin and other peripheral membrane proteins (bands 4.1, 4.2 and 6) from erythrocyte membranes caused greater than a 90% reduction in binding of erythrocyte spectrin tetramer to these stripped red cell vesicles. The remaining 5-8% of binding of erythrocyte spectrin cannot be accounted for by ankyrin and represents ankyrin-independent sites. Since brain spectrin associates with erythrocyte ankyrin with reduced affinity compared to erythrocyte spectrin (5), the binding of brain spectrin was less sensitive to residual ankyrin in extracted vesicles. Brain spectrin bound to ankyrin-depleted vesicles with an apparent capacity, estimated from a Scatchard plot, of about 15-20 pmol/mg membrane protein, corresponding to 10,000-15,000 copies/cell. This binding of brain spectrin to ankyrin-depleted vesicles is independent of ankyrin, since the $M_r=72,000$ spectrin-binding fragment of erythrocyte ankyrin failed to compete for brain spectrin binding to ankyrin-depleted erythrocyte vesicles. Furthermore, these ankyrin-independent spectrin binding sites in stripped erythrocyte vesicles are bound preferentially by brain spectrin, as determined from crossover inhibition studies where unlabeled brain spectrin was 2-3 fold more active than erythrocyte spectrin in competition for binding of

^{125}I-labeled erythrocyte spectrin to ankyrin-depleted erythrocyte vesicles.

Calmodulin Competitively and Reversibly Inhibits Association of Brain Spectrin with Synaptosomal Membrane Protein.

Little is known about the regulatory events that mediate the interactions of spectrin with spectrin-binding proteins. While spectrin is phosphorylated in vivo by cAMP-independent protein kinases, no known activity of spectrin is modulated by phosphorylation. Other modifications of proteins which can regulate activities of the protein, such as methylation and fatty-acid acylation, do not mediate binding activities of spectrin, since there has been no evidence presented to suggest that spectrin is either methylated or fatty acid-acylated. On the other hand, tissue spectrins have been shown to bind calmodulin with high affinity in a calcium-dependent manner (3,32-34). Although no functional significance has of yet been ascribed to the binding of calmodulin by spectrin, the calcium-dependent association of calmodulin-binding proteins with calmodulin modulates the activities of these proteins, such as caldesmon (35), myosin light chain kinase (36), microtubule-associated proteins (37) and adducin (38). Therefore it seemed possible that calcium/calmodulin might regulate some binding activities of brain spectrin.

Binding of ^{125}I-labeled brain spectrin to hydroxide-extracted synaptosomal membranes was inhibited by calmodulin in the presence of calcium (Fig. 3). Calmodulin, in the absence of calcium, decreased membrane binding of spectrin by only 15%, and calcium alone (from 10 nM to 50 uM) had no effect on binding of spectrin. However, in the presence of 10 uM free calcium, brain spectrin binding was decreased by greater than 75% at 5 uM calmodulin. Half maximal inhibition of binding of brain spectrin was achieved at about 1 uM calmodulin, which is well within the physiological concentration range of calmodulin in brain(estimated to be up to 25 uM) (39). Submicromolar calcium concentrations in addition to calmodulin are sufficient for inhibition of binding of brain spectrin to membranes, with half-maximal inhibition achieved at pCa=6.8-6.5 (0.16-0.3 uM) and maximal inhibition at pCa of 6.2 to 6(0.6-1 uM). Inhibition of spectrin binding by Ca^{2+}/ calmodulin is not caused by proteolysis of spectrin or membrane proteins (40) or due to alteration or denaturation of spectrin since: a) direct analysis of ^{125}I-labeled brain spectrin from pellets and supernatants of assays with Ca^{2+}/calmodulin showed brain spectrin was intact (Fig. 3B); b) NaOH-stripped synaptosomal membranes treated with calcium/calmodulin, followed by NaEGTA washes exhibited no reduction in binding compared to control membranes; c) ^{125}I-labeled brain spectrin, exposed to synaptosomal membranes in the presence of Ca^{2+}/calmodulin and subsequently treated with NaEGTA, retains an unaltered ability to bind to synaptosomal membranes.

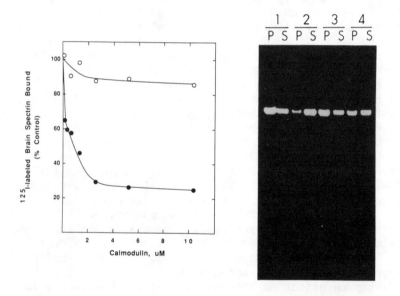

FIGURE 3.   Calmodulin inhibits brain spectrin binding to NaOH-stripped synaptosomal membranes in the presence of calcium.   A, ^{125}I-labeled brain spectrin (5.1 nM, 4.61 x 10^{5} cpm/ug) was preincubated with various concentrations of calmodulin in the presence (•) or absence (o) of 10 uM free calcium prior to addition of 8.7 ug of NaOH-extracted rat brain synaptosomal membranes for 60 min reaction at 4°C. Specific binding of brain spectrin, whether in the presence of EGTA, Ca^{2+}/EGTA, calmodulin or Ca^{2+}/EGTA/CaM, was determined by subtracting values of bound heat-treated (67°C, 15 min) ^{125}I-labeled brain spectrin from total membrane-bound spectrin.   Binding of ^{125}I-labeled spectrin

in the presence of CaM alone (o) (in EGTA-containing assay
binding buffer) was compared to spectrin binding in absence
of CaM. Spectrin binding in the presence of 10 uM Ca^{2+}/CaM
(o) was compared to membrane-bound spectrin in 10 uM Ca^{2+}
containing buffer. Binding of brain spectrin to
synaptosomal membranes in the presence of EGTA alone,
or Ca^{2+}/EGTA buffer yielding 10 uM free calcium was nearly
equivalent (±7-10%) and considered 100% control bound. B,
binding of ^{125}I-labeled brain spectrin to stripped
synaptosomal membranes was performed as in A above. The
membrane-bound spectrin-containing pellets (P) were
dissolved in 50 ul of 1 x gel electrophoresis buffer and 40
ul of the supernatant (S) was mixed with 10 ul of 5 x
electrophoresis buffer. Pellets and supernatants were then
subjected to polyacrylamide gel electrophoresis. The gels
were dried down and radiolabeled brain spectrin was
visualized by autoradiography. Samples were: lanes 1,
pellets and supernatants of ^{125}I-labeled brain spectrin
binding to NaOH-stripped synaptosomal membranes (control
binding). Lanes 2, pellets and supernatants of brain
spectrin binding in the presence of 10 uM free calcium, 5 uM
calmodulin; lanes 3, pellets and supernatants of brain
spectrin bound to synaptosomal membranes as in lanes 2
except that after 60 min, NaEGTA was added to 3 mM final
concentration, followed by 60 min of further incubation and
subsequent centrifugation; lanes 4, pellets and supernatants
containing ^{125}I-labeled brain spectrin treated as in lanes
3, above except that trifluoperazine was added instead of
Na-EGTA to a final concentration of 40 uM.

The effects of calcium/calmodulin on binding of brain
spectrin to stripped synaptosomal membranes are inhibited
and reversed by antagonists of calmodulin. Trifluoperazine,
a potent inhibitor of calmodulin function (41) completely
inhibits Ca^{2+}/calmodulin-mediated effects on spectrin
binding at 50 uM. Calcium/calmodulin inhibition of brain
spectrin binding was subsequently reversed by addition of
trifluoperazine, requiring about 120 uM trifluoperazine for
complete reversal of inhibition. Chelation of calcium with
increased NaEGTA also inhibits (not shown) and reverses
(Fig. 3B) calcium/calmodulin effects.
    Dixon plot analysis of the membrane binding of
[125]I-labeled brain spectrin revealed competitive binding
inhibition by calcium/calmodulin, with an apparent K_i=1.3uM
which is in agreement with the value obtained for half

maximal CaM inhibition of spectrin binding of 1uM(Fig. 3). Competitive inhibition of spectrin binding by calmodulin demonstrates a direct effect of calcium/calmodulin on the spectrin-membrane interaction, rather than by indirect means through other Ca/CaM-dependent processes.

Calmodulin Promotes Rapid Dissociation of Brain Spectrin from Synaptosomal Membranes.

Binding of ^{125}I-labeled brain spectrin to stripped synaptosomal membranes in the presence of calmodulin was rapidly reversed by the addition of calcium. Greater than 30% dissociation of brain spectrin occurs within 2 min of addition of calcium(the earliest experimentally measurable time point using this centrifugation assay). Subsequent reversal of binding occurred much more slowly over the next 60 min (~0.7%/min). A biphasic time course of Ca^{2+}/calmodulin inhibition of spectrin binding suggests that perhaps there are two populations of calmodulin sensitive spectrin-membrane complexes, with one type less stable and more susceptible to rapid dissociation. This experiment suggested that calcium-stimulated, calmodulin-dependent dissociation of brain spectrin from its membrane sites may occur within time constraints similar to calcium/calmodulin-mediated events occurring in vivo.

Binding of Erythrocyte Spectrin to Stripped Synaptosomal Membranes is Inhibited by Calcium/Calmodulin.

As described previously, stripped brain membranes contain specific binding sites for brain and erythrocyte spectrins, as well as sites that recognize both isoforms of spectrin. As was the case for brain spectrin, the binding of labeled erythrocyte spectrin to stripped synaptosomal membranes was also inhibited by calcium/calmodulin, with half-maximal inhibition of binding at 1.2 uM calmodulin containing 10 uM free calcium. Inhibition of membrane binding required both calcium and calmodulin, with maximal inhibition occurring at pCa=6. Unlike results obtained with brain spectrin, the binding of erythrocyte spectrin increased substantially by pCa=6 and reached a maximum (specific binding increased two fold) at 3.2 uM Ca^{2+} in the absence of calmodulin. The reason for the increased binding of erythrocyte spectrin in the presence of micromolar

calcium is not clear, although it may be due to a
calcium-binding domain in spectrin. Regardless of the
increased interactions with calcium alone, binding of
erythrocyte spectrin is dramatically reduced upon addition
of calmodulin.

Differential Regulation of RBC Spectrin-Membrane Protein
Interactions in Erythrocyte and Brain Membranes.

While binding of ^{125}I-labeled erythrocyte spectrin to
synaptosomal membranes is inhibited by calcium/calmodulin,
Ca/calmodulin (up to 5 uM) had no effect on the association
of RBC spectrin to ankyrin-containing erythrocyte membranes.
A similar insensitivity to calcium and calmodulin was
observed for association of brain spectrin with
ankyrin-containing RBC-inside-out vesicles. The results
suggest that calcium/calmodulin selectively inhibits direct
spectrin-membrane protein interactions and has no effect on
binding of erythrocyte or brain spectrin to ankyrin.
Differential regulation of spectrin-membrane interactions is
likely to exist for both brain spectrin and erythrocyte-like
spectrin in brain, suggesting the existence of a dynamic
membrane skeleton which undergoes site-directed
disassembly/reassembly of spectrin at Ca/CaM-sensitive sites
while spectrin-ankyrin linkages continuously anchor the
skeleton.

Calmodulin Inhibition of Spectrin Binding is Independent of
Association of Calmodulin with Spectrin

Erythrocyte spectrin, which binds calmodulin very
weakly (K_D=5-20uM) under denaturing conditions (42-44) is
inhibited from reassociating with stripped synaptosomnal
membranes by Ca/CaM. Moreover, binding of purified brain
spectrin beta subunit, which lacks a calmodulin-binding site
(3,33), is also inhibited by micromolar calmodulin in the
presence of 10 uM calcium, with 50% inhibition of binding of
brain spectrin at 1 uM calmodulin. These results suggest
that calmodulin-dependent inhibition of membrane binding by
spectrin is not mediated by a direct association of
calmodulin with spectrin and most likely involves
interaction of calmodulin with the membrane-binding protein.

Candidates for Spectrin-Binding Proteins from
Detergent-Solubilized Stripped Brain Membranes

Micromolar concentrations of calcium/calmodulin inhibit
spectrin-membrane protein interactions, most likely by
direct interaction of calmodulin with the spectrin-binding
proteins. Therefore, it should be possible to specifically
elute solubilized binding proteins from a spectrin affinity
column with Ca^{2+}/calmodulin. Sodium hydroxide-extracted
membranes were extracted with Triton X-100 which resulted in
a decrease in membrane binding of greater than 65% (not
shown). The reduction in binding was due to loss of high
affinity binding sites from these membranes, as determined
from Scatchard plots of binding to stripped membranes
compared to detergent-treated membranes (not shown). The
resulting detergent-solubilized proteins were radioiodinated
and applied to a RBC spectrin affinity column in an attempt
to recover active spectrin-binding proteins (Fig. 4).
Calcium alone released no column-bound proteins, and
calmodulin alone caused the elution of only a small amount
of a protein of M_r=88,000 (results not shown). Five
micromolar calmodulin/Ca^{2+} specifically eluted a polypeptide
M_r=88,000 from RBC spectrin-Sepharose. The elution of the
M_r=88,000 protein by calcium/calmodulin was highly
selective, since exposure to 0.5 M NaBr released of major
proteins with M_r=50,000, 80,000 and ~110,000-115,000 which
were still attached to the spectrin affinity column after
exposure to Ca^{2+} calmodulin. The M_r=88,000 protein eluted
by Ca^{2+}/calmodulin is a strong candidate to be a
calmodulin-sensitive binding site for spectrin, while the
NaBr-released polypeptides are likely candidates to be
calmodulin-resistant spectrin-binding proteins from stripped
brain membranes. Similar proteins were eluted with
calmodulin/calcium-utilizing a brain spectrin-Sepharose
affinity column.

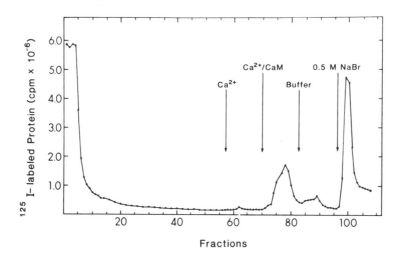

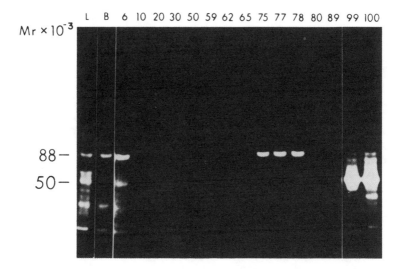

FIGURE 4. Spectrin-Sepharose affinity chromatography
of Triton X-100-solubilized proteins from NaOH-stripped
brain membranes. Ten milliliters of NaOH-extracted bovine

brain membranes (2.23 mg/ml) were extracted for 2 h at 4°C
in 10 mM sodium phosphate, 1 mM NaEGTA, 1 mM NaN$_3$, 0.5 mM
dithiothreitol, 1% (w/v) Triton X-100 buffer, pH 7.4, plus
diisopropylfluorophosphate (1:10,000), phenylmethylsulfonyl
fluoride (50 ug/ml), leupeptin (5 ug/ml), and pepstatin A (5
ug/ml). Membranes were pelleted at 30,000 x g for 45 min,
and supernatant was batchwise adsorbed to DEAE-cellulose for
60 min at 4°C. DEAE-cellulose was poured into a column and
washed sequentially with 50 ml each of 10 mM sodium
phosphate, 1 mM NaEGTA, 1 mM NaN$_3$, 0.5 mM dithiothreitol,
0.1% Triton X-100, pH 7.4 buffer; 10 mM HEPES, 1 mM NaEGTA,
1 mM NaN$_3$, 0.5 mM dithiothreitol, 0.1% Triton X-100, pH 7.4
buffer; 10 mM HEPES, 1 mM NaEGTA, 1 mM NaN$_3$, 0.1% Lubrol PX,
pH 7.4 buffer. Protein was eluted with 0.5 M NaBr, 10 mM
HEPES, 1 mM NaEGTA, 1 mM NaN$_3$, 0.1% Lubrol PX, pH 7.4, and
peak fractions typically of 0.2-0.3 mg/ml, were
radioiodinated with Na^{125}I using chloramine T as oxidant.
Free ^{125}I was separated from protein-bound ^{125}I by gel
filtration on Sephadex G-50 in 50 mM HEPES, 1 mM NaN$_3$, 0.1
mg/ml BSA, pH 6.8 buffer. ^{125}I-labeled triton solubilized
proteins ($^{\sim}10^5$ cpm/ul) were loaded onto 3 ml of RBC
spectrin-Sepharose in 50 mM HEPES, 40 mM NaCl, 1 mM EGTA, 1
mM NaN$_3$, 0.5 mM dithiothreitol, 0.1% Lubrol PX, pH 6.8,
buffer + 0.1 mg/ml BSA and washed with this buffer until
radioactivity in the eluant had reached a minimum. The
column was then washed with column buffer containing 1.2 mM
CaCl$_2$ as indicated. Calmodulin (4.8 uM) was added to the
calcium-containing column buffer and the column was eluted
as indicated ($\downarrow$). The column was washed briefly with column
buffer and finally eluted with column buffer + 0.5 M NaBr.
One milliliter fractions were collected at 5 ml/h. A,
chromatographic profile of ^{125}I-labeled protein elution from
RBC spectrin-Sepharose column. B, autoradiogram prepared
from SDS-gel electrophoresis of ^{125}I-labeled proteins eluted
from RBC spectrin-Sepharose. L, column load; B,
breakthrough fraction; numbers are column fractions.

DISCUSSION

The high affinity binding of spectrin to
ankyrin-independent sites in brain and erythrocyte membranes
may provide an important structural linkage in addition to
ankyrin-mediated interactions. A consequence of multiple
membrane linkages for spectrin is enhanced flexibility in

the placement and time of synthesis of proteins involved in spectrin-membrane interactions. Several possible arrangements of the spectrin skeleton can now be envisaged. Both ankyrin-dependent and independent linkages may occur simultaneously in the same spectrin tetramer since spectrin contains distinct binding domains for ankyrin and brain membrane proteins. Alternatively, both types of attachment of spectrin may coexist at the same time although with different spectrin molecules and/or in different regions of the cell. It is of interest in this regard that spectrin completely lines the membrane surfaces of neuronal cells (30,45), while ankyrin, as visualized by antibody against the erythrocyte isoform, colocalizes with spectrin from cell body to nerve terminal, but is absent from dendritic spines and afferent neuronal processes (46). However, while reactivity to the anti-erythrocyte isoform of ankyrin was specific for basolateral membrane domains, brain ankyrin immunoreactivity was found on all membrane surfaces in cryosections of rat kidney (47). These results suggest that there is not a simple segregation of spectrin-ankyrin (basolateral membrane domains) and direct spectrin-membrane linkages (apical membrane domains), but rather that ankyrin-mediated and ankyrin-independent linkages of spectrin to the membrane may co-exist on all membrane surfaces of cells.

Ankyrin-independent and dependent linkages of spectrin to the plasma membrane are likely to occur in the same region of the cell, but may appear at different times in assembly of the spectrin skeleton and at different stages of differentiation of erythrocytes or other cells with specialized membrane skeletons. Direct spectrin-membrane interactions could be utilized very early in assembly of the erythroid skeleton, resulting in an initial attachment of spectrin-actin complexes to the plasma membrane. Evidence supporting the existence of ankyrin-independent assembly of spectrin on the membrane is that spectrin is synthesized in nucleated erythrocyte precursors and apparently incoporated into a membrane skeleton with actin before synthesis of ankyrin and protein 4.1 (48). Spectrin also is synthesized prior to ankyrin in avian erythrocytes (49), chicken brain (50), and chicken embryo fibroblasts (51). Integral membrane protein attachment sites for spectrin would make the correlation of synthesis and assembly of spectrin and ankyrin of secondary importance, since direct spectrin-membrane linkages could exist prior to appearance of ankyrin.

Additional studies using murine erythroleukemia (MEL)
cells (52,53) show that attachment of these cells to a
fibronectin matrix is required for maturation and
differentiation into reticulocytes. Enucleated and
later-stage cells lose the ability to attach to a
fibronectin matrix due to loss of cell surface fibronectin
receptors. This detachment process is analogous to normal
release of reticulocytes from marrow into the bloodstream.
These studies suggest that synthesis, incorporation and
stabilization of the fibronectin receptor into the plasma
membrane, which is apparently required for differentiation,
may be linked to membrane skeleton assembly. Since
mammalian fibronectin receptors are associated with
cytoskeletal actin filaments via linkage to a
non-erythrocyte protein talin (54), it seems likely that the
erythrocyte fibronectin receptors will also be associated
with actin, perhaps via linkage with spectrin-actin
complexes. Such a scenario, postulating the fibronectin
receptor as an attachment protein for spectrin, would
suggest that while these sites are necessary for membrane
skeleton assembly, they would be inactive in mature
erythrocytes. Ankyrin-independent binding sites for
spectrin in mature erythrocytes may conform to these
criteria, since: 1) they exist in very small numbers; 2) are
bound preferentially by a tissue (brain) spectrin; and 3)
may be responsible for only a small percentage of attachment
of the membrane skeleton to the plasma membrane in mature
red cells, since the M_r=72,000 spectrin-binding domain of
ankyrin can inhibit nearly 95% of binding of spectrin to
inside-out vesicles. While these binding sites may be only
inactive residual sites of the initial attachment and
assembly zones in erythrocytes, they may maintain attachment
of the membrane skeleton to the membrane in nonerythroid
tissues which require attachment to the extracellular
matrix. The possiblity that association of spectrin to
ankyrin-independent membrane sites is involved in the
initial assembly and stabilization of the membrane skeleton
as described above suggests that these spectrin-binding
proteins may act as scaffolding proteins, membrane
structural proteins which are required for initiation of
construction and assembly of the membrane skeleton, but
which are removed after assembly is completed.
     An interesting consequence of an ankyrin-independent
mechanism to attach spectrin to the plasma membrane would be
that ankyrin may play an organizational role and utilize the
spectrin-actin skeleton to localize and then stabilize

integral membrane proteins to specific regions or domains of cells in addition to the structural role assumed in erythrocytes. Flexibility in skeleton assembly caused by ankyrin-independent attachment of spectrin to the membrane may reduce the immediate need for "structural" ankyrin and provide the basis for "organizational" ankyrin. Linkage of spectrin to the membrane could be maintained by direct spectrin-membrane attachment, while ankyrin-asssociated membrane proteins (perhaps associated to small cytoplasmic vesicle-bound receptors) may be inserted into specialized domains of cells by an ankyrin-dependent recognition process. Once localized to the proper membrane domain, attachment to the membrane skeleton via spectrin-ankyrin interactions would stabilize the membrane proteins. Specific localization of ankyrin and the Na/K ATPase into basolateral domains of epithelial cells (55) and ankyrin with the voltage-dependent sodium channel of Nodes of Ranvier (56) may be two examples for an organizational role of ankyrin.

Modulation of spectrin-membrane protein interactions by calmodulin suggests that spectrin can exist in a dynamic state under metabolic control and distinct from the mechanically stable membrane skeleton of erythrocytes. A consequence of independent regulation of these attachment mechanisms is that Ca^{2+}/calmodulin can dissociate direct spectrin-membrane interactions locally or regionally without disassembly of the areas of the membrane skeleton stabilized by linkage of spectrin to ankyrin. A possible physiological role for a regulated spectrin structure, suggested by Aunis and coworkers (57), could be as a lattice that separates secretory vesicles from the membrane and prevents vesicle-membrane fusion events. Calcium/calmodulin-induced disassembly of such spectrin interactions would allow access of secretory vesicles to the plasma membrane and could be an important step in regulation of exocytosis. Slower (~10 min) events such as calcium/calmodulin-dependent clearing of spectrin from regions of the plasma membrane of secretory cells (58) may also play a role in secretory vesicle recycling and in endocytosis (59-61).

Recent studies of the localization of spectrin in lymphocytes demonstrated a heterogeneous distribution with association both to the plasma membrane and to stable cytoplasmic aggregated structures (62). It was suggested that the shift in localization of spectrin from these cytoplasmic aggregates to the plasma membrane in response to hyperthermia or phorbol esters is indicative of the

maturation or functional state in the lymphocytes. The
redistribution of spectrin in lymphocytes may be analogous
to calcium-induced changes in spectrin localization in
adrenal chromaffin granules (63). In fact, calcium
participates in dissociation of spectrin-aggregated
structures (64), perhaps via calmodulin, which then enables
spectrin to redistribute and localize to the plasma membrane
where it appears in the mature cells.

An additional level of complexity results from spectrin
isoforms that coexist in the same cells. Brain spectrin
exists as two isoforms which differ in their beta subunits
and can be distinguished immunologically in chicken brain
(65) and in mouse and human brain (30,45). These spectrin
isoforms have been localized to different
membrane-cytoskeletal domains in neurons (45,66,67),
presumably to fulfill unique functions. Distinct
ankyrin-independent membrane receptor proteins for
erythrocyte and brain spectrins could provide a mechanism
for segregation of brain spectrin isoforms. Furthermore, it
is possible that Ca^{2+} effects could result in tighter
binding of an erythroctye-like spectrin isotype to its
receptors, while brain spectrin-receptor protein
interactions are unaffected. Additional binding
interactions caused by increases in calcium may play a role
in the different localizations of these spectrin isoforms
observed in brain tissues (30,45,65). The enhancement of
binding of erythrocyte spectrin by calcium most likely does
not occur in the same cellular domains that contain
calmodulin since calcium and calmodulin together strongly
inhibit RBC spectrin-brain membrane interactions.

A membrane protein of M_r=88,000 has been identified
(Fig. 4) that is dissociated from spectrin affinity columns
by calcium/calmodulin and is a candidate for the
calmodulin-sensitive spectrin-binding site in brain. An
interesting possibilty is that this spectrin-binding protein
may function as a channel for ions such as calcium or
potassium and that this channel activity could be regulated
by calcium and calmodulin in concert with the modulation of
spectrin binding. It will be important in future work to
purify this protein, determine its cellular localization,
and evaluate other functions in addition to linkage of
spectrin to membranes.

REFERENCES

1. Shotton DM, Burke BE, Branton D (1979). The molecular
    structure of human erythrocyte spectrin. J Mol Biol
    131:303-329.
2. Glenney J, Glenney P, Osborn M, Weber K (1982a).
    An F-actin and calmodulin-binding protein from isolated
    intestinal brush borders has a morphology related to
    spectrin. Cell 28:843-854.
3. Glenney J, Glenney P, Weber K (1982b). Erythroid
    spectrin, brain fodrin, and intestinal brush border
    proteins (TW 260/240) are related molecules containing
    a common calmodulin-binding subunit bound to a variant
    cell type specific subunit. Proc Natl Acad Sci USA
    79:4002-4005.
4. Glenney J, Glenney P, Weber K (1982c). F-actin-binding
    and crosslinking properties of porcine brain fodrin, a
    spectrin-related molecule. J Biol Chem 257:9781-9787.
5. Bennett V, Davis J, Fowler W (1982). Brain spectrin, a
    membrane-associated protein related in structure and
    function to erythrocyte spectrin. J Biol Chem
    257:9781-9787.
6. Speicher DW, Davis G, Yurchenco PD, Marchesi VT (1983).
    Structure of human erythrocyte spectrin. I. Isolation
    of the alpha-1 domain and its cyanogen bromide
    peptides. J Biol Chem 258:14931-14937.
7. Speicher DW, Marchesi VT (1984). Erythrocyte spectrin
    is comprised of many homologous triple helical
    segments. Nature 311:177-180.
8. Leto TL, Fortugno-Erikson D, Barton D, Yang-Feng TL,
    Francke U, Harris AS, Morrow JS, Marchesi VT, Benz EJ
    (1988). Comparison of nonerythroid alpha-spectrin genes
    reveals strict homology among diverse species. Mol Cell
    Biol 8:1-9.
9. Levine J, Willard M (1981). Fodrin:axonally transported
    polypeptides associated with the internal periphery of
    many cells. J Cell Biol 90:631-643.
10. Goodman SR, Zagon I, Kulikowski R (1981).
    Identification of a spectrin-like protein in
    nonerythroid cells. Proc Natl Acad Sci USA
    78:7570-7574.
11. Repasky E, Granger B, Lazarides E (1982). Widespread
    occurence of avian spectrin in nonerythroid cells. Cell
    29:821-833.
12. Shen BW, Josephs R, Steck TL (1986). Ultrastructure of
    the intact skeleton of the human erythrocyte membrane.

J Cell Biol 102:997-1006.
13. Byers TJ, Branton D (1985). Visualization of the protein associations in the erythrocyte membrane skeleton. Proc Natl Acad Sci USA 82:6153-6157.
14. Liu S-C, Derick LH, Palek J (1987). Visualization of the hexagonal lattice in the erythrocyte membrane skeleton. J Cell Biol 104:527-536.
15. Bennett V (1985). The membrane skeleton of human erythrocytes and its implications for more complex cells. Ann Rev Biochem 54:273-304.
16. Bennett V (1989). The spectrin-actin junction of erythrocyte membrane skeletons. Biochim Biophys Acta 988:107-121.
17. Marchesi VT (1985). Stabilizing infrastructure of cell membranes. Ann Rev Cell Biol 1:531-561.
18. Goodman SR, Zagon IS (1986). The neural cell spectrin skeleton:A review. Am J Physiol 250:C347-C350.
19. Bennett V, Stenbuck PJ (1979). Identification and partial purification of ankyrin, the high affinity membrane attachment site for human erythrocyte spectrin. J Biol Chem 254:2533-2541.
20. Bennett V, Stenbuck PJ (1980). Association between ankyrin and the cytoplasmic domain of band 3 isolated from the human erythrocyte membrane. J Biol Chem 255:6424-6432.
21. Shiffer K, Goodman SR (1984). Protein 4.1:Its association with the human erythrocyte membrane. Proc Natl Acad Sci USA 81:4404-4408.
22. Anderson RA, Lovrien RE (1984). Glycophorin is linked by band 4.1 protein to the human erythrocyte membrane skeleton. Nature 307:655-658.
23. Davis JQ, Bennett V (1984a). Brain ankyrin-Purification of a 72,000 M_r spectrin-binding domain. J Biol Chem 259:1874-1881.
24. Davis JQ, Bennett V (1984b). Brain ankyrin-a membrane-associated protein with binding sites for spectrin, tubulin, and the cytoplasmic domain of the erythrocyte anion channel. J Biol Chem 259:13550-13559.
25. Davis JQ, Bennett V (1986). Association of brain ankyrin with brain membranes and isolation of active proteolytic fragments of membrane-associated ankyrin-binidng proteins. J Biol Chem 261:16198-16206.
26. Srinivasan Y, Elmer L, Davis J, Bennett V, Angelides K (1988). Ankyrin and spectrin associate with voltage-dependent sodium channels in brain. Nature 333:177-180.

27. Steiner JP, Bennett V (1988). Ankyrin-independent membrane protein binding sites for brain and erythrocyte spectrin. J Biol Chem 263:14417-14425.
28. Steiner JP, Walke H, Bennett V (1989). Calcium/calmodulin inhibits direct binding of spectrin to synaptosomal membranes. J Biol Chem 264:2783-2791.
29. Davis JQ, Bennett V (1983). Brain spectrin-isolation of subunits and formation of hybrids with erythrocyte spectrin subunits. J Biol Chem 258:7757-7766.
30. Riederer B, Zagon I, Goodman SR (1986). Brain spectrin (240/235) and brain spectrin (240/235E):Two distinct spectrin subtypes with different locations within mammalian neural cells. J Cell Biol 102:2088-2097.
31. Bennett V (1978). Purification of an active proteolytic fragment of the membrane attachment site for human erythrocyte spectrin. J Biol Chem 253:2292-2299.
32. Davies P, Klee CB (1981). Calmodulin-binding proteins:a high molecular weight calmodulin-binding protein from bovine brain. Biochem Inter 3:203-212.
33. Kakiuchi S, Sobue K, Fujita M (1981). Purification of a 240,000 M_r calmodulin-binding protein from a microsomal fraction of brain. FEBS Lett 132:144-148.
34. Palfrey C, Schiebler W, Greengard P (1982). A major calmodulin-binding protein common to various vertebrate tissues. Proc Natl Acad Sci USA 79:3780-3784.
35. Sobue K, Muramoto Y, Fujita M, Kakiuchi S (1981b). Purification of a calmodulin-binding protein from chicken gizzard that interacts with F-actin. Proc Natl Acad Sci USA 78:5652-5655.
36. Sobue K, Morimoto K, Kanda K, Fukunaga K, Miyamoto E, Kakiuchi S (1982). Interaction of 135,000-M_r calmodulin binding protein (Myosin kinase) and F-actin: Another Ca^{2+}-and calmodulin-dependent flip-flop switch. Biochem Internat 5:503-510.
37. Kakiuchi S, Sobue K (1981). Ca^{2+}-and calmodulin-dependent flip-flop mechanism in microtubule assembly-disassembly. FEBS Lett 132:141-143.
38. Gardner K, Bennett V (1987). Modulation of spectrin-actin assembly by erythrocyte adducin. Nature 328:359-362.
39. Kakiuchi S, Yasuda S, Yamazaki R, Teshima Y, Nanda K, Kakiuchi R, Sobue K (1982). Quantitative determinations of calmodulin in the supernatant and particulate fractions of mammalian tissues. J Biochem (Tokyo) 92:1041-1048.
40. Seubert P, Baudry M, Dudek S, Lynch G (1987).

Calmodulin stimulates the degradation of brain spectrin by calpain. Synapsin 1:20-24.

41. Weiss B, Fertel R, Figlin R, Uzunov P (1974). Selective alteration of activity of multiple forms of adenosine 3-5-monophosphate phosphodiesterase of rat cerebrum. Mol Pharmacol 10:615-625.

42. Sobue K, Morimoto K, Fujita M, Kakiuchi S (1981a). Calmodulin-binding protein of erythrocyte cytoskeleton. Biochem Biophys Res Comm 100:1063-1070.

43. Burns N, Gratzer W (1985). Interaction of calmodulin with the red cell and its membrane skeleton and with spectrin. Biochem 24:3070-3074.

44. Berglund A, Backman L, Shambhag V (1986). The 240-KDa subunit of human erythrocyte spectirn binds calmodulin at micromolar calcium concentrations. FEBS Lett 201:306-310.

45. Goodman SR, Zagon IS, Riederer BM (1987). Spectrin isoforms in mammalian brain. Brain Res Bullet 18:787-792.

46. Drenckhahn D, Bennett V (1987). Polarized distribution of M_r 210,000 and 190,000 analogs of erythrocyte ankyrin along the plasma membrane of transporting epithelia, neurons, and photoreceptors. Eur J Cell Biol 43:479-486.

47. Davis J, Davis L, Bennett V (1989). Diversity in membrane binding sites of ankyrins:Brain ankyrin, erythrocyte ankyrin, and processed erythrocyte ankyrin associate with distinct sites in kidney microsomes. J Biol Chem 264, in press.

48. Hanspal M, Palek J (1987). Synthesis and assembly of membrane skeletal proteins in mammalian red cell precursors. J Cell Biol 104:1417-1424.

49. Moon, RT, Lazarides E (1984). Biogenesis of the avian erythroid skeleton:receptor mediated assembly and stabilization of ankyrin (goblin) and spectrin. J Cell Biol 98:1899-1904.

50. Nelson WJ, Lazarides E (1983). Expression of the beta subunit of spectrin in nonerythroid cells. Proc Natl Acad Sci USA 80:363-367.

51. Moon RT, Ngai J, Wold B, Lazarides E (1985). Tissue-specific expression of distinct spectrin and ankyrin transcripts in erythroid and nonerythroid cells. J Cell Biol 100:152-160.

52. Patel V, Lodish H (1986). The fibronectin receptor on mammalian erythroid precursor cells:Characterization and developmental regulation. J Cell Biol 102:449-456.

53. Patel V, Lodish H (1987). A fibronectin matrix is required for differentiation of murine erythroleukemia cells into reticulocytes. J Cell Biol 105:3105-3118.

54. Horwitz A, Duggan K, Buck C, Beckerle MC, Burridge K (1986). Interaction of plasma membrane fibronectin receptor with talin-a transmembrane linkage. Nature 320:531-533.

55. Nelson WJ, Veshnock PJ (1987). Ankyrin binding to the (Na^+K^+) ATPase and implications for the organization of membrane domains in polarized cells. Nature 328:533-535.

56. Kordeli E, Davis J, Trapp B, Bennett V (1989). An erythroid isoform of ankyrin is localized at nodes of Ranvier in myelinated axons of central and peripheral nerves. Cell, submitted for publication.

57. Perrin D, Langely OK, Aunis D (1987). Anti-alpha fodrin inhibits secretion from permeabilized chromaffin cells. Nature 326:498-501.

58. Aunis D, Bader M-F, Langely OK, Perrin D (1987). Tubulin- and actin-binding proteins in chromaffin cells. Annals NY Acad Sci 493:435-447.

59. Ceccarelli B, Hurlbut WP (1980a). Ca^{2+}-dependent recycling of synaptic vesicles at the frog neuromuscular junction. J Cell Biol 87:297-303.

60. Ceccarelli B, Hurlbut WP (1980b). Vesicle hypothesis of the release of quanta of acetylcholine. Physiol Rev 60:396-441.

61. Meldolesi J, Ceccarelli B (1981). Exocytosis and membrane recycling. Phil Trans Roy Soc London Ser B Biol Sci 296:55-65.

62. Black JD, Koury SK, Bankert RB, Repasky EA (1988). Heterogeneity in lymphocyte spectrin distribution:ultrastructural identification of a new spectrin-rich cytoplasmic structure. J Cell Biol 106:97-109.

63. Perrin D, Aunis D (1985). Reorganization of alpha-fodrin induced by stimulation in secretory cells. Nature 315:589-592.

64. Lee JK, Black JD, Repasky EA, Kubo RT, Bankert RB (1988). Activation induces a rapid reorganization of spectrin in lymphocytes. Cell 55:807-816.

65. Lazarides E, Nelson WJ (1985). Expression and assembly of the erythroid membrane-skeletal proteins ankyrin (goblin) and spectrin in the morphogenesis of chicken neurons. J Cell Biochem 27:423-441.

66. Lazarides E, Nelson WJ (1983). Erythrocyte and brain

forms of spectrin in cerebellum:Distinct
membrane-cytoskeletal domains in neurons. Science
220:1295-1296.
67. Lazarides E, Nelson WJ, Kasamatsu T (1984). Segregation
    of two spectrin forms in the chicken optic system:A
    mechanism for establishing restricted
    membrane-cytoskeletal domains in neurons. Cell
    36:269-278.

Cellular and Molecular Biology of Normal
and Abnormal Erythroid Membranes, pages 27–41
© 1990 Alan R. Liss, Inc.

LOCALIZATION OF THE ANKYRIN BINDING SITE ON THE
CYTOPLASMIC DOMAIN OF HUMAN ERYTHROID BAND 3[1]

Kevin A. Davies[*], Samuel E. Lux[+] and
Harvey F. Lodish [*#]

*Whitehead Institute, 9 Cambridge Center, Cambridge, MA
02142; +The Children's Hospital, Harvard Medical School,
Boston, MA 02115; and #Department of Biology, Massachusetts
Institute of Technology, Cambridge, MA 02139.

ABSTRACT   A non-denaturing gel shift assay has
been employed to study the interaction between ankyrin and
(i)   the cytoplasmic domain of band 3   (cdb3), and   (ii)
N-terminal peptide fragments of band 3 synthesized *in vitro*.
Early results suggest a region between amino acids 80–215 of
band 3 is primarily involved in ankyrin-binding. Further
studies using site-directed mutagenesis should allow a more
precise definition of the binding region.

INTRODUCTION

The red cell membrane skeleton is composed of two
principal structural proteins underlying the membrane,
spectrin and actin (1; and Fig.1). Protein 4.1 promotes the
interaction of spectrin tetramers with actin (2) and this
ternary complex binds to the integral membrane protein
glycophorin C.   Ankyrin, a protein of relative molecular
mass (M_r) 215,000 (215K), binds to spectrin and also to an
unknown site on the cytoplasmic domain of band 3 (cdb3) (3).
In addition, ankyrin has been shown to bind to a number of
non-erythrocyte proteins including kidney band 3 (4), the
alpha subunit of kidney Na,K-ATPase (5,6), lens cytoskeletal
proteins (7), the brain sodium channel (8), and other brain
membrane glycoproteins (9). Thus, band 3 may possess

1This work was supported by grants HL 27375 (H.F.L.) and DK
34083 (S.E.L.).   K.A.D. was supported by a postdoctoral
Fellowship from the European Molecular Biology Organization.

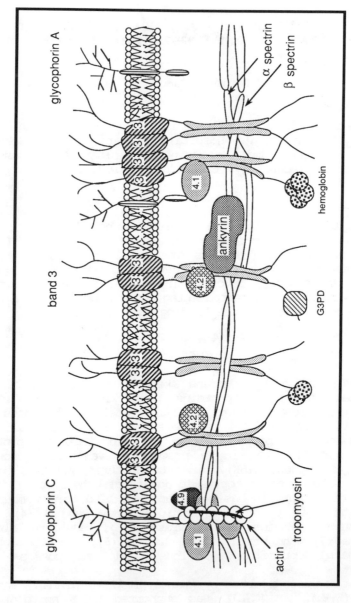

FIGURE 1. Schematic representation of the red blood cell membrane
skeleton.

a binding site for ankyrin (perhaps a contiguous stretch of amino acids) that is conserved amongst other non-erythroid ankyrin-binding proteins.

Hereditary defects in components of the red cell membrane skeleton result in abnormally shaped erythrocytes and (typically) hemolytic anemia (reviewed in reference 10). A high molecular weight variant of band 3 has recently been reported in one family with acanthocytosis and a significant reduction in the number of high-affinity ankyrin-binding sites (ABS) (11). A conformational change has been speculated to disrupt the ABS.

There exists some evidence to suggest that the ABS of band 3 may be composed of a short stretch of 21 amino acids (residues 143-163 in human erythroid band 3). Low and colleagues first proposed that the ABS is situated between a putative antigenic site and a proline-rich hinge region (reviewed in 12). This domain includes amino acids 143-163, which are highly conserved between human (13, and Lux *et al.* in preparation), murine (14) and chicken (15) band 3, as well as human (16) and murine (17) non-erythroid band 3 (Fig.2). Furthermore, it is encoded by a single exon of the mouse gene, which together with its conservation between species

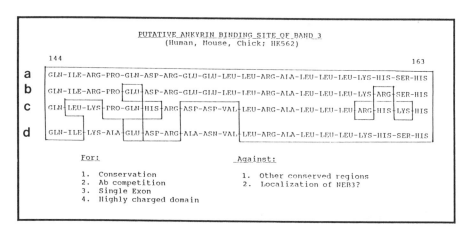

FIGURE 2. Comparison of the putative ankyrin binding sites in three erythroid and one non-erythroid band 3 species. (a) human erythroid B3 [HEB3] (13); (b) murine band 3 [MB3] (14); (c) chick band 3 [CB3] (15); (d) human non-erythroid B3 [HKB3] (16). The sequence of B3RP (17) is identical to HKB3 in this region.

implies an important functional role. A partial homology between this sequence and the alpha subunit of Na,K-ATPase has been found (6). However, it should be noted that there are three equally well conserved cytoplasmic regions on band 3, which are also good candidates for the ABS (16).

We have commenced work to define the site on band 3 which binds to ankyrin, by studying the interaction of purified ankyrin to either full-length or truncated peptides of cdb3, synthesized *in vitro* from mRNA transcripts of a human band 3 cDNA (Lux *et al.*, in preparation). Ankyrin/band 3 complexes are resolved by means of a gel-shift assay using non-denaturing polyacrylamide gel electrophoresis (ND-PAGE). In this way, it will be possible to determine the location of the ABS on band 3 by correlating binding activity with peptide sequence. ND-PAGE has been employed successfully to study the interactions of band 3 with protein 4.1 (18) and ankyrin (19), and ankyrin with spectrin (20) and Na,K-ATPase (5). The synthesis of truncated peptides by the procedure of 'run-off' transcription and translation has previously been used, in conjunction with ND-PAGE, to monitor protein-DNA interactions by gel shifts, e.g. yeast GCN4 protein (21) and *Xenopus* transcription factor TFIIIA (22). A similar method for the analysis of protein-protein interactions has been reported for the association of SV40 structural proteins (23), using a sucrose gradient sedimentation assay.

METHODS

Ankyrin/cdb3 binding assays

Ankyrin and cdb3 were prepared from red blood cell ghosts by published procedures (2,24). cdb3 was iodinated by the iodine monochloride method (25). 500ng of 125I-labeled cdb3 was incubated with increasing amounts of ankyrin at 0°C overnight. Similar incubations were performed using *in vitro* translated band 3 peptides at room temperature or 37°C. The incubation buffer was 100mM NaCl, 25mM KCl, 100ug/ml gelatin, 5mM DTT, 1mM EDTA and 20ug/ml PMSF.

Non-denaturing gel shift electrophoresis

The ankyrin/band 3 complexes were analysed on 3-8% polyacrylamide gradient gels in the following buffer: 40mM Tris HCl (pH 7.5), 40mM Na acetate and 1mM EDTA. The gels were run in the cold room for 6-16 hours, with recirculating buffer (26). Following electrophoresis, the gels were fixed and subjected to autoradiography or fluorography.

In vitro translation of N-terminal band 3 peptides

10ug aliquots of pHB3-45 DNA were linearized with each of the restriction enzymes indicated in restriction map in Fig.3. The purified templates were then used to transcribe RNA by 'run-off' transcription (21,22), using T7 polymerase according to the manufacturer's instructions (Stratagene). Approximately 250ng RNA was then added to micrococcal nuclease-treated wheat-germ extract (kindly provided by Dr. A.M. Garcia). *In vitro* translation was allowed to proceed for 2 hours at room temperature in the presence of 35S-methionine, before terminating with the addition of 2ug/ml RNase.

RESULTS

Ankyrin binds to the purified cytoplasmic domain of band 3

We firstly examined the gel shift obtained when a constant amount of 125I-labeled cdb3 was incubated with increasing quantities of ankyrin (Fig.3). As the ratio of ankyrin to cdb3 increases to greater than 1:1 (lanes 2 to 5), a new band of reduced mobility (labeled C) appears towards the top of the gel, due to complex formation. (A second complex, designated A, is also formed (lane 6), although the stoichiometries of the components are not yet known). A concomitant decrease in intensity of uncomplexed cdb3 (M) is also observed. However, when cdb3 is incubated with an excess of heat-denatured ankyrin or when the incubation is performed in the presence of excess unlabeled cdb3, no shift in radioactivity is observed. Thus, cdb3 specifically binds to ankyrin *in vitro*.

This result is also obtained when incubations are conducted in the presence of 20% (v/v) wheat-germ extract, simulating the experimental conditions to be described below (result not shown). Thus there are no components in the extract which might interfere with the binding assay. Incubating 125I-labeled cdb3 for 2 hours in a wheat germ translation reaction does not abolish binding to ankyrin, ruling out phosphorylation effects upon binding activity.

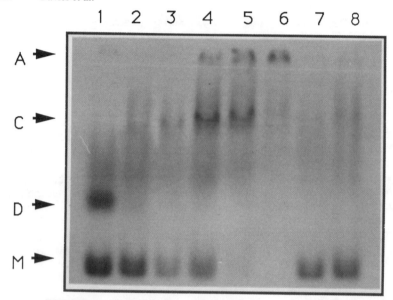

FIGURE 3. Ankyrin binding to the cytoplasmic domain of band 3 results in a gel-shift *in vitro*. 500ng 125I-labeled cdb3 were incubated at 0°C overnight with the following molar ratios of ankyrin: lane (1) no ankyrin; (2) 1:5; (3) 1:2; (4) 1:1; (5) 2:1; (6) 4:1; (7) heat-denatured ankyrin (2:1), and (8) 2:1 ankyrin + fourfold excess unlabeled cdb3. The gel was run for 16 hours at 4°C, before autoradiography.

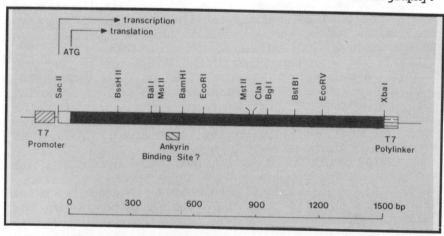

FIGURE 4. Restriction map of band 3 cDNA, pHB3-45.

In vitro transcription and translation of human band 3
cytoplasmic polypeptides

Three overlapping cDNA clones encompassing the entire
5'-untranslated and coding region of human band 3 have been
isolated (Lux *et al.* in preparation). We constructed a cDNA
clone, pHB3-45, which possesses a 1.56kb SacII-XbaI insert
(Fig.4) encoding 60bp of the 5'-untranslated region, the
entire cytoplasmic domain (60-1260bp) extending to the EcoRV
site, and two membrane-spanning domains (1261-1500bp).

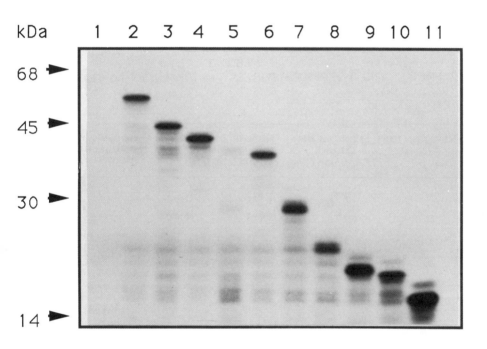

FIGURE 5. *In vitro* translation of N-terminal band 3
peptides in a wheat germ extract. 250ng RNA was translated
in 50ul wheat germ extract for 2 hours at 23°C, in the
presence of 35S-methionine. 5ul reaction aliquots were run
out on a 7% Laemmli gel. Restriction enzymes used to
linearize the pHB3-45 template are indicated. Lane (1) no
RNA control; (2) XbaI; (3) EcoRV; (4) BstBI; (5) BglI; (6)
ClaI; (7) EcoRI; (8) BamHI; (9) MstII; (10) BalI; and (11)
BssHII. Protein molecular weight standards are indicated.

pHB3-45 DNA was linearized with ten restriction enzymes prior to performing 'run-off' transcription and translation in wheat germ extract, chosen in preference to reticulocyte lysate to avoid any possible associations due to the presence of mammalian cytoskeletal proteins in the medium.

The synthesis of the N-terminal band 3 peptides is shown in Fig.5. In each case except for the smallest peptide (BssHII), the observed molecular weight agrees well with that predicted from the cDNA sequence (13; see Table 1). For example, RNA transcribed from EcoRV-digested pHB3-45 DNA produced a pure 45K, full-length peptide. (This peptide contains 25 additional C-terminal amino acids as compared to the chymotrypsin-cleaved cdb3). A few minor

TABLE 1

N-TERMINAL BAND 3 PEPTIDES SYNTHESIZED FROM pHB3-45 TEMPLATE

RESTRICTION ENZYME	LENGTH OF CODING FRAGMENT (bp)	NO. OF AMINO ACIDS	PREDICTED MOLECULAR WEIGHT (Da)	OBSERVED MOLECULAR WEIGHT (kDa)
XbaI	1500	483	61 450	60.0
EcoRV	1200	385	49 075	46.5
BstBI	1080	343	43 074	43.0
BglI	950	300	38 161	37.0
ClaI	880	276	35 120	35.0
EcoRI	700	216	27 331	26.0
BamHI	600	182	23 322	21.5
MstII	490	146	19 949	19.0
BalI	450	132	16 706	18.0
BssHII	290	79	9 820	16.0

bands of lower molecular weight are also observed, which may be due to limited proteolysis, or false initiation at internal methionine residues. Approximately 2ng protein was synthesized in a 50ul reaction volume. Thus, there is a panel of nine progressively truncated human band 3 peptides with which to assay for ankyrin binding.

Binding of *in vitro* translated band 3 fragments to ankyrin

5ul aliquots of newly-synthesized band 3 peptide in wheat germ extract were mixed with various concentrations of ankyrin in a 20ul volume and incubated overnight, before analyzing the products by ND-PAGE. When the identical conditions to those used for cdb3 binding to ankyrin in Fig.3 were employed, no binding was detected, i.e. incubation of ankyrin with the EcoRV peptide at 0°C did not result in complex formation or a gel shift. However, upon repeating the incubation step at 37°C overnight, a standard gel shift was observed (Fig.6). A complex of lower mobility was formed between the EcoRV peptide and ankyrin, resulting in a shift in the labeled band 3. Binding was abolished, however, if the ankyrin was heat-denatured beforehand. The only significant difference between the experiments using either cdb3 or *in vitro* translated peptide was the concentration of the band 3 fragment – there was at least a one hundred-fold reduction using the wheat germ product. Further results suggest that the next four N-terminal peptides in order of decreasing size (BstBI, BglI, ClaI and EcoRI), truncated back to the EcoRI site (i.e. containing a minimum of the N-terminal 215 amino acids only) all retain ankyrin-binding activity. However, the shortest peptide (BssHII) which possesses 79 amino acids, shows no binding activity. Experiments are in progress to repeat and corroborate these findings. However, there is some evidence that the ABS is situated between residues 80-215, in agreement with previously published models (6,12,14-17).

DISCUSSION

A number of assumptions were made at the outset of this project. Firstly, although cdb3 specifically binds to ankyrin, it remained to be demonstrated whether an N-terminal fragment of band 3, synthesized *in vitro* in the absence of the membrane-spanning domain, could adopt the

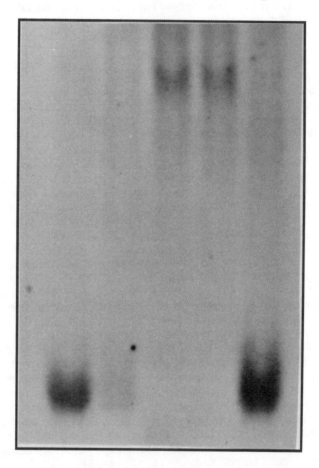

FIGURE 6. Gel shift between ankyrin and EcoRV band 3 cytoplasmic peptide, translated *in vitro*. 5ul of 35S-labeled EcoRV band 3 peptide (in wheat germ extract) was incubated in a 20ul total volume with varying quantities of ankyrin, at 37°C overnight, prior to ND-PAGE. Lane (1) peptide alone; (2) + 200ng ankyrin; (3) + 800ng ankyrin; (4) + 800ng ankyrin, without binding buffer; and (5) + 800ng heat-denatured ankyrin.

correct conformation to bind to ankyrin. Furthermore, the effects of truncating the cytoplasmic peptides might disrupt the tertiary structure and destroy the conformation of the binding site. However, due to the elongated structure of cdb3 in solution (12) and the predicted absence of significant tertiary structure (Lux *et al.*, in preparation) it was believed that *in vitro* translated N-terminal band 3 peptides would adopt the native conformation.

We initially characterized the association between ankyrin and iodinated cdb3 using ND-PAGE, before repeating the analysis with the *in vitro* translated peptides. The results of our gel-shift experiments are similar to those obtained by Tao's group (20), although we note that all the labeled cdb3 appears to become complexed with ankyrin. We also observe two complexes of differing mobilities (labeled C and A in Fig.3), but the second complex seen at the origin of the gel is more likely to be a non-specific aggregate caused by the excess of ankyrin present, and not due to an altered ankyrin conformation. In the first lane two bands are seen (labeled M and D in Fig.3), suggestive of monomer and dimer conformations. (The monomer band is in fact a doublet caused by chymotrypsin cleavage to produce 41K and 43K species). It is interesting to note that the dimer band disappears first, as soon as a trace of ankyrin is added. This may be indicative of ankyrin preferentially binding to, or promoting the dissociation of, the dimer. We tend to favour the latter possibility, especially since Willardson and Low (this volume) have shown that cross-linking cdb3 abolishes ankyrin binding. Also in agreement with this finding, Bennett isolated the ankyrin/band 3 complex and found the components to be monomers in a 1:1 ratio (27).

The successful binding of the EcoRV peptide to ankyrin suggests that (a) synthetic band 3 <u>can</u> adopt the correct conformation to bind ankyrin in the absence of the transmembrane domain; (b) the concentration of band 3 in the reaction is not a critical factor; (c) the success of elevating the temperature in driving the formation of the ankyrin/band 3 complex may signify a possible hydrophobic (entropic) association between the two proteins. Band 3 exists predominantly as a dimer or tetramer in the erythrocyte membrane, but it is not clear what effect this has upon ankyrin binding activity.

These results suggest that at least part of the ankyrin binding site is located between residues 80-215 of human band 3. This data agrees with that obtained by two other groups using antibodies to specific regions of band 3

to compete with ankyrin for binding.   Davis *et al.* (28) found
that residues 175–186 were most likely to participate in the
ABS.   Willardson and Low (this volume) discovered three
regions that are implicated in the ABS: residues 191–204, a
region including cysteine 317, and the N-terminus.   Both
groups downplay the significance that has been attached to
residues 143–163, even though a partial homology of this
sequence to the alpha subunit of Na,K-ATPase has recently
been noted (6).

Knowledge of the interaction between band 3 and
ankyrin will be important not only for our understanding of
the precise structure of the erythrocyte cytoskeleton, but
also in discovering other interactions in non-erythroid
cells, where increasing numbers of erythrocyte membrane
protein homologues are being discovered.   We intend to
characterize the binding domain in detail, and to examine
mutations of the binding-site *in vivo*.   Four principle areas
of investigation are proposed:

Precise characterization of the ankyrin binding site.
We are extending the analysis with the eight C-terminal
truncated peptides (Fig.3) to determine at which point
ankyrin-binding activity is lost.   Loss of binding activity
will provisionally indicate the location of the ABS, which
will be further studied by creating N-terminal deletions.
Once defined, specific amino acids in the ABS will be
mutated using site-directed mutagenesis to examine the effect
on ankyrin-binding.

Localization of additional binding sites of band 3.
The same techniques will be willl be used to examine the
binding of band 3 to erythrocyte proteins 4.1 and 4.2, and
to glycolytic enzymes such as glyceraldehyde-3-phosphate
dehydrogenase (GAPDH).   There are four highly conserved
domains between human, mouse and chicken band 3, three of
which are encoded by single exons (Lux *et al.*, in preparation),
that are good candidates for binding sites.

Ankyrin binding in band 3 homologues.   It will be of
considerable interest to examine whether non-erythroid band
3 homologues (16,17) also bind to ankyrin, and to correlate
such binding with their localization within the cell.   For
example, there are two classes of band 3 in the renal tubule
epithelial cells.   Kidney band 3 (KB3) (29) – a
differentially transcribed product of the single-copy
erythroid gene (30,31) – has been colocalized with ankyrin
at the basolateral surface of tubule intercalated cells (4).
However, B3RP (17), murine non-erythroid band 3, is present
in the apical membrane and appears not to be bound to

ankyrin (32). Yet B3RP does contain the short stretch of conserved amino acids that has been proposed to constitute the ABS (16). Using cDNAs for both murine KB3 and B3RP (17,29) it will be possible to synthesize cytoplasmic peptides by 'run-off' transcription and translation and subsequently to determine which species can bind to ankyrin.

The effect of ankyrin/band 3 binding in differentiation of erythroleukemia cells. To complement the *in vitro* binding studies of band 3 and ankyrin, it would be of great interest to examine the physiological consequences of binding-site mutations *in situ*. Murine erythroleukaemia (MEL) cells can be induced to differentiate synchronously in culture with dimethylsulphoxide. If grown on fibronectin-coated dishes, they enucleate and form reticulocytes over a seven-day period (35). The fate of normal or mutated human band 3 transfected into such cells could be followed on the mouse background.

REFERENCES

1. Bennett V (1985). The membrane skeleton of human erythrocytes and its implications for more complex cells. Ann Rev Biochem 54:273.
2. Cohen CM and Foley SF (1984). Biochemical characterization of complex formation by human erythrocyte spectrin, protein 4.1 and actin. Biochemistry 23:6091.
3. Bennett V and Stenbuck PJ (1980). Association between ankyrin and the cytoplasmic domain of band 3 isolated from the human erythrocyte membrane. J Biol Chem 255:6424.
4. Drenckhahn D, Schluter K, Allen DP and Bennett V (1985). Colocalisation of band 3 with ankyrin and spectrin at the basal membrane of intercalated cells in the rat kidney. Science 230:1287.
5. Nelson WJ and Veshnock PJ (1987). Ankyrin binding to (Na+K)ATPase and implications for the organisaton of membrane domains in epithelial cells. Nature 328:533.
6. Morrow JS, Cianci CD, Ardito T, Mann AS and Kashgarian M (1989). Ankyrin links fodrin to the alpha sububit of Na,K-ATPase in Madin-Darby kidney cells and in intact renal tubule cells. J Cell Biol 108:455.
7. Allen DP, Low PS, Dola A and Maisel H (1987). Band 3 and ankyrin homologues are present in eye lens: evidence for all major erythrocyte membrane components in same

non-erythroid cell.   Biochem Biophys Res Comm 149:266.

8. Srinivasan Y, Elmer L, Davis J, Bennett V and Angelides
    K (1988). Ankyrin and spectrin associate with voltage-
    dependent sodium channels in brain.   Nature 333:177.

9. Davis JQ and Bennett V (1986). Association of brain
    ankyrin with brain membranes and isolation of active
    proteolytic fragments of membrane-associated ankyrin-
    binding protein(s).   J Biol Chem 261:16198.

10. Davies KA and Lux SE (1989). Hereditary disorders of the
    red cell membrane skeleton. Trends in Genetics (in
    press).

11. Kay MMB, Bosman GJ and Lawrence C (1988). Functional
    topography of band 3: specific structural alteration
    linked to functional aberrations in human erythrocytes.
    Proc Natl Acad Sci USA 85:492.

12. Low PS (1986). Structure and function of the cytoplasmic
    domain of band 3: center of erythrocyte membrane-
    peripheral protein interactions.   Biochem Biophys Acta
    864:145.

13. Tanner M, Martin PG and High S (1988). The complete
    amino acid sequence of the human erythrocyte membrane
    anion-transport protein deduced from the cDNA sequence.
    Biochem J 256:703.

14. Kopito RR and Lodish HF (1985). Primary structure and
    transmembrane orientation of the murine anion exchange
    protein.   Nature 316:234.

15. Kim H-RC, Yew NS, Ansorge W, Voss H, Schwager C,
    Vennstromm B, Zenke M and Engel JD (1988). Two
    different RNAs are transcribed from a single genomic
    locus encoding the chicken erythrocyte anion transport
    proteins (band 3).   Mol Cell Biol 8:4416.

16. Demuth DR, Showe LC, Ballantine M, Palumbo A, Fraser PJ,
    Cioe L, Rovera G and Curtis PJ (1986). Cloning and
    structural characterization of a human non-erythroid
    band 3-like protein.   EMBO J 5:1205.

17. Alper SL, Kopito RR, Libresco SM and Lodish HF (1988).
    Cloning and characterization of a murine band 3-related
    cDNA from kidney and from a lymphoid cell line.   J Biol
    Chem 263:17092.

18. Pasternack GR, Anderson RA, Leto TL and Marchesi VT
    (1985). Interactions between protein 4.1 and band 3.
    J Biol Chem 260:3676.

19. Lu P-W, Soong C-J and Tao MJ (1985). Phosphorylation of
    ankyrin decreases its affinity for spectrin tetramer.
    J Biol Chem 260:14958.

20. Soong C-J, Lu P-W and Tao M (1987). Analysis of

band 3 cytoplasmic domain phosphorylation and association with ankyrin. Arch Biochem Biophys 254:509.

21. Hope IA and Struhl K (1985). GCN4 protein, synthesized in vitro, binds HIS3 regulatory sequences: implications for general control of amino acid biosynthetic genes in yeast. Cell 43:177.

22. Vrana KE, Churchill MEA, Tullius TD and Brown DD (1988). Mapping functional regions of transcription factor TFIIIA. Mol Cell Biol 8:1684.

23. Gharakhanian E, Takahashi J, Clever J and Kasamatsu H (1988). In vitro assay for protein-protein interaction: Carboxyl-terminal 40 residues of simian virus structural protein VP3 contain a determinant for interaction with VP1. Proc Natl Acad Sci USA 85:6607.

24. Bennett V (1983). Proteins involved in membrane-cytoskeleton association in human erythrocytes: spectrin, ankyrin and band 3. Meth Enzymol 96:313.

25. Goldstein JL, Basu SK and Brown MS (1983). Receptor-mediated endocytosis of low-density lipoprotein in cultured cells. Meth Enzymol 98:241.

26. Morrow JS and Haigh WB, Jnr. (1983). Erythrocyte membrane proteins: detection of spectrin oligomers by gel electrophoresis. Meth Enzymol 96:299.

27. Bennett, V. (1982). Isolation of an ankyrin-band 3 oligomer from human erythrocyte membranes. Biochem Biophys Acta 689:475.

28. Davis L, Lux SE and Bennett V (1989). Mapping the ankyrin-binding site of the erythrocyte anion exchanger. (Submitted).

29. Alper SL, Kopito RR and Lodish HF (1987). A molecular biological approach to the study of ion transport. Kidney Int 32 suppl 23:S117.

30. Kopito RR, Andersson M and Lodish HF (1987). Structure and organization of the murine band 3 gene. J Biol Chem 262:8035.

31. Kopito RR, Andersson MA and Lodish HF (1987). Multiple tissue-specific sites or transcriptional initiation of the mouse anion antiport gene in erythroid and renal cells. Proc Natl Acad Sci USA 84:7149.

32. Alper SL, Brosius FG III, Garcia AM, Davies KA, Gluck S, Brown D and Lodish HF (1989). Two gene products encoding putative anion exchangers of the distal nephron. Anal NY Acad Sci (in press).

33. Patel V and Lodish HF (1987). A fibronectin matrix is required for differentiation of murine erythroleukemia cells into reticulocytes. J Cell Biol 105:3105.

**Cellular and Molecular Biology of Normal
and Abnormal Erythroid Membranes, pages 43–59**
© **1990 Alan R. Liss, Inc.**

MEMBRANE SKELETAL PROTEIN 4.1 OF HUMAN ERYTHROID AND NON-ERYTHROID CELLS IS COMPOSED OF MULTIPLE ISOFORMS WITH NOVEL SIZES, FUNCTIONS AND TISSUE SPECIFIC EXPRESSION

Tang K. Tang[2,3,5], Zhi Qin[4], Thomas Leto[4,6]
Vincent T. Marchesi[4], and Edward J. Benz, Jr.[2,3]

Departments of Internal Medicine[2], Human Genetics[3],
Pathology[4], School of Medicine, Yale University,
New Haven, CT 06510

ABSTRACT   Protein 4.1 is an important cytoskeletal protein present in many cell types. We have demonstrated that many isoforms of protein 4.1 arise from a single gene by alternative mRNA splicing at least 5 positions, or sequence motifs along the mRNA molecule. One motif is expressed specifically in erythroid cells; we have shown that this motif is induced during erythroid maturation, and that it is required for binding to erythroid spectrin/actin. Two mRNA splicing events in the 5' end can, if they occur in concert, create a new translation start site and open reading frame in the 5' untranslated region, causing production of a 135 kd protein that is abundant in the nucleus. Protein 4.1 isoforms thus comprise a complex protein family expressed in most cell types. Alternate mRNA splicing events thus generate isoforms with novel sizes, functions and cell type specific patterns of expression.

---

[1]This work was supported by NIH grants HL24385, AM28376, and GM21714.
[5]Present address: Institute of Biomedical Sciences, Academia Sinica, Taipei 11529,Taiwan, ROC
[6]Present address: National Institute of Allergy and Infectious Diseases, National Institutes of Health, Bethesda, MD 20892

INTRODUCTION

Protein 4.1 is an 80 kd sulfhydryl rich phosphoprotein originally isolated from cytoskeletal preparations of mature human red cells. Protein 4.1 is important for maintenance of the structural integrity and flexibility of the red cell membrane and its underlying cytoskeleton (1,2). Defects in the quantity or structure of protein 4.1 are associated with congenital hemolytic anemias (3,4).

Erythrocyte protein 4.1 has been characterized in considerable detail. In erythrocytes it serves as a linking molecule, attaching the spectrin/actin cytoskeletal scaffold to the lipid bilayer by means of the cytoplasmic domains of trans-membrane proteins. Limited chymotryptic digestion (Figure 1) yields four fragments (5). The amino terminal 30 kd domain appears to bind the trans-membrane protein glycophorin in the presence of triphos-phoinositides (TPI). The 10 kd domain contains the sites for binding to complexes of erythroid spectrin and actin (5).

Immunologically cross-reactive forms of protein 4.1 can be found in most tissues. These isoforms exhibit remarkable diversity with regard to the numbers of discrete molecular weight forms present in each tissue, and their intracellular localization (6-14). In non-erythroid tissues protein 4.1 appears to be prominent in the nucleus (Tang et al., to be submitted) in intracytoplasmic fibrillar networks (6) or in perinuclear region (13) as well as in the subplasmalema. These findings suggest that erythroid protein 4.1 is the prototype of either a large gene family or a large protein family arising from a single gene by alternative processing of mRNA and/or protein products. Recently, Conboy et al (15) reported the cDNA sequence encoding a protein 4.1 isolated from a reticulocyte cDNA library. We (14) and others (16,17) have subsequently presented evidence that non-erythroid and erythroid protein 4.1 exhibited discrete regional differences in mRNA structure that most likely arise by alternate mRNA splicing.

We now present new information suggesting that many isoforms are generated by mRNA splicing. At least one of these motifs is expressed in a tissue-specific manner, in which it is required for spectrin/actin binding. We also discuss recent findings suggesting that modification of the 5' untranslated region of the mRNA alters the translation potential of the mRNA in such a way that a higher molecular weight peptide exhibiting prominent nuclear staining is produced.

RESULTS

Diverse Structures of cDNA Clones Encoding Multiple Forms of
Protein 4.1 in Erythroid and Lymphoid Cells.

    Figure 1 shows a molecular model for the structure of
the prototypical erythroid protein 4.1 species, based on
mRNA sequence, partial amino acid sequence data, and
functional analysis[5]. The regions of the putative
glycophorin and spectrin/actin binding sites are indicated.

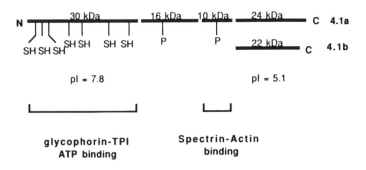

Molecular model of human erythrocyte protein 4.1

Figure 1.   A molecular model of human erythrocyte
protein 4.1 deduced from limited proteolytic digestions and
chemical degradation studies (5).

    Figure 2 diagrams the structure of several repre-
sentative cDNAs obtained from erythroid and non-erythroid
sources.   Sequence differences were limited to five regions
ranging in size from 17 to 105 nucleotides. (Most recently
we have identified 2-4 additional motifs.)   These are
indicated as the blocks labeled Motifs I - V in Figure 2.

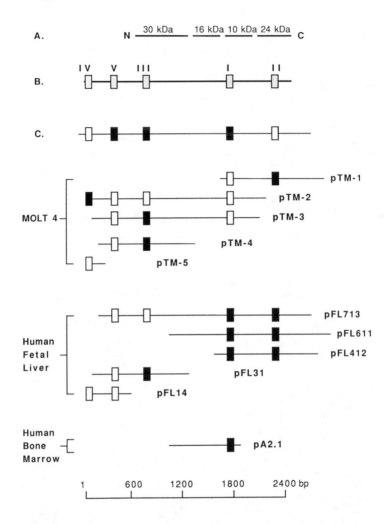

Figure 2.   Summary of the diverse protein 4.1 cDNA
clones isolated from the cDNA libraries of different source
of tissues. (A) Structural domains of human erythrocyte
protein 4.1. (B) Five different nucleotide sequence motifs
(I to V) identified in protein 4.1 mRNAs. (C) Diverse
structure of protein 4.1 cDNA clones isolated from human
lymphoid (MOLT 4), fetal liver, and bone marrow cDNA
libraries. An open block indicates the sequence is absent in
the cDNA clones; a black block indicates that the sequence
is present.

Since Southern blot analysis of genomic DNA reveals one or at most a very few copies of the 4.1 gene (our unpublished results; 4,16,17) there are clearly not enough gene loci to account for the diversity of mRNA sequences we observed. However, sequence variation is confined to a few discrete blocks (Figure 2). Both of these considerations strongly support the notion that the array of cDNA's we encountered arose by alternative mRNA splicing.

We have named the five sequence blocks Motifs I-V, in the order of their discovery (Figures 3). MOTIF I is 63 nucleotides long, encoding a 21 amino acid segment within a 10 kd spectrin/actin binding domain. MOTIF II (102 nucleotides) encodes a 34 amino acid segment near the carboxyl end of the 22/24 kd domain. MOTIF III (105 nucleotides) encodes a 35 amino acid peptide near the amino terminal end of the 30 kd domain. MOTIF IV is 17 bases long in the 5' untranslated region. MOTIF V, also located in the 5' untranslated region, is 80 bases long.

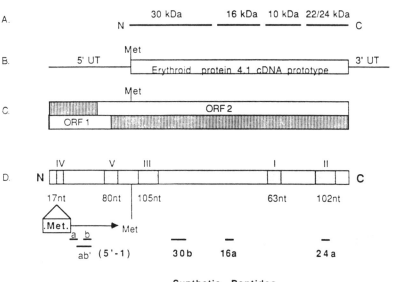

Figure 3. Diverse forms of erythroid and non-erythroid protein 4.1 and alignment of synthetic peptides used for generation of site specific antibodies. (A) Structural domains of human erythrocyte protein 4.1. (B) Erythroid protein 4.1 cDNA clone reported by Conboy et al., (1986b).

(C) Two open reading frames (ORF 1 and 2) found in erythroid 4.1 sequence. (D) Variable motifs (I to V) defined by comparison of erythroid (Conboy et al., 15) and lymphoid cDNA sequence. Synthetic peptides, 5'-1, 30b, 16a, and 24a, are described in detailed in the Results section.

The unique features of MOTIF's IV and V merit further preliminary comment (Figure 3). These motifs can exert complex effects on the structure and translational function of protein 4.1 mRNA. The 5' untranslated sequence of the prototypical protein 4.1 mRNA contains a long open reading frame (ORF-1) contiguous with the ORF-2 in the figure. In erythrocyte protein 4.1 ORF-2 is translated from the indicated initiator methionine codon into an 80 kd polypeptide. Upstream of this initiator codon, all three reading frames are "closed" by a cluster of termination codons located 40 - 300 bases upstream of the initiator methionine. There is no other initiator methionine in the 5' untranslated sequence. However, some of the cDNA's that we isolated possessed an additional motif at the extreme 5' end (MOTIF IV) and also lacked an 80 base motif (MOTIF V), located between MOTIF IV and the erythrocyte initiator AUG. Removal of the 80 bases within MOTIF V deletes several termination codons. Retention of MOTIF IV in the mRNA introduces a methionine codon surrounded by a strong consensus translation initiation signal (18). Moreover, the combination of a 17 base insert (MOTIF IV) and an 80 base deletion (MOTIF V) shifts the reading frame; counting from the A of the AUG of the new upstream methionine codon in MOTIF IV, there are no termination codons encountered between this methionine and the initiator methionine of the 80 kd protein. The reading frame is thus continuous and in phase with that beginning with the erythrocyte initiator AUG.

Concerted retention of MOTIF IV and deletion of MOTIF V can generate a new protein 4.1 isoform having a higher molecular weight. This additional coding sequence adds 209 amino acids to the amino terminal end of the prototypical 4.1 (80 kd) molecule. Initiation at the upstream methionine creates a larger protein within which the C-terminal 80 kd represents the prototypical 80 Kd 4.1 molecule.

The cDNA's we have characterized establish the structure of several distinctive protein 4.1 mRNAs and predict the existence of many heterogeneous isoforms. Moreover, the identification of these five sequence motifs provide the structural bases for at least 32 mRNAs, from which 16 distinct protein isoforms can be generated. (Since MOTIF IV and MOTIF V must act in concert to generate additional protein isoforms, there can be more mRNAs than proteins.)

Expression of Multiple Protein 4.1 mRNAs in Erythroid and Non-Erythroid Cells.

In order to detect protein 4.1 mRNAs expressed in various tissues and species, we developed nucleic acid probes for mRNAs containing or lacking specific motifs. Poly A^+ mRNA and total RNA were isolated from human erythroid and non-erythroid cells and analyzed either by Northern blot hybridization (Figure 4) or RNase protection analysis (Figure 5). Northern blots were analyzed with lymphoid 4.1 cDNA probe (PTM-1). RNase protection analysis was performed with synthetic RNA probes containing the appropriate motifs. mRNA is containing or lacking the particular motif thus generate "protected" (RNA'se resistant) fragments of different lengths.

One major mRNA band, at about 6.6 kb was detected in the RNAs prepared from HEL, K562, MOLT 4, and HeLa cell lines as well as in a CML patient (Figure 4). A minor species at 4.4 kb was also detected. Protein 4.1 mRNA's from bovine (BAE), mouse (MEL), and sheep (SR) cells, migrate as bands of distinctive size, but, the hybridization signal is retained even after stringent washing conditions. These results suggest that protein 4.1 mRNA sequences are highly conserved across species, but that significant size differences, possibly in the untranslated regions, exist.

Expression of Protein 4.1 mRNA's in Erythroid Cells.

We have previously reported (14) that protein 4.1 mRNA levels increase after DMSO induction of erythroid maturation in mouse erythroleukemia cells (MELC); Figure 4 shows a representative result. As indicated by Figure 5, MOTIF I is expressed only in erythroid cell mRNA; indeed, we have previously shown that expression of MOTIF I is induced in MELC by DMSO (data not shown, 14). Figure 6 shows the results of RNase protection analysis of MOTIF IV expression in erythroid and non-erythroid cells. As shown in Figure 6A, at least two types of protein 4.1 mRNAs (one containing, and one lacking MOTIF IV) were produced from MOLT 4 and HEL cells. About two thirds of the protein 4.1 mRNA contains MOTIF IV in MOLT 4 cells. In sharp contrast (Figure 6), human reticulocytes (HR) show almost no mRNA that retains this motif. Note the multiple banding pattern shown in Figure 6A. This could arise from nuclease digestion artifacts, or indicate potential additional motifs in that region. Interestingly, the MOTIF IV signal in HeLa cells is very weak (Figure 6A). Similar results were found when the probes spanning MOTIF II (Figure 6C) or III (Figure 6B) were used. These results might represent a lesser content of protein 4.1 mRNA in HeLa cells.

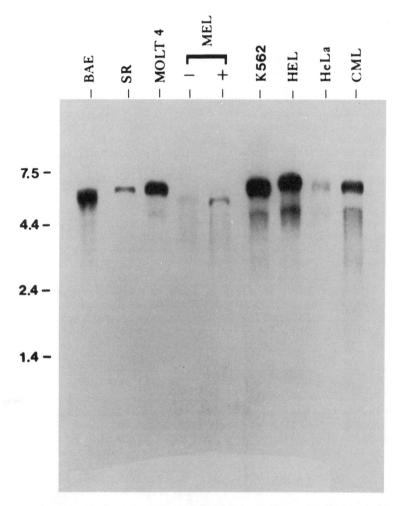

Figure 4. RNA blot analysis of erythroid and non-erythroid mRNAs. 5ug Poly A$^+$ mRNAs isolated from BAE (Bovine arotical endothelial cells, a gift from Dr. J. Madri, Yale University), SR (Sheep reticulocyte), MOLT 4 (a human T cell leukemia line), - MEL (uninduced mouse erythroleukemia line), + MEL (dimethyl sulfoxide induced), K562 and HEL (human erythroleukemia lines), HeLa (human epitheloid carcinoma line), and leukocytes of CML (chronic myelogenous leukemia) patients were hybridized with the pTM-1 cDNA probe (Figure 2C). Standards used for size estimates were RNA ladder markers (kilobase).

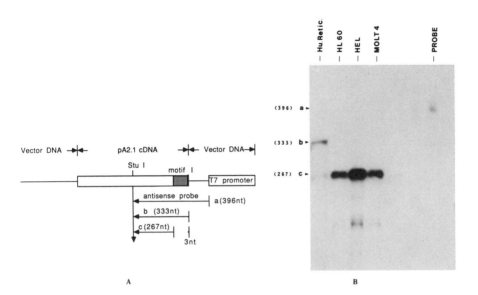

Figure 5. Erythroid specific expression of MOTIF I by an RNase protection assay. Specific antisense probes were designed by constructing sequence specific cDNA clones that contain specific motifs. The cDNA inserts of these clones were subcloned into a pGEM-4 or -7Z vectors, which contains SP6 or T7 RNA polymerase promoters. Antisense RNAs were generated from the T7 promoter within the vector. Total RNA's (30mg) were hybridized to the antisense probe spanning MOTIF I. The sizes of the nuclease resistant bands expected for undigested probe (396nt), RNA containing MOTIF I (333nt), RNA lacking MOTIF I (267nt) are shown. See figures for cell types.

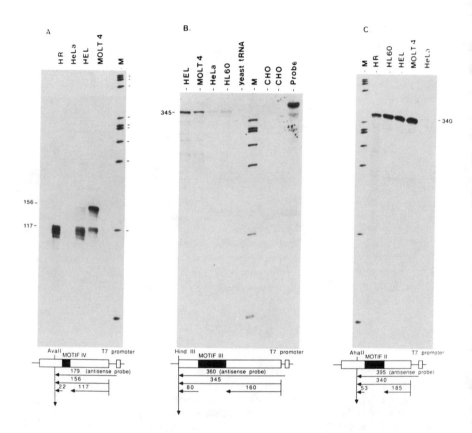

Figure 6. Detection of erythroid and non-erythroid protein 4.1 mRNAs by RNase protection assay. Total RNAs (30ug) from different tissues or cell lines were hybridized to the antisense probes which span MOTIF IV (A), MOTIF III (B), or MOTIF II (C). HR, human reticulocyte; HL60, human promyelocytic leukemia line; CHO, Chinese hamster ovary line; HEL, human erythroleukemia line; MOLT 4, human T cell leukemia line; HeLa, human epitheloid carcinoma line. Bars denote φX174 Hae III-digested DNA size markers (M). The positions of size markers are indicated in nucleotide.

In contrast to the distribution of MOTIF IV, mRNA containing Motifs III (the protected fragment is 345nt) or II (340nt) represent well over 90% of the mRNA found in both erythroid and non-erythroid cells (Figure 6B and 6C).

Expression of Protein Isoforms in Non-Erythroid Cells.

Analysis of non-erythroid protein 4.1 mRNAs (Figure 6A) suggested that the majority of the mRNA contains MOTIF IV, and thus possess the potential for translation into a higher molecular weight isoform. We sought to identify this higher molecular weight protein in intact cells by raising antisera against peptides encoded by specific splicing events. Synthetic peptides derived from the deduced amino acid sequences of the 30 kd (30b), 16 kd (16a), and 24 kd (24a) were prepared as well as a synthetic peptide mixture, 5'-1, which is a mixture of 3 peptides a, b, and ab' shown in Figure 3. The 5'-1 peptides were derived from the predicted amino terminal translated sequence of the larger 4.1 isoform, whose synthesis begins with the methionine within the 17 base MOTIF IV. Polyclonal antisera were raised against these peptides, purified, and characterized.

Figure 7 shows immunoblot analysis of 4.1 proteins from MOLT 4 cells. Isoforms corresponding to peptide chains of approximately 135 kd and 80 kd were identified in MOLT 4 cells. Both proteins strongly react with antibodies against intact erythroid protein 4.1 and anti-30b, 16a, and 24a antibodies. Interestingly, higher molecular weight forms were also detected on the blot with some of these antibodies. The anti 5'-1 antibody detected only the 135 kd protein, suggesting that the high molecular weight form predicted by cDNA sequence analysis was expressed in intact cells. Immunofluorescent analysis of nucleated cells (data not shown; Tang, et al., submitted, 1989) has shown that inclusion of MOTIF IV and deletion of MOTIF V generate a novel high molecular weight protein 4.1 isoform that is at least partially localized in the nucleus.

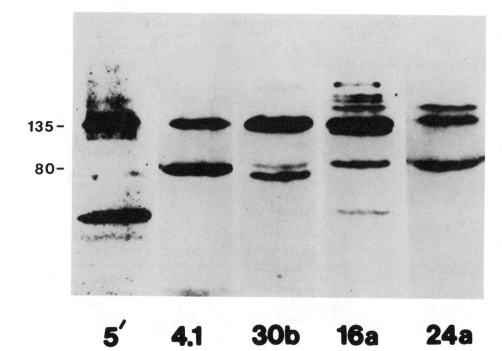

Figure 7.   Immunoblot analysis of lymphoid protein 4.1
isoforms. Solubilized proteins from MOLT 4 cells were
separated by NaDodSO4/PAGE and blotted onto nitrocellulose
as described (14).   Blotted proteins were probed with
polyclonal anti intact erythroid 4.1, anti 5'-1, -30b, -16a,
and -24a antibodies, and detected by ^{125}I-labeled
Staphylococcus protein A (14). The numbers shown on the left
are in kilodalton.

Functional Importance of the "Erythroid-Specific" Motif,
MOTIF I.

    MOTIF I encodes 21 amino acids at the aminoterminus of
the 10 kd domain. Correas, et al. (19,20) had previously
presented evidence that the 10 kd domain bound efficiently
to spectrin actin complexes. Therefore, we hypothesized
that MOTIF I was an essential component of this binding
activity. This hypothesis is teleologically appealing
because of the apparent confinement of MOTIF I expression to
erythroid cells and the presence in erythrocytes of a unique
form of spectrin, erythrocyte spectrin.
    In order to evaluate the spectrin/actin binding
properties of MOTIF I, we constructed cDNA's encoding 2
protein 4.1 isoforms identical in all respects except for
the presence or absence of MOTIF I (data not shown). The
cDNA's were inserted into pGEM vectors so that they could be
transcribed into mRNA and then translated into ^{35}S labeled
protein in cell-free extracts.
    The assay used to evaluate binding consisted of
incubating spectrin/actin mixtures with the ^{35}S labeled
protein 4.1, followed by ultracentrifugation. Native
erythrocyte protein 4.1 forms a ternary complex with
spectrin and actin and pellets. However, in reaction with
spectrin alone or actin alone is more limited; no pelletable
material is formed.

    Spectrin/actin and protein 4.1 containing MOTIF I
formed pelletable complexes (data not shown). In contrast,
protein 4.1 lacking MOTIF I formed no complexes. Therefore,
we conclude that the tissue-specific expression of MOTIF I
in erythroid cells endows these forms of protein 4.1 with
spectrin/actin binding properties appropriate to the
particular type of cytoskeleton formed in red cells.

DISCUSSION

Previous studies have provided indirect evidence for the existence of multiple isoforms of protein 4.1 (12,14,15,16) that are immunologically cross-reactive, expressed in many tissues, and heterogeneous with respect to size and relative abundance of size classes. Moreover, localization of protein 4.1 by immunocytochemical methods suggested that these isoforms might be distributed in and around the nucleus (Tang et al., submitted), and along stress fibers (6), as well as under the cytoplasmic membrane. We have described studies that establish the existence of multiple isoforms and provide a genetic basis for many of these forms. Protein 4.1 appears to be a protein family arising from a multiplicity of messenger RNAs generated by alternative mRNA processing.

A novel result of our studies, not anticipated by previous work, was the existence of a high molecular weight class of protein 4.1 isoforms generated from the same gene by the alternate splicing events discussed in the Results section. The protein can be uniquely identified by an anti-peptide antibody that we have designed on the basis of novel amino terminal peptides translatable into protein only if the appropriate mRNA splicing events occur. The size of the protein isolated from whole cells agrees closely with the predicted size. This high molecular weight protein is abundant in the nucleus (Tang et al, submitted). We postulate that protein 4.1 isoforms are important for assembly and integrity of skeletal structures within the nucleus, as well as the cytoplasm.

Erythroid cells (human reticulocytes and MELC) exhibited unique patterns of protein 4.1 mRNA expression. These cells contain almost no mRNA encoding the larger isoform (Figure 6) but are the only cells to produce isoforms expressing MOTIF I (14; Figure 5).

Protein 4.1 is a bifunctional protein, attaching to the cytoplasmic domain of trans-membrane proteins (glycophorin 3) at its amino terminal end, and to cytoskeletal structures (spectrin/actin complexes) by means of the 10 kd domain. It is important to note that the assignments of functions to specific domains have been accomplished only for erythroid forms of the protein 4.1 - in systems employing membrane and cytoskeletal elements derived from erythroid cells. The function of isoforms expressed in non-erythroid tissues remains an open question. Our results suggest that retention of MOTIF I is important for binding of the molecule to erythroid spectrin/actin complexes. This may account for its unexpected intracellular distribution. The sequence motifs that we have identified might subserve novel functions of the protein.

ACKNOWLEDGMENTS

We thank C. E. Mazzucco and S. Pleasic for technical assistance. We also thank Ms. Phoebe Barron for expert manuscript preparation. Figure 4 reproduced from Reference 14, with permission.

REFERENCES

1. Marchesi VT (1985). Stabilizing infrastructure of cell membranes. Annu Rev Cell Biol 1:531.
2. Bennett V (1985). The membrane skeleton of human erythrocytes and its implications for more complex cells. Annu Rev Biochem 54:273.
3. Conboy J, Mohandas N, Tchernia G, Kan YW (1986). Molecular basis of hereditary elliptocytosis due to protein 4.1 defficiency. N Engl J Med 315:680.
4. Tchernia G, Mohandas N, Shohet SB (1981). Deficiency of cytoskeletal membrane protein band 4.1 in homozyous hereditary elliptocytosis: implications for erythrocyte membrane stability. J Clin Invest 68:454.
5. Leto TL, Correas I, Tobe T, Anderson RA, Horne WC (1986). Structure and function of human erythrocyte cytoskeletal protein 4.1. In Bennett V, Cohen CM, Lux SE, Palek J, (eds): "Membrane Skeletons and Cytoskeletal Membrane Associations," New York: Alan R. Liss, p. 201.

6. Cohen CM, Foley SF, Korsgren C (1982). A protein immunologically related to erythrocyte band 4.1 is found on stress fibers of non-erythroid cells. Nature 299:648.

7. Spiegel JE, Beardsley DS, Southwick FS, Lux SE (1984). An analogue of the erythroid membrane skeletal protein 4.1 in nonerythroid cells. J Cell Biol 99:886.

8. Aster JC, Welsh MJ, Brewer GJ, Maisel H (1984). Identification of spectrin and protein 4.1-like proteins in mammalian lens. Biochem Biophys Res Commun 119:726.

9. Baines AJ, Bennett V (1985). Synapsin I is a spectrin-binding protein immunologically related to erythrocyte protein 4.1. Nature 315:410.

10. Davies GE, Cohen CM (1985). Platelets contain proteins immunologically related to red cell spectrin and protein 4.1. Blood 65:52.

11. Goodman SR, Casoria LA, Coleman DB, Zagon IS (1984). Identification and isolation of brain 4.1. Science 224:1433.

12. Granger BL, Lazarides E (1984). Membrane skeletal protein 4.1 of avian erythrocytes is composed of multiple variants that exhibit tissue-specific expression. Cell 37:595.

13. Leto TL, Pratt BM, Madri JA (1986). Mechanisms of cytoskeletal regulation: modulation of aortic endothelial cell protein band 4.1 by the extracellular matrix. J Cell Physiol 127:423.

14. Tang TK, Leto TL, Correas I, Alonso MA, Marchesi VT, Benz Jr EJ (1988). Selective expression of an erythroid-specific isoform of protein 4.1. Proc Natl Acad Sci USA 85:3713.

15. Conboy J, Kan YW, Shohet SB, Mohandas N (1986). Molecular cloning of protein 4.1, a major structural element of the human erythrocyte membrane skeleton. Proc Natl Acad Sci USA 83:9512.

16. Conboy JG, Chan J, Mohandas N, Kan YW (1988). Multiple protein 4.1 isoforms produced by alternative splicing in human erythroid cells. Proc Natl Acad Sci USA 85:9062.

17. Ngai J, Stack JH, Moon RT, Lazarides E (1987). Regulated expression of multiple chicken erythroid membrane skeletal protein 4.1 variants is governed by differential RNA processing and translational control. Proc Natl Acad Sci USA 84:4432.

18. Kozak M (1984). Compilation and analysis of sequences upstream from the translational start site in eukaryotic mRNAs. Nucl Acids Res 12:857.

19. Correas I, Leto TL, Speicher DW, Marchesi VT (1986). Identification of the functional site of erythrocyte protein 4.1 involved in spectrin-actin association. J Biol Chem 261:3310.

20. Correas I, Speicher DW, Marchesi VT (1986). Structure of the spectrin-actin binding sites of erythrocyte protein 4.1. J Biol Chem 261:13362.

**Cellular and Molecular Biology of Normal
and Abnormal Erythroid Membranes, pages 61–74
© 1990 Alan R. Liss, Inc.**

PROTEIN 4.1 mRNA STRUCTURE IN NORMAL AND
ABNORMAL ERYTHROID MEMBRANES[1]

John G. Conboy

Cancer Research Institute, University of
California, San Francisco, CA 94143

ABSTRACT. Protein 4.1 is a multi-functional
structural protein located in the erythrocyte
membrane skeleton and in many nonerythroid
cells. Rapid cloning of protein 4.1 mRNA by a
modification of the polymerase chain reaction
(PCR) has facilitated sequence analysis of
4.1 in normal and abnormal erythrocyte
membranes. In normal human reticulocytes, we
characterized multiple closely-related
protein 4.1 mRNAs that appear to be derived
by alternative mRNA splicing of exons from a
single complex gene. This finding raises the
possibility that the many binding functions
ascribed to protein 4.1 may reside in
distinct structural isoforms. In a patient
with hereditary elliptocytosis and shortened
protein 4.1, molecular cloning by PCR
revealed an internal deletion involving 80
amino acids (aa) in the spectrin/actin
binding region.

INTRODUCTION

The specialized mechanical and morphological
properties of the erythrocyte membrane are
maintained by an extensive and highly organized
network of structural proteins, collectively
termed the membrane skeleton, that underlies the
plasma membrane on its cytoplasmic side (1-3). By

---

[1]This work was supported by NIH grant DK 32094.

classical biochemical studies of purified skeletal
proteins from normal individuals and patients with
inherited membrane abnormalities, a reasonable
model of this important cellular structure has
emerged. Now, molecular biological analysis of the
genes encoding red cell membrane skeletal proteins
is proceeding in earnest, with the recent cloning
of cDNAs for protein 4.1(4,5), α- and β-spectrin(6-
9), band 3(10), glycophorins A(11) and C(12,13),
and ankyrin(15,16). These studies are revealing
more and more diversity in the structure and
expression of the membrane skeletal proteins in
various cell types, due to expression of
homologous nonerythroid genes (16-18) and to
alternative splicing of pre-mRNA derived from a
single multi-exon gene(19). The latter mechanism
can generate a family of mRNAs that encode
multiple "spliceoforms" of important cellular
structural proteins.

We are studying the structure and expression
of the protein 4.1 gene in erythroid and
nonerythroid cells. Using cloned human reticulocyte 4.1 cDNA, we previously deduced the entire
primary amino acid sequence of a prototype protein
4.1 polypeptide and investigated expression of 4.1
mRNA in other human tissues by Northern blot-
ting(4). We also determined that erythroid protein
4.1 is encoded by a single copy gene on chromosome
1(20). In this paper I will focus on some recent
unexpected findings regarding the complexity of
expression of the protein 4.1 gene. We have used a
reverse transcriptase/polymerase chain reaction
(PCR) protocol to clone and characterize multiple
species of protein 4.1 mRNA from human erythroid
and nonerythroid cells. Three major applications
of this approach are addressed: (1) analysis of
alternative splicing in normal human reticulocyte
RNA, (2)characterization of 4.1 mutations using
4.1 mRNA from HE patients, and (3)analysis of
nonerythroid 4.1 expression and structure.

ALTERNATIVE RNA SPLICING

Transcription of a complex multi-exon gene
produces a single species of pre-mRNA that is the

substrate for all subsequent splicing reactions. This pre-mRNA retains the original organization of the gene and is composed of introns, constitutively expressed exons, and alternatively expressed exons. Formation of mature mRNAs requires removal of introns by splicing events that join together the coding sequences in adjacent exons. Constitutive exons are always represented in the final product, whereas alternative exons can be spliced in or out by a sophisticated RNA processing machinery. The end result is production of a population of mature cytoplasmic mRNAs that are identical except for small insertions and deletions of these exon "cassettes." Translation of such mRNAs results in synthesis of a family of protein "spliceoforms" that differ by the presence or absence of small peptides within an otherwise identical framework (reviewed in 21).

CHARACTERIZATION OF MULTIPLE ERYTHROID PROTEIN 4.1 mRNAs

Two cloning techniques have been utilized to study the structure of many different 4.1 mRNAs that are present in normal human reticulocyte mRNA: traditional cDNA cloning, and the more recent polymerase chain reaction (PCR) methodology for enzymatic amplification of RNA sequences. We have found a number of insertions and deletions among this population of protein 4.1 mRNAs. This information allowed us to deduce an alternative splicing "map" of the complicated multi-exon protein 4.1 gene.

Analysis by Traditional cDNA Cloning

Sequence comparison of several 4.1 cDNA clones isolated from human reticulocyte (4,19) and human T-lymphocyte (5) cDNA libraries revealed differences characteristic of alternatively spliced mRNAs. That is, the cDNAs from these two libraries were identical except for three cassettes of sequence: the reticulocyte cDNA

encoded peptides of 21 amino acids (aa) (in the
spectrin/actin binding region) and 35aa (in the
30kD domain) that were not present in the
lymphocyte cDNA, and conversely, the lymphocyte
clone encoded a 34aa peptide (in the C-terminal
domain) not found in the reticulocyte cDNA.

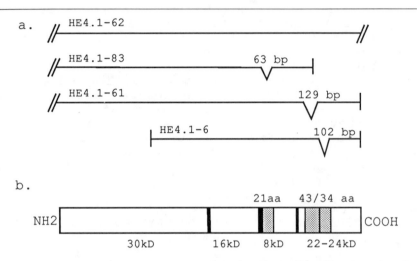

Figure 1a. Structure of alternatively spliced protein 4.1
isoforms detected by cDNA cloning. 1b. Structural model of
protein 4.1 from reference 22.

Alternative splicing was also detected among
cDNAs from a single cell lineage. Figure 1
illustrates four different types of protein 4.1
cDNAs isolated from the reticulocyte cDNA library.
Panel a shows the location of splicing differences
among these mRNAs. The number of nucleotides in
each cassette is an integral multiple of three, so
that deletion or insertion of any combination will
not alter the downstream reading frame.
Panel b shows a structural model of
erythrocyte protein 4.1, derived from biochemical
studies of total erythrocyte protein 4.1 (22).
Superimposed on this protein model, we show the
size and location of the three peptides whose
expression was variable among these four
reticulocyte 4.1 cDNAs. Four protein 4.1
polypeptides can be produced that are identical

except for the precise in-frame deletion or insertion of these peptides.

Analysis by Reverse Transcriptase/Polymerase Chain Reaction.

      This surprising heterogeneity in protein 4.1 structure was found by analysis of only a dozen or so cDNAs. Because this approach may well have overlooked less abundant isoforms, we decided to conduct a more systematic and thorough search. Protein 4.1 mRNA sequences were amplified in a two-stage reaction involving synthesis of single-stranded DNA catalyzed by reverse transcriptase, followed by amplification using standard PCR techniques with specific oligonucleotides and the thermal stable DNA polymerase from *Thermus aquaticus* (23-25; Figure 2). Alternatively spliced mRNAs possessing insertions or deletions within the limits of the amplified region yield different sized DNA fragments. These isoform-specific DNA fragments can be resolved by polyacrylamide gel

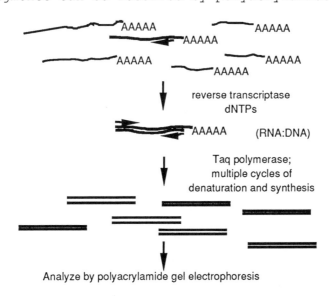

Figure 2. Scheme for PCR analysis of 4.1 mRNA

electrophoresis and purified for DNA sequence
analysis.
     Analysis of 4.1 mRNA sequences spanning the
entire spectrin/actin binding domain, including
the alternatively expressed 21aa peptide, was
performed using oligonucleotides A and B (Fig. 3).
Based on the previous cDNA cloning studies, the
expected products should be 441 bp ("+21aa") and
381 bp ("-21aa"). Amplified 4.1 mRNA sequences
yielded two DNA bands with appropriate mobilities
(lane 2). DNA sequence analysis showed that the
441bp product actually consisted of two
molecularly distinct species: a predominant
product encoding the entire 8kD spectrin/actin
binding domain(26), including the 21aa peptide;
and a minor component encoding a novel peptide of
19aa substituted for the 21aa at exactly the same
position in the polypeptide chain. The smaller DNA
amplification product of 378nt encodes the
expected -21aa isoform.
     Amplification of the C-terminal coding region
of 4.1 mRNA was accomplished similarly using

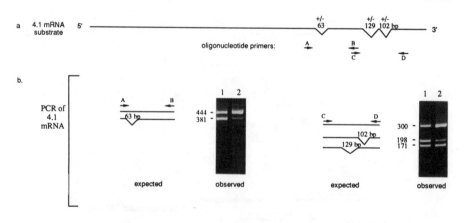

Figure 3.

oligonucleotides C and D (Fig. 3, right, lane 1).
The three DNA bands produced in this reaction were
sequenced and shown to correspond exactly to the
three isoforms observed by cDNA cloning: a 300bp

band that includes sequences encoding both alternatively expressed 43 and 34aa peptides; a 198bp fragment encoding the -34aa isoform; and a 171bp fragment encoding the -43aa isoform.

Finally, we examined the 30kD and 16kD domains of 4.1 mRNA. In the 30kD domain, the major amplified DNA fragments were identical to the published reticulocyte 4.1 sequence (4). Additionally, two minor products were observed, corresponding to polypeptides having deletions of 35 and 73aa, respectively (not shown). The 35aa peptide is the same sequence that was deleted in the lymphocyte 4.1 cDNA (5). In contrast to the other three domains of protein 4.1, analysis of the 16kD region did not reveal any evidence of alternative splicing.

PCR analysis of protein 4.1 mRNA has thus revealed considerable variation within the framework of the 80kD erythroid 4.1 polypeptide. A total of 6 alternatively expressed peptides have been characterized: 2 in 30kD, 2 in the spectrin/actin binding domain, and 2 in the C-terminal region. Taking into account the possibility of various splicing combinations among the exons encoding these peptides, a large family of closely related 4.1 isoforms can potentially be encoded by a single gene. The relative abundance of specific spliceoforms can be estimated based on their relative frequency in our cDNA library and on the 'time course' of production of specific DNAs in the PCR reaction. Several isoforms are relatively common, i.e., those with the deletions of 35aa (in the 30kD domain) and 43aa (in the C-terminal domain). Others are quite rare, including the 73aa deletion (30kD domain) and the 19aa insertion (spectrin/actin binding domain).

Alternative splicing in the 5' region of protein 4.1 mRNA.

The published reticulocyte 4.1 cDNA had a long 5'untranslated sequence of approximately 800 bases. It contains two overlapping open reading frames of 100 (ORF1) and 170aa (ORF2), respectively (Figure 4). ORF1 is contiguous with the authentic downstream 4.1 sequence, but contains no AUG translation start site to drive its synthesis; ORF2 extends farther upstream, but is out of frame with the authentic 4.1 sequence. Although these sequences could not be translated in the context of this mRNA, it seemed unlikely that ORFs of such great length could exist by chance. Recently, PCR analysis of this region has revealed the presence of spliced 4.1 mRNAs that may utilize these ORF sequences to encode higher molecular weight 4.1 polypeptides.

One strategic splicing change fuses ORF1 and ORF2 with the downstream 4.1 sequence, creating a contiguous ORF extending about 100-200aa (in different spliceoforms) upstream of the normal NH_2-terminus. Fusion is effected by deleting a block of 80 nucleotides located upstream of the normal AUG, in the region of overlap between ORF1 and ORF2. This critical splicing difference removes stop codons at the end of ORF1 and joins it to ORF2. The resulting mRNA has an open reading frame extending >200aa upstream of the normal NH_2-terminus. In two less abundant but related mRNAs, more extensive deletions were observed, initiating at the same 80nt and extending 3' past the normal AUG by an additional 54 or 159nt (not shown). These latter mRNA species not only encode a potential NH_2-terminal extension, but also have deletions of the first 18 or 53aa found in the 80kD 4.1 polypeptide.

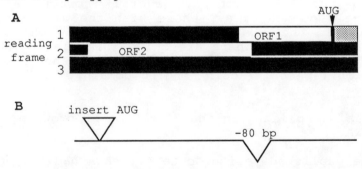

Figure 4. Translation potential in the 5' region of 4.1 mRNA.

A second alternative splicing event is required in order for these mRNAs to be expressed, namely, introduction an upstream AUG in the 5' ORF sequence (Figure 4B). Genomic DNA analysis has identified, at the 5' end of a large upstream exon, a potential AUG that can be spliced into or out of mature 4.1 mRNA by alternative usage of 3' splice acceptor sites(not shown).

Deletion of the normal AUG and utilization of the upstream AUG appear very rare in reticulocytes. However, we believe these structures are bona fide reticulocyte isoforms rather than an in vitro PCR artifacts, because cDNAs with identical sequences have recently been isolated from the reticulocyte cDNA library. The upstream AUG provides an attractive mechanism whereby high molecular weight 4.1 variants may be synthesized in other cells. In fact, an upstream translation initiation site has been reported in a lymphocyte 4.1 cDNA(27).

CHARACTERIZATION OF PROTEIN 4.1 MUTATIONS

Altered expression of protein 4.1 has, in several patients, been associated with hereditary elliptocytosis (HE). Patients with this disorder exhibit red cells with abnormal elliptical morphology and decreased mechanical stability. At least three distinct protein 4.1 phenotypes have been implicated in HE: complete deficiency(28), elongated protein 4.1(29), and shortened protein 4.1(29,30).

Previous studies of these mutants were focussed on DNA and protein, since in the past these substrates were more amenable to analysis than was RNA. However, RNA studies have a decided advantage in that any mutation can be sequenced in rapid and unambiguous fashion, allowing one to completely deduce the structure of the mutant protein. Thus, the current strategy of choice for characterization of 4.1 mutations is to clone and sequence the abnormal 4.1 mRNA by the reverse transcriptase/PCR method.

Figure 5 outlines the strategy being used to analyze mutant 4.1 mRNAs from each of the phenotypic classes mentioned above. In the patient with complete 4.1 deficiency, RNA and DNA analysis showed that affected reticulocytes express a shortened 4.1 mRNA that appears to have a deletion near the 5' end (20). In the case of the qualitatively altered 4.1 species, extensive studies by Sally Marchesi showed that both protein abnormalities were localized to the spectrin actin binding domain(31).

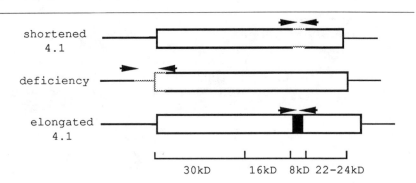

Figure 5. Strategy for PCR-cloning of mutant 4.1 mRNA from patients with hereditary elliptocytosis. Dotted lines indicate approximate limits of deletions; the black box represents inserted sequence.

Using the oligonucleotide primers indicated in the diagram, we have recently determined that the shortened 4.1 mRNA has a deletion of 240 nucleotides encoding 80 amino acids. This deletion encompasses virtually all of the spectrin/actin binding domain and part of the carboxy-terminal domain as well.

NONERYTHROID PROTEIN 4.1

Many nonerythroid tissues express RNAs that cross-hybridize with erythroid 4.1 cDNA in Northern blots(4). Similarly, proteins that crossreact immunologically with antibodies to erythroid 4.1 have also been detected in several nonerythroid tissues(32); some of the latter have very heterogeneous molecular weights. As a first step toward characterization of these related polypeptides, we have again used the reverse transcriptase/PCR technique to begin analysis of nonerythroid 4.1 mRNAs. When amplification of the spectrin/actin binding domain of 4.1 mRNA from liver, reticulocytes, and lymphocytes was performed, the predominant PCR product in reticulocytes, again, was the "+21aa" isoform. In contrast, lymphocytes and liver expressed predominantly the "-21aa" isoform (not shown). Furthermore, sequence analysis of the liver fragment showed nucleotide substitutions that may indicate the existence of a second protein 4.1 gene expressed in certain nonerythroid cells.

DISCUSSION

Several closely related erythrocyte protein 4.1 cDNAs have been characterized by analysis of cloned reticulocyte cDNAs and by PCR amplification of reticulocyte mRNA sequences. The existence of multiple protein 4.1 isoforms in a single cell type was unexpected and it raises important new questions regarding both the function of these proteins and the molecular biology of protein 4.1 gene expression. Previous studies have defined functional interactions between protein 4.1 and several other components of the skeleton, including spectrin and actin, band 3, and glycophorin (34,35). These interactions are dynamic in nature, regulated by phosphorylation (36), by phospho-inositide co-factors (37), and by calcium/calmodulin binding (38,39). The results presented here raise the possibility that individual binding sites or regulatory sites may reside in the variably expressed peptides, i.e., that different isoforms have different functions in the membrane. Alternatively, the family of 4.1 isoforms may exhibit a range of binding affinities for other membrane skeletal proteins important in the dynamics of the erythrocyte membrane.

Genetic evidence indicates that only a single protein 4.1 gene is expressed in human erythrocytes(28). Preliminary analysis of the protein 4.1 gene by genomic southern blotting and cloning experiments suggests that the gene is composed of multiple constitutive and alternative exons spread over at least 100kb(unpublished data). Complex regulation of pre-mRNA splicing events appears to modulate both tissue-specific expression of protein 4.1 isoforms as well as expression of multiple polypeptides within a single cell type-reticulocytes. Protein 4.1 thus joins a growing group of structural proteins for which alternative splicing is utilized to generate structural heterogeneity within the protein products of a single genomic gene (21). Previous studies have shown also that avian nucleated erythrocytes contain multiple protein 4.1 isoforms (40) that may be produced by alternative splicing.

Finally, the PCR amplification technique represents a powerful method to characterize 4.1 mRNA from various nonerythroid cell types and from normal and abnormal red cells. We have demonstrated its utility in characterization of 4.1 mutations from patients with hereditary elliptocytosis, and expect that many more mutations will be sequenced in the future. Preliminary work has also revealed heterogeneity in 4.1 structure from nonerythroid mRNA, presenting us with the opportunity to study 4.1 structure and function in nonerythroid cells.

ACKNOWLEDGEMENTS

I would like to thank Drs. N. Mohandas and Y.W. Kan for their support and encouragement during this project. Special thanks for outstanding technical assistance also are due to Jeff Chan.

REFERENCES

1. Evans EA, Hochmuth RM (1977). J Membr Biol 30: 351-362.
2. Chasis JA, Mohandas N (1986). J Cell Biol 103: 343-350.
3. Waugh RE (1982) Biophys J 39: 273-278.
4. Conboy J, Kan YW, Shohet SB, Mohandas N (1986). Proc Natl Acad Sci USA 83: 9512-9516.

5. Tang TK, Leto TL, Correas I, Alonso MA, Marchesi VT, Benz EJ (1988). Proc Natl Acad Sci USA 85: 3713-3717.
6. Curtis PJ, Palumbo PJ, Ming J, Fraser P, Cioe L, Meo P, Shane S, Rovera G(1985). Gene 36: 357-362.
7. Linnenbach AJ, Speicher DW, Marchesi VT, Forget BG (1986). Proc Natl Acad Sci USA 83: 2397-2401.
8. Prchal JT, Morley BJ, Yoon S-H, Coetzer TL, Palek J, Conboy JG, Kan YW (1987). Proc Natl Acad Sci USA 84: 7468-7472.
9. Winkelmann JC, Leto TL, Watkins PC, Shows TB, Linnenbach AJ, Sahr KE, Kathuria N, Marchesi VT, Forget BG (1988). Blood 72: 328-334.
10. Tanner MJA, Martin PG, High S (1988). Biochem J 256: 703-712.
11. Siebert PD, Fukuda M (1986). Proc Natl Acad Sci USA 83: 1665-1669.
12. High S, Tanner MJA (1987). Biochem J 243: 277-280.
13. Colin Y, Rahuel C, London J, Romeo PH, d'Auriol L, Galibert, Cartron JP (1986). J Biol Chem 261: 229-233.
14. Lux S, John K, Shaler O, Forget B, Chilote R, Marchesi S, McIntosh S, Harris P, Watkins P, Bennett V (1988). Blood 72: Suppl 1, 93a.
15. Lambert S, Lawler J, Yu HI, Speicher DW, Prchal JT, Palek J (1988). Blood 72: Suppl 1, 30a.
16. McMahon AP, Giebelhaus DH, Champion JE, Bailes JA, Lacey S, Carritt B, Henchman SK, Moon RT (1987). Differentiation 34: 68-78.
17. Watkins PC, Eddy R, Forget BG, Chang JG, Rochelle R, Shows TB (1988). Amer J Human Genet (Suppl) A161.
18. Chan J, Conboy JG, Kan YW, Mohandas N (1989). J Cell Biol 107: 24a.
19. Conboy J, Chan J, Mohandas N, Kan YW (1988). Proc Natl Acad Sci USA 85: 9062-9065.
20. Conboy J, Mohandas N, Tchernia G, Kan YW (1986). N Engl J Med 315: 680-685.
21. Breitbart RE, Andreadis A, Nadal-Ginard B (1987). Ann Rev Biochem 56: 467-495.
22. Leto TL, Marchesi VT (1984). J Biol Chem 259: 4603-4608.
23. Scharf SJ, Horn GT, Erlich HA (1986). Science 233: 1076-1078.

24. Chehab FF, Doherty M, Cai S, Kan YW, Cooper S, Rubin EM (1987). Nature 329: 293.
25. Kogan SC, Doherty M, Gitschier J (1987). N Engl J Med 317: 985-990.
26. Correas I, Speicher DW, Marchesi VT (1986). J Biol Chem 261: 13362-13366.
27. Tang TK, Mazzucco CE, Leto TL, Benz E, Marchesi VT (1988). Clin Res 36: 405a.
28. Tchernia G, Mohandas N, Shohet S B (1981). J Clin Invest 68: 454-460.
29. McGuire M, Smith BL, Agre P (1988). Blood 72: 287-293.
30. Alloisio N, Dorleac E, Delauney J, Girot R, Garland C, Boivin P (1982). Blood 60: 265-267.
31. Marchesi S, Letsinger JT, Agre PA, McGuire M, Speicher DW (1988). Blood 72: Suppl 1, 36a.
32. Anderson RA, Correas I, Mazzucco C, Castle JD, Marchesi VT (1988). J Cellular Biochem 37: 269-284.
33. Ruiz-Opazo N, Nadal-Ginard B (1987). J Biol Chem 262: 4755-4765.
34. Branton D, Cohen CM, Tyler J (1983). Cell 24: 24-32.
35. Bennett V (1985). Ann Rev Biochem 54: 273-304.
36. Eder PS, Soong C-J, Tao M (1986). Biochemistry 25: 1764-1770.
37. Anderson R, Marchesi V (1985). Nature 318: 295-298.
38. Takakuwa Y, Mohandas N (1988). J Clin Invest 82: 394-400.
39. Anderson J, Morrow J (1987). J Biol Chem 262: 6365-6372.
40. Granger BL, Lazarides E (1985). Nature 313: 238-241.

Cellular and Molecular Biology of Normal
and Abnormal Erythroid Membranes, pages 75–87
© 1990 Alan R. Liss, Inc.

THE ERYTHROCYTE Rh POLYPEPTIDES[1]

Peter Agre,[2] Barbara L. Smith, Ali M. Saboori,
Bradley M. Denker, and Marcel P. de Vetten

Departments of Medicine and Cell Biology/Anatomy,
Johns Hopkins University School of Medicine,
Baltimore, Maryland 21205

ABSTRACT A M_r 32,000 integral membrane protein can
be surface labeled on intact Rh(D) positive
erythrocytes and immunoprecipitated with anti-D IgG.
This "Rh polypeptide" was purified from SDS-
solubilized membranes by hydroxylapatite
chromatography and analyzed by two dimensional
iodopeptide maps. Rh polypeptides isolated from Rh(D)
positive and negative erythrocytes were nearly
identical, although a consistently detectable
polymorphism was evident. Polypeptides related to the
Rh polypeptide were isolated similarly from membranes
prepared from nonhuman erythrocytes, but the latter
were found to lack the extracellular domain shared
amongst all human Rh isoforms. An acylation/
deacylation mechanism was found to covalently and
reversibly attach ^{3}H-palmitic acid to a approximately
six erythrocyte membrane proteins, and the major
substrate of this mechanism is the Rh polypeptide.
The physiologic function of the Rh polypeptide
remains to be established, but a role in the
organization of membrane phospholipid is considered
likely.

---

[1]This work was supported in part by NIH grant R01
HL33991 and NATO research grant 0556/88.
[2]Established Investigator of the American Heart
Association.

INTRODUCTION

Despite their large clinical importance, the erythrocyte Rh antigens have remained a biochemical enigma until recently (1,2). The Rh antigens are defined by specific agglutination with antisera from sensitized individuals, but it has not been possible to directly identify the biochemical structures which produce this surface immunoreaction. Two European groups independently demonstrated the presence of an integral membrane protein of approximately M_r 32,000 which could be surface labeled with ^{125}I and immunoprecipitated with Rh specific antibodies (3,4). The M_r 32,000 Rh polypeptide is certain to be a key component of the Rh antigen, however the isolated polypeptide nolonger reacts with Rh IgG in solution or on immunoblots. The Rh polypeptide is associated with the membrane skeleton (5,6). The physiologic function of the Rh polypeptide has not been identified, and only small amounts of the Rh polypeptide have been isolated by immunological methods (7-9).

We review here selected biochemical features of the Rh polypeptides which have recently been uncovered in our laboratory. Together these data indicate that the Rh polypeptide is a fundamental structural protein which plays a role in normal membrane lipid organization.

RESULTS

Identification of the Rh polypeptide.

Intact erythrocytes from individuals with known Rh types were surface labeled with $Na^{125}I$, and membranes were analyzed by SDS-PAGE autoradiography (Figure 1). Seven bands were labeled including the glycophorins and band 3. As previously reported by others (3,4), the presence of a M_r 32,000 membrane protein was seen below glycophorin A, and the intensity of the band reflected the presence of Rh(D), the major Rh antigen. DD cells had the strongest labeling, Dd were intermediate, and dd cells were the weakest although labeling was detectable.

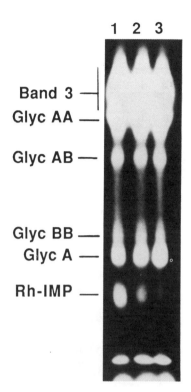

Figure 1. Surface ^{125}I-labeling of membranes from DD, Dd, and dd erythrocytes (lanes 1-3 respectively). Intact erythrocytes were shaken in glass vials coated with Iodogen (Pierce) also containing 1 mCi of Na^{125}I. Membranes were prepared by hypotonic lysis and analyzed by SDS-PAGE autoradiography. Reprinted with permission from J. Biol. Chem. (10).

The Rh polypeptide was immunoprecipitated from each of these preparations with anti-D IgG. The M_r 32,000 polypeptides were dramatically immunoprecipitated from the DD and Dd preparations. Although more weakly labeled, none of the Rh polypeptide in the dd preparation was precipitated (Figure 2, left panel). Of note, band 3 was nonspecifically precipitated from all preparations. In addition, another weaker band of M_r 64,000 was apparent in lanes 1 and 2 (arrow), and this was assessed to be a dimer of the Rh polypeptide. Furthermore, when the immunoprecipitates and supernatants for the DD and dd preparations were compared, it was apparent that the M_r 32,000 Rh polypeptide was nearly quantitatively precipitated from the former (Figure 2, right panel).

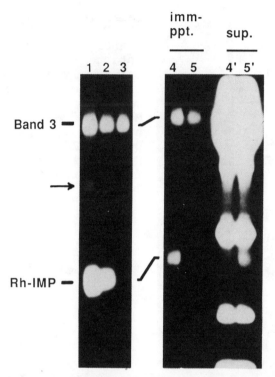

Figure 2. Immunoprecipitation of Rh polypeptide from DD, Dd, and dd erythrocytes (lanes 1-3 respectively). The ^{125}I-labeled erythrocytes were incubated with anti-D IgG; membranes were prepared and solubilized in Triton X-100; immune complexes were isolated by adsorption onto protein A bearing Staphylococci (Pansorbin, Calbiochem) and analyzed by SDS-PAGE autoradiography. The precipates and supernatants from DD (lanes 4 and 4') and dd erythrocytes (lanes 5 and 5') were compared. Reprinted with permission from J. Biol. Chem. (10).

Isolation of the Rh polypeptide.

The immunoprecipitated surface ^{125}I-labeled Rh polypeptide was further purified by preparative SDS-PAGE and utilized as a radiochemically pure probe for large-scale purification of the Rh polypeptide. Due to the

difficulty is solubilizing the Rh polypeptide, it was
necessary to employ SDS solubilized membrane vesicles as a
starting material. SDS leads to permanent denaturation of
the proteins and will interfere with most standard
chromatographic methods. Nevertheless, hydroxylapatite
chromatography in SDS effectively permitted isolation of
the Rh polypeptide in nearly pure form (Figure 3). The
final stages of hydroxylapatite chromatography were pooled
and further purified by preparative SDS-PAGE. The product
was assessed to be > 99 % pure, and the recovery was
nearly 20 %. When calculated back, the overall
purification was approximately 180 fold.

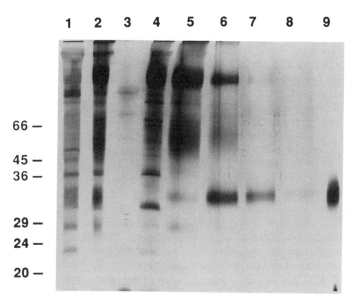

Figure 3. Isolation of Rh polypeptide evaluated by
silver stained SDS-PAGE. Membranes and KI-extracted
vesicles were prepared from two units of DD erythrocytes
and were solubilized in SDS (lanes 1,2) and applied to a
hydroxylapatite column. The presence of Rh polypeptide was
monitored by the addition of a tracer of immunoprecipitated surface ^{125}I-labeled Rh polypeptide. This was
eluted with 0.3 M sodium phosphate (lane 3), gradients of
0.3-0.5 M (lane 4) and 0.5-0.8 M sodium phosphate (lanes
5-8). Peak fractions were combined and further purified by
preparative SDS-PAGE (lane 9). Reprinted with permission
from Proc. Natl. Acad. Sci. USA (11).

Comparison of purified Rh polypeptides.

Rh polypeptides were isolated similarly from pints of blood obtained from several individuals with several different Rh types including DD and dd. The purified Rh polypeptides were indistinguishable by one dimensional SDS-PAGE. Moreover the N-terminal amino acid sequences were identical and unique when compared to computer sequence banks.

S S K Y P R S V R R X L P L W A L T L E A A

The same N-terminal amino acid sequence was independently determined by two other laboratories who analyzed Rh polypeptide isolated by immunoprecipitation with monoclonal antibodies to D (9,12).

Rh polypeptides purified from DD and dd erythrocytes by hydroxylapatite chromatography were compared by two dimensional mapping of chymotryptic iodopeptides, and a striking polymorphism was apparent (Figure 4). It was clear that at least two central iodopeptides were uniquely absent in all of five dd preparations but were present in all of 12 DD and Dd preparations. More recent work was pursued by Drs. Dominique Blanchard and Christian Bloy in the laboratory of Dr. Jean-Pierre Cartron in Paris and in collaboration with our group. Employing monoclonals specific for c, D, or E, the corresponding Rh polypeptides were isolated from a single donor of the cDE/cDE type and were compared by two dimensional iodopeptide analysis (13). The c, D, and E peptides were clearly demonstrated to be homologous but specific differences were notable (data not shown). The c, D, and E antigens are therefore associated with related but distinct polypeptides.

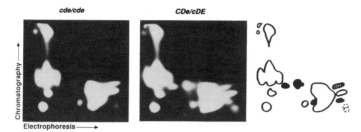

Figure 4. Two dimensional iodopeptide maps comparing Rh polypeptides purified from dd (left) and DD erythrocytes (middle). The purified Rh polypeptides were oxidized with chloramine T, labeled with I^{125}, and isolated from preparative SDS-PAGE gels and digested extensively with alpha chymotrypsin. The digests were analyzed in two dimensions. The composite (right) compares the iodopeptide spots: open figures are common to both, solid figures are unique to the DD preparations. Reprinted with permission from Proc. Natl. Acad. Sci. USA (11).

Nonhuman analogs of the Rh polypeptide.

The Rh antigens are known to be restricted to human erythrocytes, although the higher primates have a blood group which is related. Nevertheless the Rh antigens are not present on the erythrocytes of the rhesus monkey, and the name of the Rh system is therefore a misnomer. The hydroxylapatite method was employed to isolate putative Rh polypeptides from erythrocytes obtained from four nonhuman species known to lack Rh immunoreactivity (rhesus monkey, cow, cat and rat). The product of these purifications was found to be very similar to the M_r 32,000 Rh polypeptide isolated from human erythrocytes. Nevertheless, when compared by two dimensional iodopeptide maps, it was clear that only a limited amount of homology exists (Figure 5). Of note, none of the nonhuman preparations contained the iodopeptide known to be surface ^{125}I-labeled on human erythrocytes (labeled "S" on the top right panel). Also, while the different species had a variety of other iodopeptides which co-migrated with the human iodopeptides, only two were present in the preparations of all five species (marked with arrows).

82   Agre et al.

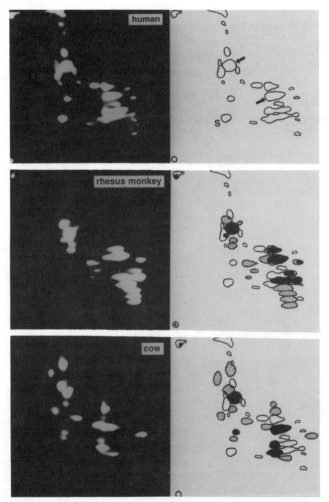

Figure 5. Two dimensional iodopeptide maps of analogs to Rh polypeptides isolated by hydroxylapatite chromatography from rhesus monkey, cow, cat, and rat erythrocytes. The composite drawings (right) compare the iodopeptides. Open figures are the human iodopeptides; cross-hatched figures are the nonhuman iodopeptides; solid figures are found in human and nonhuman iodopeptides. "S" indicates the surface ^{125}I-labeled iodopeptide found in the extracellular domain of the human Rh polypeptide. Arrows identify iodopeptides shared amongst all species. Reprinted with permission from J. Clin. Invest. (14).

Fatty acid acylation of the Rh polypeptide.

It has been thought that the Rh polypeptide may have a phospholipid component (15,16). Initial efforts to solubilize the Rh polypeptide were frustrated by the extreme hydrophobicity of the polypeptide, even though the amino acid composition was similar to several other integral membrane proteins. A post-translational fatty acid acylation was considered a possible explanation for this behavior and was evaluated by incubating intact erythrocytes with ^{3}H-palmitic acid prior to SDS-PAGE fluorography (17). Approximately six membrane proteins were found to be labeled, including one major band of M_r 32,000 (Figure 6). None of the bands corresponded to the known membrane proteins, bands 1-7 or the glycophorins. Analysis of membranes from dd and DD erythrocytes were similar. Analysis of membranes from Rh$_{mod}$ erythrocytes (a rare phenotype deficient in all C/c, D, and E/e antigens) demonstrated that the M_r 32,000 band was not labeled. The M_r 32,000 band was immunoprecipitated with anti-D IgG from the DD but not from the dd erythrocytes. The ^{3}H-palmitic acid labeling was found to be a covalent thioester linkage which formed independent of protein synthesis (not shown). In other studies the labeling of the intact erythrocytes was stopped and a chase with unlabeled palmitic acid was undertaken. Interestingly the labeling of all bands was found to be completely reversed with the chase (Figure 7). Thus an ongoing acylation/deacylation mechanism was found for which the Rh polypeptide is the major substrate.

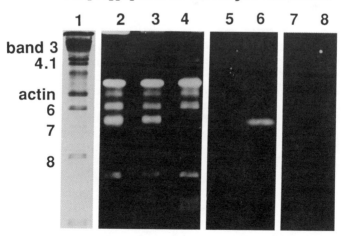

Fig. 6 (legend on page 84).

Figure 6 (at bottom of previous page). Labeling of erythrocyte membranes with ^{3}H-palmitic acid. Intact dd (lanes 2, 5, and 7) DD (lanes 3, 6, and 8) or Rh$_{mod}$ erythrocytes (lane 4) were incubated for 24 hours in minimum essential medium containing 5 mM pyruvate and 2 mCi of ^{3}H-palmitic acid. Membranes were prepared and analyzed by SDS-PAGE after Coomassie staining (lane 1) or fluorography (lanes 2-8). Reprinted with permission from J. Biol. Chem. (17).

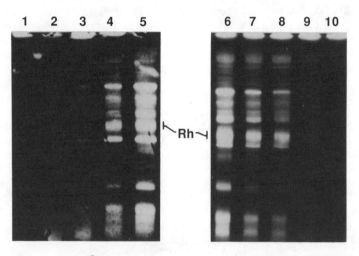

Figure 7. ^{3}H-Palmitic acid labeling of erythrocytes increases with time but is reversible. Intact erythrocytes were incubated with ^{3}H-palmitic acid for 0.5, 1.5, 4.5, 12, and 24 hours (corresponding to lanes 1-5) prior to preparation of membranes and SDS-PAGE fluorography. In a separated experiment, erythrocytes were incubated with ^{3}H-palmitic acid for 5 hours prior to chase with unlabeled palmitic acid for 0, 1, 3, 9, and 19 hours (corresponding to lanes 6-10). Reprinted with permission from J. Biol. Chem. (17).

DISCUSSION

Application of current methods in membrane biology have permitted isolation of a M_r 32,000 integral membrane protein which is the site of a polymorphism linked to the Rh phenotype. To date, the relationship between the Rh polypeptide and the Rh antigens is incompletely understood, since the isolated polypeptide nolonger reacts with Rh specific IgG. This may result from irreversible denaturation of the Rh polypeptide during isolation, but the existence of a specific membrane conformation or the existence of additional subunits or cofactors cannot be ruled out.

The Rh polypeptide is an extremely hydrophobic molecule. It has a single tyrosine-containing domain protruding outside of the cell and approximately eleven additional tyrosines which are presumably located within the lipid bilayer or intracellularly. The surface labeling of the extracellular domain is most dramatic for the D polypeptide. The c and E polypeptides appear to be homologous to D although less efficiently iodinated, presumably due to a difference in surface conformation. The isolation from nonhuman erythrocytes of polypeptides which are related to the Rh polypeptide indicates that the Rh polypeptide is a fundamental structural molecule which is conserved amongst diverse species. It is therefore likely that the Rh polypeptide plays an important physiologic function. Interestingly, the nonhuman Rh analogs all appear to lack the extracellular tyrosine-containing domain, indicating that the domain of the molecule probably associated with Rh antigenicity is not required for the normal functioning of the molecule.

The long held concept that Rh antigens are somehow related to membrane lipid was underlined by the studies which demonstrated prominent and reversible covalent fatty acid acylation. It seems likely that this acylation is related to the organization of membrane phospholipid, and this may be an important function of the Rh polypeptide.

Future studies need to determine the entire amino acid sequence and gene organization of the Rh polypeptide. This may establish whether the differences in the c, D, and E antigens and polypeptides result from gene duplication or alternate splicing of mRNA. It is currently unclear whether the Rh polypeptides are expressed in nonerythroid tissues. Existing antibodies are not reactive on immunoblots, and antipeptide antibodies and

86   Agre et al.

ribonucleoprobes are needed. Additional biochemical characterization of the fatty acid acylation and expression of the Rh cDNA may permit the clear elucidation of the normal function of this interesting molecule.

The authors thank Ms. Rosetta S. Shirey and Dr. Peter Issitt for blood samples, reagents, and helpful suggestions. In addition, we thank our colleagues Drs. Christian Bloy, Dominique Blanchard, and Jean-Pierre Cartron at the CNTS in Paris for numerous discussions and scientific inspirations.

1. Cartron J-P (1988). Recent advances in the biochemistry of blood group Rh antigens. In Rouger P, Salmon C (eds): "Monoclonal antibodies against human red blood cell and related antigens," Paris: Arnette, p 69.
2. Gahmberg CG (1988). Molecular characteristics of the blood group Rho(D) molecule. In Harris JR (ed): "Subcellular Biochemistry," vol. 12, New York: Plenum Press, p 95.
3. Moore S, Woodrow CF, McClelland DBL (1982). Isolation of membrane components associated with human red cell antigens Rho(D), (c), (E) and Fy^a. Nature 295:529.
4. Gahmberg CG (1983). Molecular characterization of the human red cell Rho(D) antigen. EMBO J 2:223.
5. Gahmberg CG, Karhi KK (1984). Association of Rho(D) polypeptides with the membrane skeleton in Rho(D) - positive human red cells. J Immunol 133:334.
6. Ridgwell K, Tanner MJA, Anstee DH (1984). The rhesus (D) polypeptide is linked to the human erythrocyte cytoskeleton. FEBS Lett 174:7.
7. Bloy C, Blanchard D, Lambin P, Goossens D, Rouger P, Salmon C, Cartron J-P (1987). Human monoclonal antibody against Rh(D) antigen: partial characterization of the Rh(D) polypeptide from human erythrocytes. Blood 69:1491.
8. Suyama K, Goldstein J (1988). Antibody produced against isolated Rh(D) polypeptides reacts with other Rh-related antigens. Blood 72:1622.

9. Avent ND, Ridgwell K, Mawby J, Tanner MJA, Anstee DJ, Kumpel B (1988). Protein-sequence studies on Rh-related polypeptides suggest the presence of at least two groups of proteins which associate in the human red-cell membrane. Biochem J 256:1043.

10. Agre P, Saboori AM, Asimos A, Smith BL (1987). Purification and partial characterization of the M_r 30,000 integral membrane protein associated with the erythrocyte Rh(D) antigen. J Biol Chem 262:17497.

11. Saboori AM, Smith BL, Agre P (1988). Polymorphism in the Mr 32,000 Rh protein purified from Rh(D)-positive and negative erythrocytes. Proc Natl Acad Sci USA. 85:4042.

12. Bloy C, Blanchard D, Dahr W, Beyreuther K, Salmon C, and Cartron JP (1988). Determination of the N-terminal sequence of human red cell Rh(D) polypeptide and demonstration that the Rh(D), (c) and (E) antigens are carried by distinct polypeptide chains. Blood 72:661.

13. Blanchard D, Bloy C, Hermand P, Cartron J-P, Saboori A, Smith BL, Agre P (1988). Two-dimensional iodopeptide mapping demonstrates erythrocyte Rh D, c, and E polypeptides are structurally homologous but nonidentical. Blood 72:1424.

14. Saboori AM, Denker BM, Agre P (1989). Isolation of proteins related to the Rh polypeptides from nonhuman erythrocytes. J Clin Invest 83:187.

15. Green F (1972). Erythrocyte membrane lipids and Rh antigen activity. J Biol Chem 247:881.

16. Kuypers F, Van Linde-Sibenius-Tripp M, Roelofsen B, Tanner MJA, Anstee DJ, Op den Kamp JAF (1984). Rh_{null} human erythrocytes have an abnormal membrane phospholipid organization. Biochem J 221:931.

17. de Vetten MP, Agre P (1988), The Rh polypeptide is a major fatty acid-acylated erythrocyte membrane protein. J Biol Chem 263:18193.

Cellular and Molecular Biology of Normal
and Abnormal Erythroid Membranes, pages 89–112
© 1990 Alan R. Liss, Inc.

PHOSPHORYLATION MEDIATED ASSOCIATIONS OF THE RED
CELL MEMBRANE SKELETON

Carl M. Cohen, Bipasha GuptaRoy and Richard
Fennell

Dept. of Biomedical Research
St. Elizabeth's Hospital
736 Cambridge Street
Boston, MA   02135

ABSTRACT

All of the major red cell membrane skeletal
proteins (with the exception of actin) are
phosphorylated by one or several of the endogenous
red cell protein kinases. These skeletal proteins
apparently are subject to an ongoing, steady-state
turnover of PO_4 via the concerted action of kinases
and phosphatases. In this article we review the
possible roles for skeletal protein phosphorylation
during erythroid development, in the mature normal
red cell and in certain disease states. We also
review and summarize the known effects of
phosphorylation on all skeletal associations
studied to date, and present new information on the
effects of protein kinase C phosphorylation on
skeletal stability. Finally, we present a summary
of key questions which will need to be answered in
order to fully appreciate the role of skeletal
protein phosphorylation for red cell physiology.

I.   INTRODUCTION

While the red cell is not generally thought
of as being a particularly dynamic cell, it
probably is subject to more mechanical stress and
deformation than any other cell in the body. The
remarkable mechanical strength of the red cell

membrane is widely held to be due to the network of proteins which adheres tightly to the inner surface of the plasma membrane. This membrane skeletal network forms a self-assembled two-dimensional array which is tightly anchored to the membrane via multiple protein-protein, and possibly protein-lipid associations, and provides the necessary strength to the otherwise fragile lipid bilayer.

The assembly of the skeletal network from the various proteins of which it is comprised via binary, ternary and more complex interactions has been the subject of intense scrutiny (see 1,2 for reviews). The high affinity of some of these associations (3) is consistent with our qualitative expectations for the strength of the skeletal network. However, recent observations have led us to question whether the biochemical parameters measured in vitro truly reflect the properties of these associations in situ. Some of these concerns have arisen from the simple observation that all of the proteins of the membrane skeleton (with the exception of actin) are phosphorylated, and it is well known that phosphorylation can dramatically alter the interactions and properties of proteins. Other proteins, particularly adducin, may bind calmodulin (4,5) and may be subject to in vitro regulation by Ca^{++} as a result (6). Still other associations such as that between band 4.1 and glycophorin may be subject to modulation via the level of membrane triphosphoinositide (7). Agents, such as intracellular 2,3-diphosphoglycerate (8,9) or other metabolic intermediates, and hemoglobin, or its breakdown products (10), may also play important roles in modifying skeletal protein associations.

As a consequence of the above it is critical that we evaluate our concepts of cytoskeletal assembly by asking two questions. 1: To what degree do the biochemical parameters of the key skeletal associations measured in vitro reflect their actual in vivo values? If we are to take seriously the significance of the above mentioned post-translational modifications then there is a strong likelihood that many of the Kds and other parameters which have been measured in vitro may

be far different from those which apply _in vivo_.
2: Is the membrane skeleton a passive network which
provides mechanical strength only on the basis of
un-regulated associations? Or, rather, are some
or all of the key network associations modulated
by the post-translational alterations mentioned
above?

II. POSSIBLE FUNCTIONS OF SKELETAL PROTEIN PHOSPHORYLATION

The notion that red cell mechanical
properties or shape can be affected by
physiological signals or agents has little
experimental support. It is known that a wide
variety of exogenous non-physiological agents can
dramatically alter cell shape and stability, as can
a variety of membrane or metabolic defects.
However, there are very few examples of changes in
any red cell membrane mechanical properties or
their biochemical antecedents such as skeletal
phosphorylation, in response to physiological
stimuli. Nevertheless, several circumstances in
which changes in skeletal protein phosphorylation
may be important can be envisioned. These include
the following:

A. Modulation During Erythroid Development

Skeletal protein phosphorylation may be
important to the dramatic changes in cellular
organization which occur during erythroid
development. Membrane and membrane skeletal
proteins are synthesized asynchronously during
mammalian hematopoiesis, with spectrin being
synthesized at earliest times, and band 3 at later
times (11,12,13,14). During early stages of
synthesis, when the membrane density of the
skeletal proteins is low, it is not at all clear
how newly synthesized proteins associate with the
membrane or with each other. Without the full
complement of ankyrin, band 4.1 and band 3 it is
difficult to imagine how stable skeletal complexes
are assembled and maintained. One possibility is

that the newly synthesized proteins are not phosphorylated and have a very low Kd of association, which facilitates the formation of stable complexes, even when proteins are at low density. Once the proteins achieve sufficient density on the membrane and the cell nears full maturation, such low Kds may be inappropriate. Increased phosphorylation of skeletal proteins at that time may be a mechanism by which the cell can effect a maturation-triggered adjustment in skeletal protein associations to a level appropriate for the mature erythrocyte.

An additional role for phosphorylation during erythroid development relates to the dramatic re-arrangements which must take place in nucleated erythroid precursors during cytokinesis and, finally, enucleation. It may be that skeletal protein associations need to be temporally modulated in order for these events to take place. Transient changes in the phosphorylation of spectrin, band 4.1, ankyrin and other proteins may facilitate the membrane remodeling required for such alterations. We are currently testing this hypothesis using synchronized cultures of murine erythroleukemia cells.

B.   Steady State Regulation of Membrane Mechanical Properties

Phosphorylation may in fact play a central role in maintaining the mechanical properties of the membrane skeleton in the mature cell, even though kinase activates and phosphorylation levels are presumably at steady state and do not change perceptibly. This may be thought of as regulation by "steady-state" phosphorylation. The idea behind this proposal comes from the observation that most or all of the skeletal proteins will undergo phosphorylation in unstimulated intact red cells (detected by incubating cells with $^{32}PO_4$ to label intracellular γ-^{32}P-ATP). Under these conditions, $^{32}PO_4$ incorporation represents steady state turnover of protein phosphate, presumably due to the concerted action of endogenous phosphatases and kinases.   In principle, the activity of these enzymes should be such that the steady state level of PO$_4$ on the skeletal proteins is kept at some appropriate value. At steady state, most of the skeletal proteins are not maximally phosphorylated as can be seen from the increased phosphate incorporation brought about by stimulating protein kinase C, c-AMP dependent kinase, and others in the intact cell (15,16,17,18). Coupled steady-state systems of phosphatases and kinases have been shown to provide the potential for very sensitive and dynamic response to physiological stimuli (19). For example, the presence of very low concentrations of kinase activators plus phosphatase inhibitors can result in a multiplicative or synergistic effect by comparison with the effects on either agent acting alone.

In order to ascertain the consequences of steady state phosphorylation additional information is needed. For example, we need to know the levels of PO$_4$ on skeletal proteins in intact cells. Moreover, in light of evidence showing selective effects of specific kinases on protein functions (20), we also need to know which sites or domains are phosphorylated within these proteins in vivo. Until this information is available the extent to which steady state phosphorylation levels affect protein-protein associations in situ will remain speculative.

C.   Response to Shear or Mechanical Stress

Despite the lack of supporting evidence, the possibility that the levels of red cell skeletal protein phosphorylation can change in response to extra- or intracellular signals or other environmental conditions must be considered. It is possible for example that the levels of skeletal protein phosphorylation change transiently under conditions of high shear stress, or extreme deformation. For example, under conditions of high fluid shear tighter skeletal protein associations may limit cell deformation and fragmentation. Conversely, under conditions of extreme deformation more relaxed associations may facilitate flow and reduce the chances of an obstruction. How the cell might regulate phosphorylation levels in response to such situations is also speculative. However, some type of response sensitive to membrane stretching or bending, possibly using the skeletal network itself as a transducing mechanism, may be possible. Stretch or deformation sensitive activation of intracellular kinases has in fact been observed in certain cell types. For example, stretching induces a 40-70% increase in the phosphorylation of the 20kDa myosin light chain in rat uterine smooth muscle (21), and arterial smooth muscle (22,23) in the absence of any other stimulants. This phosphorylation results in the production of spontaneous active tension upon release of the stretch. Evidence suggests that the increase in phosphorylation is triggered by the stretch-induced release of Ca^{++} from intracellular Ca^{++} stores (23). It is not inconceivable that a similar stretch or deformation sensitive response could occur in red cells leading to the phosphorylation of red cell myosin (24,25,26) or other skeletal proteins.

While there is no direct evidence that skeletal protein phosphorylation can control the mechanical properties of normal red cell membranes, recent measurements of the osmotic and filterability characteristics of malaria parasite infected red cells are highly suggestive (27). Murine red cells infected with plasmodium berghei were tested for their ability to pass repeatedly through 3μm pore size filters, as well as for their ability to withstand mild osmotic stress without lysis. It was found that the cells most able to survive these tests also showed a substantially enhanced phosphorylation of a variety of membrane proteins (probably including some membrane skeletal proteins) as well as of an unidentified prominent 43 kDa membrane-associated phosphoprotein. These intriguing observations make it of great interest to identify these proteins with enhanced phosphorylation. It is also critical to determine whether malarial or red cell kinases are the causative agents, as well as to define the mechanism(s) of kinase activation in the infected cells. One intriguing possibility is that enhanced phosphorylation of skeletal proteins is used by the cell as a mechanism to keep the cells as deformable as possible, in an attempt to minimize circulatory obstruction by parasite infected cells.

III. SPECIFIC EFFECTS OF PHOSPHORYLATION ON
      SKELETAL PROTEIN ASSOCIATIONS

A.   Spectrin-actin-band 4.1 Complex Formation

        Numerous studies have provided clear documentation that phosphorylation of several membrane or membrane skeletal proteins can significantly affect their properties. Table I summarizes some of the principal red cell membrane protein associations known or suspected of being affected by phosphorylation, as well as the kinases which affect or may affect these associations. There are a large number of associations which may be affected by protein phosphorylation, and the list of associations for which effects have been documented is growing rapidly. However, in all cases studied, phosphorylation has the effect of decreasing the extent of association or affinity of binding.
        Of the associations studied, our group has been particularly interested in the ternary complex formed when band 4.1 promotes the tenacious binding of spectrin to F-actin (3,9). This complex is one of the key protein associations of the skeletal network and modulation of its stability may provide a mechanism for the regulation of cellular mechanical properties. Binding of band 4.1 to spectrin has been shown to be sensitive to the state of band 4.1 phosphorylation by casein kinase A (CKA), a membrane-associated cAMP-independent kinase (MAK), protein kinase C (PKC), and cAMP-dependent kinase (PKA) (41,42). In addition, band 4.1 stimulated binding of spectrin to actin has been shown to be dramatically reduced following phosphorylation by either PKA or PKC (41). In the latter case, incorporation of between 2 and 3 moles PO_4/mole band 4.1 can reduce complex formation by 70-80%. While it is at present unknown to what extent band 4.1 is phosphorylated by PKC, PKA or MAK in vivo, even a small degree of phosphorylation

TABLE I

ERYTHROCYTE KINASES AND THEIR EFFECTS ON MEMBRANE SKELETAL PROTEINS

PHOSPHORYLATED PROTEIN	ERYTHROCYTE KINASES WHICH ACT ON THE PROTEIN	ASSOCIATION OR FUNCTION WHICH MAY BE SUBJECT TO REGULATION	EFFECT OF PHOSPHORYLATION ON ASSOCIATION OR FUNTION
ADDUCIN	PROTEIN KINASE C (RBC-PKC I)* (17,18,67)	SPECTRIN-ACTIN BINDING	------
	Ca^{++}-STIMULATED KINASE (RBC-PKC II) (17)	MEMBRANE ASSOCIATION	------
	cAMP-DEPENDENT KINASE (PKA) (15,52) (?)		
ANKYRIN	MAK (28) (?)	BAND 3 BINDING	REDUCTION BY MAK AND CKA (38)
	cAMP-DEPENDENT KINASE (28,30)	SPECTRIN BINDING	REDUCTION BY MAK AND CKA (39,40)
		BAND 4.2 BINDING	------
BAND 4.1	PROTEIN KINASE C (RBC-PKC I) (17,18,32)	SPECTRIN BINDING	REDUCTION BY PKC,PKA,CKA AND MAK (41,42)
	cAMP-DEPENDENT KIANSE (16,28)	SPECTRIN-ACTIN-BAND 4.1 COMPLEX FORMATION	REDUCTION BY PKC,PKA (41)
	MAK (16)	BAND 3 BINDING	REDUCTION BY PKC (20)
	Ca^{++}-STIMULATED KIANSE (RBC-PKC II) (17)	GLYCOPHORIN BINDING	------
BAND 4.9	PROTEIN KINASE C (RBC-PKC I) (17,18,32)	ACTIN BUNDLING	REDUCTION BY PKA (43)
	Ca^{++}-STIMULATED KINASE (RBC-PKC II) (17)	MEMBRANE BINDING	REDUCTION BY PKA (44)
	cAMP-DEPENDENT KINASE (PKA) (15)		

*Abbreviations used:
MAK: human red cell membrane-associated cAMP-independent kinase, referred to in some cases as casein kinase (37)
PKC: protein kinase C
PKC I: red cell cytosolic TPA-stimulated protein kinase C
PKC II: red cell membrane-associated protein kinase C - see Discussion
CKA: casein kinase, type A
TYR-kinase: tyrosine kinase
a ? indicates that there is some question as to the identity of the kinase or substrate in the cited study

TABLE I (CONTINUED)

ERYTHROCYTE KINASES AND THEIR EFFECTS ON MEMBRANE SKELETAL PROTEINS

PHOSPHORYLATED PROTEIN	ERYTHROCYTE KINASES WHICH ACT ON THE PROTEIN	ASSOCIATION OR FUNCTION WHICH MAY BE SUBJECT TO REGULATION	EFFECT OF PHOSPHORYLATION ON ASSOCIATION OR FUNCTION
BAND 3	MAK (16,28,29) TYROSINE KINASE (33,34,35)	ANKYRIN BINDING BAND 4.1 BINDING BAND 4.2 BINDING GLYCOLYTIC ENZYME BINDING	------ ------ ------ REDUCTION BY TYR-KINASE (45)
GLYCOPHORIN	MAK (36)	BAND 4.1 BINDING	------
SPECTRIN (β CHAIN)	MAK (29,37)	BAND 4.1 BINDING ANKYRIN BINDING TETRAMER OR OLIGOMER FORMATION	------ ------ ------

*Abbreviations used:
MAK: human red cell membrane-associated cAMP-independent kinase, referred to in some cases as casein kinase (37)
PKC: protein kinase C
PKC I: red cell cytosolic TPA-stimulated protein kinase C
PKC II: red cell membrane-associated protein kinase C -see Discussion
CKA: casein kinase, type A
TYR-kinase: tyrosine kinase
a ? indicated that there is some question as to the identity of the kinase or substrate in the cited study

leading to as little as a 10% effect on ternary complex formation, could in principle have a major effect on the rheological properties of the cell.

B.   Membrane Association of Band 4.1

In addition to promoting the binding of spectrin to F-actin, band 4.1 also may participate in anchoring the skeletal network to the membrane. Three types of band 4.1-membrane association have been documented. These are: (1) Association of band 4.1 with the cytoplasmic domain of glycophorin (46). (2) Association of band 4.1 with the cytoplasmic domain of band 3 (47), and (3) Association with anionic lipids (48,49). Of these associations only the second has been shown to be sensitive to the state of band 4.1 phosphorylation. We have shown (20) that phosphorylation of band 4.1 by protein kinase C virtually abolishes the binding of band 4.1 to the cytoplasmic domain of band 3 on the membrane, as well as to the isolated 43 kDa cytoplasmic domain in solution (R. Fennell and C.M. Cohen, unpublished data). By contrast, phosphorylation of band 4.1 by PKA had no effect on its association with band 3, and phosphorylation by either kinase has no apparent effect on binding to glycophorin (20). To date, there is no evidence to suggest that phosphorylation of either glycophorin or the cytoplasmic domain of band 3 affects their association with band 4.1, although phosphorylation of band 3 by tyrosine kinase has been shown to affect binding of glycolytic enzymes (45). Such effects will require further investigation.

C.   Ankyrin Binding to Band 3 and Spectrin

Phosphorylation of ankyrin by CKA or MAK reduces by about half its stoichiometry of binding to the 43 kDa cytoplasmic domain of band 3 (38). By contrast, phosphorylation of the 43 kDa domain of band 3 by CKA had no effect on this association (38). Since there are apparently multiple phosphorylation sites within the cytoplasmic domain of band 3 (50) it will be of interest to determine whether other kinases, especially tyrosine kinase (33,34,35,45), affect its associations with ankyrin. Similarly, phosphorylation of ankyrin with CKA or MAK results in a decreased affinity for spectrin (39,40). Interestingly, the decrease is selective for binding to spectrin tetramers, and oligomers; binding to spectrin dimers was unaffected by ankyrin phosphorylation. Phosphorylation of spectrin by CKA or MAK was not found to have any effect upon the Kd of spectrin-ankyrin binding (40). These results suggest that alterations in the state of ankyrin phosphorylation may have profound effects on numerous red cell properties. It will be of great interest to determine whether ankyrin phosphorylation changes in response to exogenous stimuli or is altered in abnormal red cells.

D.   Band 4.9 Phosphorylation

While band 4.9 is a prominent skeletal phosphoprotein its function in the red cell is far from clear. In vitro band 4.9 causes the bundling of actin filaments (51), and it is commonly held to have some, as yet undocumented, association with actin in the mature red cell. Band 4.9 also associates with some integral component of the membrane, since it remains behind on inside-out vesicles when spectrin and actin are eluted at low ionic strength and binds to alkalai-stripped inside-out vesicles (44). Recently, it has been shown that phosphorylation of band 4.9 by PKA reversibly abolishes the actin bundling activity of the protein in vitro (43). By contrast, phosphorylation by PKC had no effect (although substantially lower amounts of PO_4 were incorporated into band 4.9 by this kinase). Preliminary studies have also shown that phosphorylation of band 4.9 by PKA (but not PKC) abolishes the associations of this protein with its membrane binding site (44). These results show that in vitro, the associations of band 4.9 can be highly regulated by phosphorylation. It is interesting to note that while band 4.9 is a

prominent skeletal substrate for PKC, neither of
the functions discussed above appear sensitive to
PKC phosphorylation.

E.   Red Cell Membrane Skeletal Stability

        The results summarized above suggest that
phosphorylation of any one or several skeletal
components in situ should have the effect of
loosening specific skeletal connections, presumably
leading to a less stable skeleton or more flexible
network.   A direct test of this hypothesis is
complicated by several factors. First, the exact
state of phosphorylation of the various skeletal
proteins in situ is unknown. Second, in our hands
it   has   been   difficult   to   stimulate   the
incorporation of more than a fraction of a mole of
PO_4 per mole of protein (e.g. band 4.1) in either
intact cells or ghosts via PKC or PKA. As a
result, it is unclear by what percent the overall
level of PO_4 incorporation is increased upon
stimulation of specific kinases.   With these
limitations in mind, we have attempted to measure
the effect of protein phosphorylation on skeletal
stability in a simplified in vitro system.
        Figure 1 shows an experiment in which we
tested whether phosphorylation of red cell
membranes by red cell protein kinase C would affect
skeletal   stability.   Phosphorylation   was
accomplished by pre-treating intact red cells with
12-o-tetradecanolylphorbol 13-acetate (TPA) in
order to activate protein kinase C (17,18). Ghosts
were prepared from these cells, and phosphorylation
by membrane-associated protein kinase C was
initiated by addition of ATP. Next, the ghosts
were extracted with Triton X-100 to prepare
membrane skeletons. These skeletons were incubated
in increasing concentrations of Tris-HCl, an agent
which induces skeletal disassembly at high
concentrations (53).   Skeletal stability was
assessed by measuring the release of band 4.1
protein from cytoskeletons following high speed
centrifugation. Figure 1 shows that skeletons from
cells pretreated with TPA showed greater release
of band 4.1 at all concentrations of Tris than

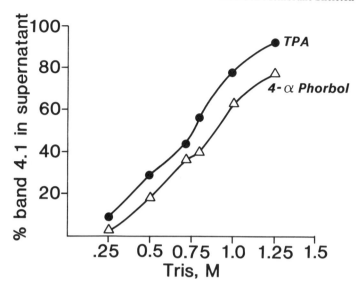

Figure 1. Tris-induced dissociation of red cell membrane skeletons. Whole blood was washed three times in phosphate buffered saline (PBS) and incubated at 37°C with 1 μM TPA or 1 μM 4-α-phorbol for 30 min. Cells were then washed twice with PBS and lysed in 20 volumes of ice cold lysis buffer (5 mM sodium phosphate with 0.5 mM EGTA, pH 8.0). Red cell ghosts were sedimented at 15,000 rpm for 15 min in a Sorval SS34 rotor and washed in lysis buffer until white. Ghosts were phosphorylated in 5 mM sodium acetate pH 6.5, 1 mM EGTA, 4 mM NaF, 2 mM PMSF, 1 μg/ml leupeptin, 10 mM $MgCl_2$ and 20 μM γ-^{32}P-ATP (100-200 cpm/pmole, used to monitor PO_4 incorporation). After incubation at 30°C for 40 min ghosts were washed with ice cold lysis buffer containing 2 mM PMSF and 1 μg/ml leupeptin (lysis buffer A). Washed ghosts were then extracted with ice cold 1% Triton X-100 in phosphate buffer in the presence of 1 M KCl for 20 min. followed by sedimentation at 18,000 rpm in a Sorval SS34 rotor for 20 min. The pellet (Triton shells) was washed once with lysis buffer A and resuspended in the same buffer. Triton shells were then incubated in increasing concentrations of Tris-HCl pH 8.0,

ranging from 0.25 M to 1.5 M at 4°C for 20 min and centrifuged as above. The supernatant was removed and the pellet was resuspended in the same volume of lysis buffer A as the supernatant. Equal volumes of the supernatant and pellet were subjected to electrophoresis in the presence of SDS. Gels were stained with Coomassie blue and the amount of band 4.1 in the supernatant and pellet was quantified using an LKB ultroscan XL Laser densitometer. The amount of band 4.1 in the supernatant is expressed as a percentage of the total. ●-● Triton shells from TPA treated red cells. △-△ Triton shells from 4-α-phorbol treated red cells.

---

skeletons from cells treated with the inactive phorbol ester 4-α-phorbol. These results do not pinpoint any single protein as being responsible for skeletal instability, since band 4.1, 4.9 and adducin all showed increased phosphorylation under these conditions. However, the results do show, as expected, a generalized decrease in the stability of the skeletons from TPA treated cells. While the difference between the TPA and 4-α-phorbol curves under these conditions is not great, two points must be noted: 1) as noted above the molar PO_4 incorporation in such studies is generally low, typically approximately 0.2 moles PO_4/mole of band 4.1 are incorporated. This, of course, is above whatever undetermined level of endogenous PO_4 the protein posseses; and 2) even quite small changes in the overall mechanical stability of the skeleton may have pronounced effects on the deformation characteristics or stability of the intact cell. Measurements of the mechanical properties of single cells under conditions designed to alter protein phosphorylation would be most revealing.

IV. PERSPECTIVES AND DISCUSSION

The above results as well as the published data listed in Table I show clearly that phosphorylation is likely to have profound effects on almost every key skeletal protein association studied to date. There are many questions which need to be addressed in order for us to understand in detail whether and to what extent these effects are relevant in the intact red cell. These include:

A. Do red cells respond to hormones or other extracellular agents by altering the level of skeletal protein phosphorylation? Intriguing early results of Allen and Rasmussen (54) showing prostaglandin and epinephrine induced changes in red cell filterability need to be followed up using more sensitive single-cell measurement techniques in conjunction with simultaneous measurement of phosphorylation. Some evidence for adrenergic stimulation of red cell protein phosphorylation has been presented (55), and red cells may contain large amounts of epinephrine or nonepinephrine in their membranes (56). Effects of other hormones such as insulin, for which the red cell has receptors (57) need also to be examined in light of reports suggesting effects of this hormone on red cell filterability and other properties (58,59) including phosphorylation (60).

B. Do the absolute amounts of the various red cell kinases change during erythroid development? The red cell is quite efficient at expelling a wide variety of intracellular components, membrane proteins and receptors during the maturation process. The fact that numerous kinases are retained to maturity suggests a priori that their function is important in the mature red cell. Nevertheless, quantitative measurements of the amounts of each of the kinases listed in Table I during progressive stages of cell maturity would show whether particular types of kinases are selectively retained while others are excluded.

C. Are there other kinases active in red cell besides those listed in Table I? The most notable absence from Table I is a calcium-calmodulin dependent kinase, an enzyme which is widely distributed in many cells and tissues. We previously reported that red cells contained a membrane-associated kinase activity which required only micromolar Ca^{++} for activation (17). This kinase appeared distinct from red cell protein kinase C because a) it was membrane-associated in the absence of TPA, and did not require TPA for activation b) unlike the TPA-activated kinase, it did not appreciably phosphorylate band 4.9 and c) this kinase was unaffected by extracellular digestions which caused a reduction in PKC activity. In addition to this, the kinase activity was inhibitable by the calmodulin inhibitor trifluoperazine, and its activity was lost when membranes were treated with 0.1 mM EGTA, a treatment which elutes calmodulin from red cell membranes.

In spite of the above, several attempts to purify a Ca^{++}-calmodulin dependent kinase from red cell membranes were unsuccessful. However, we did find that there was a kinase activity associated with red cell membranes which was extractable with 0.1 mM EGTA and which when partially purified by ion exchange chromatography, gel filtration and phenyl sepharose chromatography had all of the characteristics of protein kinase C. (E. Ling, R. Fennell, and C.M. Cohen, unpublished data). We are currently in the process of characterizing this enzyme in greater detail, but our results thus far suggest that it is an isozyme of protein kinase C distinct from the cytosolic enzyme, and which is constitutively membrane-associated (we have referred to this enzyme as PKC II in Table I). Because it apparently has a distinct substrate specificity from the cytosolic enzyme as well as distinct activation requirements, it may represent a novel regulatory pathway for red cells. Since the enzyme needs only micromolar Ca^{++} for activation it may also be involved with the many Ca^{++} dependent alterations which have been described in red cells and red cell membranes.

In addition to the above, the role of the tyrosine kinase which acts on the cytoplasmic domain of band 3 clearly warrants more attention. It will be important to determine whether phosphorylation of band 3 by this kinase affects its association with membrane skeletal proteins, particularly ankyrin and band 3. It is also essential to determine whether this kinase is subject to activation by external agents, or whether its activity is altered in young, old or abnormal cells.

D. What role do phosphatases play in regulating skeletal protein associations? The fact that red cell skeletal proteins can incorporate $^{32}PO_4$ from $\gamma-^{32}P$-ATP in intact cells under steady state conditions suggests that at least some skeletal protein phosphates are undergoing continual turnover. It seems likely that endogenous phosphatases play a role in this turnover. Several types of phosphatases have been described in red blood cells (61,62,63,64,65,66). Spectrin phosphatase activity was found in red cell cytosol, and could be resolved into four distinct molecular weight phosphatase species (61). Low molecular weight phosphatases have also been reported (62). In addition, red cells possess cytosolic and membrane-associated phosphotyrosyl phosphatase activity (63,64,65). Interestingly, the only red cell substrate identified for this phosphatase to date is the phosphotyrosine on the cytoplasmic domain of band 3 (64,65). At this time it is not known which of the above phosphatases act on proteins such as band 4.1, ankyrin, band 4.9 or adducin. In principle it is likely that alterations or regulation of phosphatase activity would have just as important implications for skeletal associations as changes in kinase activity. The properties and behavior of red cell phosphatases is an important area for further investigation.

E. Finally, can methods be developed to measure transient changes in red cell skeletal protein phosphorylation levels during deformation or mechanical stress? Such measurements are likely to be challenging since these changes may be small and rapidly reversible. Nevertheless, in light of our knowledge of the effects of phosphorylation on skeletal associations there is some reason to believe that changes in PO_4 levels may be an important part of the cells' response to the different circulatory environments and stresses which it experiences.

Acknowledgements: The authors thank Ms. Lucille
Paul for her expert typing of the manuscript.   This
work was supported by N.I.H. grants HL 24382 and
HL 37462.

V.   REFERENCES

1.   Cohen CM (1983). The molecular organization
        of the red cell membrane skeleton. Semin
        Hematol 20:141.
2.   Bennett V (1985). The membrane skeleton of
        human erythrocytes and its implications for
        more complex cells. Ann Rev Biochem 54:272.
3.   Ohanian V, Wolfe LC, John KM, Pinder JC, Lux
        SE, Gratzer WB (1984).   Analysis of the
        ternary interaction of the red cell membrane
        skeletal proteins spectrin, actin, and 4.1.
        Biochem 23:4416.
4.   Agree P, Gardner K, Bennett, V (1983).
        Association   between   human   erythrocyte
        calmodulin and the cytoplasmic surface of
        human erythrocyte membranes.   J Biol Chem
        258:6258.
5.   Gardner K, Bennett V (1986).   A new
        erythrocyte membrane-associated protein with
        calmodulin binding activity.   J Biol Chem
        261:1339.
6.   Mische SM, Mooseker MS, Morrow JS (1987).
        Erythrocyte adducin: a calmodulin-regulated
        actin-bundling   protein   that   stimulates
        spectrin-actin   binding.   J   Cell   Biol
        105:2837.
7.   Anderson RA, Marchesi VT (1985). Regulation
        of the association of membrane skeletal
        protein   4.1   with   glycophorin   by   a
        polyphosphoinositide. Nature 318:295.
8.   Sheetz   MP,   Casaly   J   (1980).   2,3-
        diphosphoglycerate and ATP dissociate
        erythrocyte membrane skeletons. J Biol Chem
        255:9955.
9.   Cohen CM, Foley SF (1984).   Biochemical
        characterization of complex formation by

human erythrocyte spectrin, protein 4.1 and actin. Biochemistry 23:609

10. Liu SC, Zhai S, Lawler J, Palek J. (1985). Hemin-mediated dissociation of erythrocyte membrane skeletal proteins. J Biol Chem 260:12234.

11. Chang H, Langer PJ, Lodish HF (1976). Asynchronous synthesis of erythrocyte membrane proteins. Proc Nat Acad Sci USA 73:3206.

12. Koch PA, Gartrell JE, Gardner FH, Carter JR Jr. (1975). Biogenesis of erythrocyte membrane proteins in in vivo studies of anemic rabbits. Biochim Biophys Acta 389:162.

13. Hanspal M, Palek J (1987). Synthesis and assembly of membrane skeletal proteins in mammalian red cells precursors. J Cell Biol 105:1417.

14. Lehnert ME, Lodish HF (1988). Unequal synthesis and differential degradation of α and ß spectrin during murine erythroid differentiation. J Cell Biol 107:413.

15. Thomas E, King L, Morrison M (1979). The uptake of cyclic AMP by human erythrocytes and its effect on membrane phosphorylation. Arch Biochem Biophys 196:459.

16. Plut DA, Hosey MM, Tao M (1978). Evidence for the participation of cytosolic protein kinases in membrane phosphorylation in intact erythrocytes. Eur J Biochem 82:333.

17. Cohen CM, Foley SF (1986). Phorbol ester- and Ca^{2+}-dependent phosphoryaltion of human red cell membrane skeletal proteins. J Biol Chem 261:7701.

18. Palfrey HC, Waseem A (1985). Protein kinase C in the human erythrocyte. J Biol Chem 260:16021.

19. Schacter E, Chock PB, Stadtman ER (1984). Regulation through phosphorylation/de-phosphorylation cascade systems. J Biol Chem 259:12252.

20. Cohen CM, Danilov Y, Fennell R, Gupta-Roy B (1989). Phosphorylation mediated associations of the red cell membrane skeleton. J Cell Biochem 13B:209.

21.   Csabina S, Barany M, Barany K (1986).
        Stretch-induced myosin light chain
        phosphorylation in rat uterus. Arch Biochem
        Biophys 249:374.
22.   Barany K, Ledvora RF, Mougios V, Barany M
        (1985). Stretch-induced myosin light chain
        phosphorylation and stretch-release-induced
        tension development in arterial smooth
        muscle. J Biol Chem 260:7126.
23.   Vander Mealen DL, Barron JT, Barany M
        (1983). Stretch-induced phosphorylation of
        the 20,000-dalton light chain of myosin in
        arterial smooth muscle. J Biol Chem
        258:14080.
24.   Fowler VM, Davis JQ, Bennett V (1985).
        Human erythrocyte myosin: identification and
        purification. J Cell Biol 100:47.
25.   Matovcik LM, Groschel-Stewart V, Schrier SL
        (1986). Myosin in adult and neonatal human
        erythrocyte membranes. Blood 67:1668.
26.   Wong AJ, Kiehart DP, Pollard YD (1985).
        Myosin from human erythrocytes. J Biol Chem
        260:46.
27.   Yuthavong Y, Limpaiboon T (1987). The
        relationship of phosphorylation of membrane
        proteins with the osmotic fragility and
        filterability of plasmodium berghei-infected
        mouse erythrocytes. Biochim Biophys Acta
        929:278.
28.   Hosey MM, Tao M (1976). An analysis of the
        autophosphorylation of rabbit and human
        erythrocyte membranes. Biochemistry
        15:1561.
29.   Avruch J, Fairbanks G. (1974).
        Phosphorylation of endogenous substrates by
        erythrocyte membrane protein kinases. I. A
        monovalent cation-stimulated reaction.
        Biochemistry 13:5507.
30.   Fairbanks G, Avruch J (1974).
        Phosphorylation of endogenous substrates by
        eythrocyte membrane protein kinases. II.
        Cyclic adenosine monophosphate-stimulated
        reactions. Biochemistry 13:5514.
31.   Ling E, Sapirstein V (1984). Phorbol ester
        stimulates the phosphorylation of rabbit
        erythrocyte band 4.1. Biochem Biophys Res

Commun 120:291.

32. Faquin WC, Chahwala SB, Cantley LC, Branton D (1986). Protein kinase C of human erythrocytes phosphorylates bands 4.1 and 4.9. Biochim Biophys Acta 887:142.

33. DeKowski SA, Rybicki A, Drickamer K (1983). A tyrosine kinase associated with the red cell membrane phosphorylates band 3. J Biol Chem 258:2750.

34. Phan-Dinh-Tuy F, Henry J, Rosenfield C, Kahn A (1983). Characterization of a human red blood cell tyrosine kinase. Nature (London) 305:435.

35. Mohamed AH, Steck TL (1986). Band 3 tyrosine kinase. J Biol Chem 261:2804.

36. Hosey MM, Tao M (1977). Differential phosphoryaltion of band 3 and glycophorin in intact and extracted erythrocyte membranes. J Supramolec Struct 6:61.

37. Fairbanks G, Avruch J, Dino JE, Patel VP (1978). Phosphorylation and dephosphorylation of spectrin. J Supramolec Struct 9:97.

38. Soong C-J, Lu P-W, Tao M (1987). Analysis of band 3 cytoplasmic domain phosphorylation and association with ankyrin. Arch Biochem Biophys 254:509.

39. Cianci CD, Giorgi M, Morrow JS (1988). Phosphorylation of ankyrin down-regulates its cooperative interaction with spectrin and protein 3. J Cell Biochem 37:301.

40. Lu P-W, Soong CJ, Tao M (1985). Phosphorylation of ankyrin decreases its affinity for spectrin tetramer. J Biol Chem 260:14958.

41. Ling E, Danilov YN, Cohen CM (1988). Modulation of red cell band 4.1 function by cAMP-dependent kinase and protein kinase C phosphoryaltion. J Biol Chem 263:2209.

42. Eder PS, Soong C-J, Tao M (1986). Phosphorylation reduces the affinity of protein 4.1 for spectrin. Biochemistry 25:1764.

43. Husain-Chishti A, Levin A, Branton D (1988). Abolition of actin-bundling by phosphorylation of human erythrocyte protein

4.9. Nature 334:718.

44. Husain-Chishti A, Branton D (1989). Phosphorylation abolishes the interaction of protein 4.9 with human erythrocyte membranes. J Cell Biochem 13B:210.

45. Low PS, Allen DP, Zioncheck TF, Chari P, Willardson BM, Glahlen RL, Harrison ML (1987). Tyrosine phosphorylation of band 3 inhibits peripheral protein binding. J Biol Chem 262:4592.

46. Anderson RA, Lovrien RE (1984). Glycophorin is linked by band 4.1 protein to the human erythocyte membrane skeleton. Nature 307:665.

47. Pasternack GR, Anderson RA, Leto TL, Marchesi VT (1985). Interactions between protein 4.1 and band 3. J Biol Chem 260:3676.

48. Cohen AM, Liu SC, Lawler J, Derick L, Palek J (1988). Identification of the protein 4.1 binding site to phosphatidylserine vesicles. Biochem 27:614.

49. Sato SB, Ohnishi S (1983). Interaction of a peripheral protein of the erythrocyte membrane, band 4.1, with phosphatidylserine-containing liposomes and erythrocyte inside-out vesicles. Eur J Biochem 130:19.

50. Drickamer LK (1976). Fragmentation of the 95,000-dalton transmembrane polypeptide in human erythrocyte membranes. J Biol Chem 251:5115.

51. Siegel DL, Branton D (1985). Partial purification and characterization of an actin-bundling protein, band 4.9, from human erythrocytes. J Cell Biol 100:775.

52. Fairbanks G, Palek J, Dino JE, Liu PA (1983). Protein kinases and membrane protein phosphorylation in normal and abnormal human erythrocytes: variation related to mean cell age. Blood 61:850.

53. Ohanian V, Gratzer W (1984). Preparation of red-cell-membrane cytoskeletal constituents and characterization of protein 4.1. Eur J Biochem 144:375.

54. Allen JE, Rasmussen H (1971). Human red blood cells: prostaglandin E2, epinephrine,

and isoproterenol alter deformability. Science 174:512.

55. Nelson MJ, Ferrell JE, Huestis WH (1979). Adrenergic stimulation of membrane protein phosphorylation in human erythrocytes. Biochem Biophys Acta 558:136.

56. Hagiwara H, Hollister AS, Carr RK, Inagami T (1988). Norepinephrine and epinephrine in human erythrocyte plasma membranes. Biochem Biophys Res Commun 154:1003.

57. Im JH, Meezan E, Rackley CE, Kim HD (1983). Isolation and characterization of human erythrocyte insulin receptors. J Biol Chem 258:5021.

58. Juhan E, Buonocore M, Juove R, Vague P, Moulin JP, Vialettes B (1982). Abnormalities of erythrocyte deformability and platelet aggregation in insulin-dependent diabetics corrected by insulin in vivo and in vitro. The Lancet 535.

59. Dutta-Roy AK, Ray TK, Sinha AK (1985). Control of erythrocyte membrane microviscosity by insulin. Biochim Biophys Acta 816:187.

60. Hesketh JE (1986). Insulin inhibits the phosphorylation of the membrane cytoskeletal protein spectrin in pig erythrocytes. Cell Biol Int Rep 10:623.

61. Usui H, Kinohara N, Yoshikawa K, Imazu M, Imaoka T, Takeda M (1983). Phosphoprotein phosphatases in human erythrocyte cytosol. J Biol Chem 258:10455.

62. Clari G, Monet V (1981). Partial purification and characterization of phosphoprotein phosphatase from human erythrocyte hemolysate. Biochem Int 2:509.

63. Clari G, Brunati AM, Moret V (1986). Partial purification and characterization of phosphotyrosyl-protein phosphatase(s) from human erythrocyte cytosol. Biochem Biophys Res Commun 137:566.

64. Boivin P, Galand C (1986). The human red cell acid phosphatase is a phosphotyrosine protein phosphatase which dephosphorylates the membrane protein band 3. Biochem Biophys Res Commun 134:557.

65.   Clari G, Brunati AM, Moret V (1987). Membrane-bound phosphotyrosyl-protein phosphatase activity in human erytrhocytes. Dephosphoryaltion of membrane band 3 protein. Biochem Biophys Res Commun 142:587.
66.   Kiener PA, Carrol D, Roth BJ, Westhead EV (1987). Purification and characterization of a high molecular weight type 1 phosphoprotein phosphatase from the human erythrocyte. J Biol Chem 262:2016.
67.   Ling E, Gardner K, Bennett V (1986). Protein kinase C phosphorylates a recently identified membrane skeleton-associated calmodulin-binding protein in human erythrocytes. J Biol Chem 261:13875.

Cellular and Molecular Biology of Normal
and Abnormal Erythroid Membranes, pages 113–130
© 1990 Alan R. Liss, Inc.

MULTIPLE KINASES PHOSPHORYLATE SPECTRIN.

Sheenah M. Mische and Jon S. Morrow

Yale University School of Medicine, Laboratory of Pathology
310 Cedar Street, New Haven, CT. 06510

ABSTRACT   Erythrocyte spectrin is a multiply phosphorylated protein.   As isolated, spectrin co-
purifies with several kinase activities, including
those that are cAMP independent (casein kinase),
cAMP dependent, and those that require calcium and
calmodulin.   Ion exchange HPLC isolated beta and alpha spectrin subunit which was free of kinase activity.   Reassociation of alpha and beta spectrin to
form the heterodimer did not restore activity,
demonstrating that spectrin itself is not a kinase.
On average, spectrin was found to incorporate four
moles of [^{32}P] phosphate per mole beta spectrin   in
vivo, whereas, in vitro, the incorporation of approximately one mole of phosphate per mole of
spectrin was achieved with several different
kinases.   These results suggest that spectrin phosphorylation may be under multiple control.   The differences between   in vivo and in vitro phosphorylation suggest that the local environment or state of
spectrin in the cytoskeleton may also influence its
ability to be phosphorylated.

INTRODUCTION

The human erythrocyte provides a unique opportunity to
study protein phosphorylation of membrane skeletal proteins,
as the majority of these proteins are multiply phosphorylated (1,2).   The human erythrocyte contains a number of
protein kinases.   They are distinguished by their substrate
specificity, regulation, and cellular distribution.   The
kinases that have been identified are predominantly as

sociated with the plasma membrane, similar to their counter-parts in other cell systems (3). Four major types of protein kinases are recognized in the erythrocyte: cAMP in-dependent or casein kinases (membrane and soluble forms) (4-6), cAMP dependent kinase (types I and II) (2,3,7,8); calmodulin dependent protein kinase (9), and protein kinase C (10-13).

Spectrin is one of the major phosphoproteins in the human erythrocyte (2,14). The phosphorylation of spectrin, as well as a number of other erythrocyte proteins, was first demonstrated by in-vivo labeling of intact erythrocytes with ortho [^{32}P] phosphate by Palmer and Verpoorte in 1971 (15). Subsequently, Avruch and Fairbanks demonstrated that phos-phorylation of beta spectrin results from the activity of a membrane bound salt-stimulated cAMP independent casein kinase (16). A cAMP independent kinase extracted from the cytosol also phosphorylated spectrin in-vitro (2), and spectrin has been postulated to autophosphorylate itself (17).

The structural characterization of beta spectrin has localized all of the phosphorylation sites (with literature values ranging from 4-6 moles phosphate/mole dimer) (2,14,18) to a C-terminal 17 kD peptide generated by CNBr cleavage of the beta chain (14,19). Both phosphoserine and phosphothreonine have been identified (14). Typical litera-ture values of in-vitro phosphate incorporation for spectrin are less than 1 mole phosphate/mole dimer (14,20,21), al-though higher values have been reported (2). It is not known whether spectrin is reversibly phosphorylated, al-though presumably it is since phosphatases have been demonstrated to be active towards spectrin, but are less well characterized (22,23).

In order to further characterize the kinases respon-sible for spectrin phosphorylation, both in vivo and in vitro phosphorylation studies have been performed, using both dimer and isolated beta spectrin as substrate. The en-dogenous kinase activity of spectrin was studied and preparations of kinase-free spectrin were obtained. In vitro studies were performed with casein kinase (both soluble and membrane), cAMP dependent kinases isolated from human erythrocytes, and calcium-calmodulin dependent protein kinase type II prepared from bovine brain.

METHODS

Spectrin preparation: Spectrin was prepared from fresh
human erythrocyte ghost membranes (24).   Spectrin dimer,
tetramer, and higher oligomers were prepared by gel filtration using Sephadex CL-4B (Pharmacia) (25).   Beta spectrin
was separated from alpha spectrin using a modification of
the method of Yoshino and Marchesi (26).   Briefly, spectrin
(as a low salt extract from ghosts), in either 20 mM Tris-
HCl, pH 7.6, 1 mM EDTA, or isoKCl buffer (20 mM Tris-HCl pH
7.6, 130 mM KCl, 10 mM NaCl, 1 mM EDTA 0.05 mM PMSF) was
diluted 1:1 by the addition of a 2x solution of buffer A (6M
urea, 40 mM Tris-HCl, pH 7.6, 0.3 M NaCl, 2 mM EDTA, 1 mM
2-mercaptoethanol). HPLC ion exchange chromatography was
used to separate the alpha and beta spectrin, as well as the
other protein components present in the low salt extract. A
DEAE-TSK 5PW column (75 x 7.5 mm) (BioRad Laboratories,
Richmond, CA) equilibrated in buffer A (3 M urea, 0.15 M
NaCl, 20 mM Tris-HCl, pH 7.6, 1 mM EDTA) was used at a flow
rate of 1.2 ml/minute and monitored at 280 nm.   Approximately 5 mg of protein was the standard load for each
analysis. The protein was eluted with a step gradient of 12%
buffer B (3 M urea, 0.5 M NaCl, 20 mM Tris-HCl, pH 7.6, 1 mM
EDTA) followed by 18% buffer B and finally 40% buffer B.

Kinase preparations: Casein kinase (membrane bound) was
prepared by the   method of Tao et al (5).   The method of
Simkowski and Tao was used for the preparation of soluble
casein kinase,   and the method of Rubin was used for the
isolation of cAMP dependent kinases I and II (4,7).   The
method of McGuinness et al. was used to purify the calmodulin dependent type II kinase from bovine brain (27).

Kinase assays: Column fractions and enzyme preparations
were assayed for kinase activity using buffer conditions of
Tao et al. and the method of Cook et al. (5,28).

Quantitation of specific activity: The method of Fenner et
al.   was used to quantitate the amount of protein analyzed
by gel electrophoresis,   and the method of Tishler and
Epstein was used to quantitate the incorporation of ^{32}P incorporated (29,30).   Quantitation of inorganic phosphate was
performed by the method of Duck-Chong (31).

Other methods: Sodium dodecyl sulfate polyacrylamide gel

electrophoresis (SDS PAGE) was performed following the procedure of Laemmli (32). Nondenaturing gel electrophoresis was performed using the method of Morrow and Haigh (33).

RESULTS

Spectrin extracts contain multiple kinases.

Spectrin was isolated from human erythrocytes by standard procedures using a low salt extract of ghost membranes. Following precipitation with ammonium sulfate and dialysis into isoKCl buffer, the protein solution was applied to a Sephadex CL4-B column. The results of one such separation are shown in Figure 1A.

Peak fractions were pooled and analyzed by SDS PAGE, as shown in the inset of Figure 1A. Gel filtration of crude spectrin separates spectrin oligomers, tetramers, and dimers, designated as O, T, and D respectively. In addition to the oligomer forms of spectrin, a low molecular weight peak (K) elutes after dimer spectrin. Analysis by SDS PAGE (see inset) shows that this peak contains spectrin, adducin, protein 4.1, protein 4.9, actin, and several other erythrocyte membrane proteins which elute from the membrane with spectrin under low salt conditions.

CL4-B column fractions were assayed for several different kinase activities. As can be seen, the low salt extract contains considerable activity for each kinase. Most of these activities are present in the K peak, with casein kinase the predominant kinase present. There is also considerable kinase activity for casein associated with each of the spectrin species. Calcium-calmodulin dependent kinase (Figure 1C) and cAMP dependent kinase (Figure 1D) are also present in this region of the elution profile, but show little correlation with the spectrin elution.

These results demonstrate that there is kinase activity which copurifies with spectrin, and there are at least three different kinases present in crude, unfractionated spectrin. Since spectrin is a substrate for both the casein kinases, (4,5), and, since the majority of the kinase associated with spectrin is casein kinase, this activity was studied in more detail than the others.

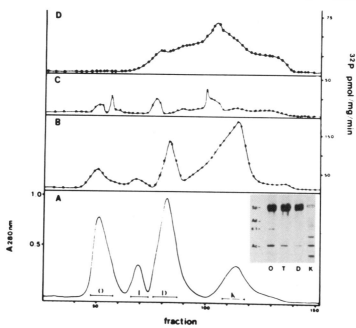

FIGURE 1 *Spectrin co-purifies with several kinases.*
A) Gel filtration chromatography of crude erythrocyte
spectrin. Fractions were pooled as indicated. (inset) pooled
fractions (O, T, D, K). B) Casein kinase activity was as-
sayed with casein (50 ug) as the substrate.   C) Kinase as-
say for cAMP dependent kinase. Histone (25 ug) was used as
the substrate, and values reflect cAMP (30 uM) stimulatable
kinase activity.   D) Kinase assay of calmodulin stimulated
kinase activity was assayed in the presence of CaCl$_2$ (100
uM) and 10 uM calmodulin (bovine brain). Synapsin (5 ug)
was used as the substrate. 50 ul of alternate fractions
were used (specific activity (^{32}P-gamma ATP) was 240
cpm/pmol). The points on each graph represent the average
of two separate gel filtrations experiments each assayed in
triplicate.

Spectrin oligomers, tetramers, and dimers (O,T,D, and
K CL4-B pools) were used as substrates for casein kinase in
the presence of ^{32}P-ATP. The SDS PAGE and autoradiogram
are shown in Figure 2. Spectrin is the major phosphoprotein
present. In addition, proteins with apparent molecular
weights of 46 kD, 105 and 100 kD, and 80 kD, which cor

respond to protein 4.9, adducin, and protein 4.1 are also phosphorylated. These results indicate that there are multiple protein substrates for casein kinase in column purified spectrin.

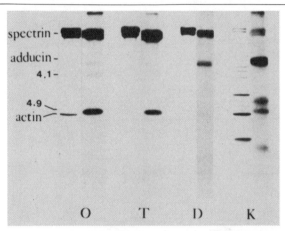

FIGURE 2   *Spectrin CL-4B pools contain numerous substrates for casein kinase. Samples O, T, D, and K were incubated at 37° C for 5 minutes in the presence of casein kinase (100 units) and ^{32}P-gamma ATP (specific activity 410 cpm/pmole). The reaction was stopped with the addition of electrophoresis solubilizing buffer and analyzed by SDS PAGE.*

Spectrin does not autophosphorylate.

Because considerable kinase activity remained with spectrin dimer, further purification of spectrin was necessary. Previous studies have suggested that spectrin itself has kinase activity (2,17). Tao and coworkers have demonstrated that casein kinase binds tightly to spectrin under physiological salt conditions, but this binding is reduced with higher salt conditions (5). In order to separate casein kinase from spectrin, as well as to purify kinase-free beta spectrin for structural and phosphorylation studies, HPLC ion exchange chromatography was used and is shown in Figure 3.

In 3M urea, 0.15M NaCl, the low molecular weight proteins which are present in crude spectrin (adducin, protein 4.1, protein 4.9, actin and several others) elute in the first peak from the column (peak 1). A step gradient of 0 to 12% B (0.150 M to 0.192 M NaCl) elutes beta spectrin (peak 2), followed by a peak which contains a mixture of alpha and beta spectrin (peak 3). A second step gradient of 16% to 18% B (0.192 M to 0.21 M NaCl) elutes alpha spectrin (peak 4). The final peak (peak 5) elutes in a step gradient of 18% to 40% B (0.21 M to 0.3 M NaCl) and contains what appears to be a population of proteins present in a stable cytoskeletal complex.

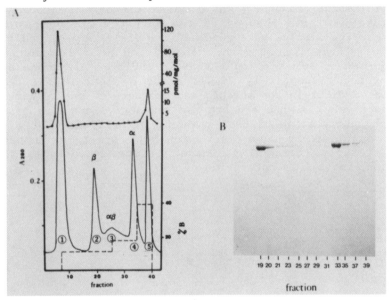

FIGURE 3 *Isolated beta or alpha spectrin has no kinase activity. A.) DEAE HPLC ion exchange chromatography of crude spectrin (4 mg), as described in Methods. Aliquots (50 ul) of alternate fractions were assayed for casein kinase activity after a 1:4 dilution to reduce urea concentration. Casein was used as the substrate (specific activity of ^{32}P-gamma ATP = 157 cpm/pmol). B.) SDS PAGE analysis of HPLC fractions.*

As can be seen from the plot of casein kinase activity in Figure 3, greater than 90% of the kinase activity applied to the DEAE column is eluted from the column in the first peak. A second peak of kinase activity is found with peak 5. However, there is no casein kinase activity associated with either alpha or beta spectrin. These results suggest

that the kinase activity previously attributed to spectrin
is presumably casein kinase tightly bound to spectrin.

    In order to exclude the possibility that the dissocia-
tion of alpha and beta spectrin destroyed an intrinsic
kinase activity, alpha and beta spectrin were reassociated
and assayed for kinase activity.   Alpha spectrin, beta
spectrin, and equal mixtures of each were dialyzed against a
common buffer containing 20 mM Tris-HCl, pH 7.5, 5 mM $MgCl_2$,
1 mM EDTA, 1.8 mM 2-mercaptoethanol, 130 mM KCl, 20 mM NaCl.
Casein kinase (25 units) was added to one of the alpha-beta
mixtures.   Three changes of the buffer were made over 3
hours.   The samples were removed from dialysis and incubated
at 37° C for 1 hour with the addition of ^{32}P-gamma ATP.
(Figure 4).   Lanes a and b contain purified alpha and beta
spectrin, respectively. Lanes c and d contain the reassociated dimer in the absence and presence of casein kinase,
respectively.   Lanes e-h are the respective autoradiograms.
No phosphorylation of beta spectrin either before or after
reassociation is seen,   although beta spectrin is phos-
phorylatable (Lane h).   These results demonstrate that
spectrin itself is not a kinase.

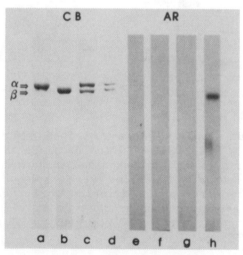

FIGURE 4   *Reassociated spectrin heterodimer contains
no kinase activity. SDS PAGE analysis of alpha spectrin
(a), beta spectrin (b), reassociated alpha-beta spectrin
without (c) and with (d) casein kinase. The phosphorylation
reaction was stopped with the addition of a 5X
electrophoresis solubilizing buffer and analyzed by SDS
PAGE.   The corresponding autoradiograms (e-h) are shown for
a-d, respectively.*

Quantitation of spectrin phosphorylation.

Purified beta spectrin or beta spectrin associated with alpha spectrin in dimer form was used as a substrate for a number of kinases, either from erythrocytes (casein kinase, membrane and soluble forms, cAMP dependent kinases I and II), or other sources (calcium-calmodulin dependent kinase II from bovine brain, cAMP dependent kinase I from skeletal muscle). Phosphorylation of beta spectrin in the heterodimer was quantitated from gel slices cut from Coomassie blue stained gels, as described in METHODS. The results of these phosphorylation assays are shown in Figure 5.

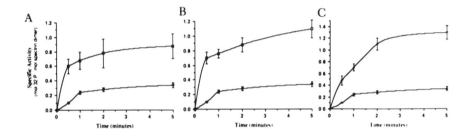

FIGURE 5 *Kinetics of <u>in-vitro</u> phosphorylation of spectrin dimer by A) membrane casein kinase, B) soluble casein kinase, and C) calcium-calmodulin dependent kinase ( ), and cAMP dependent protein kinase ( ). 250 ug of spectrin dimer was incubated at 37° C with (closed symbols) or without (open symbols) added kinase and ^{32}P-gamma ATP (640 cpm/pmol). At the times indicated, aliquots from each reaction mixture were taken. The reaction was stopped with the addition of 5X solubilizing buffer and analyzed by SDS PAGE. Beta spectrin specific activity was calculated as described in METHODS. Assays were done in triplicate.*

Beta spectrin is the only spectrin subunit phosphorylated under these conditions, and is phosphorylated by all of the kinases studied, with the exception of the cAMP dependent kinases. This kinase failed to incorporate additional phosphate into spectrin. An average of one mole phosphate was incorporated per mole of spectrin dimer by the membrane casein kinase as compared to spectrin phosphorylation without the addition of casein kinase (Figure

5A). These results are in agreement with values reported in the literature for in-vitro phosphorylation of spectrin (2). The soluble casein kinase incorporated about 0.8 moles of phosphate per mole of spectrin dimer and the curve of the time course is shown in Figure 5B. Also shown in Figure 5A and B is the endogenous level of kinase activity associated with spectrin dimer. Calmodulin dependent kinase (calcium dependent purified from bovine brain) catalyzed the incorporation of 1.2 moles of phosphate per mole of spectrin dimer (Figure 5C). Also shown in Figure 5C is the time course of spectrin phosphorylation by cAMP dependent kinase (type I). As can be seen, the amount of ^{32}P incorporated into spectrin is comparable to the levels of ^{32}P incorporated by endogenous kinase activity associated with spectrin dimer (see Figure 5A and B).

Purified spectrin dimer also contains a number of additional proteins which are phosphorylated under the conditions used for phosphorylating spectrin, complicating ^{32}P analysis of spectrin. Figure 6A shows a Coomassie Blue stained gel and corresponding autoradiogram of spectrin dimer labeled with ^{32}P by casein kinase. It can be easily seen that the trace amount of adducin, protein 4.1, protein 4.9 and other minor proteins which copurify with spectrin dimer from CL4-B gel filtration contain a considerable amount of ^{32}P label. In contrast, Figure 6B contains a Coomassie blue stained gel and autoradiogram of purified beta spectrin phosphorylated under the same conditions.

Purified beta spectrin is phosphorylated to about the same extent as beta spectrin present in the heterodimer form by the membrane casein kinase (Figure 7A), with an average of 0.8 moles phosphate per mole of beta spectrin. Phosphorylation of beta spectrin by soluble casein kinase (Figure 7B) or calmodulin dependent kinase in the presence of calcium (Figure 7C) is approximately 50% of the amount of phosphate incorporated into spectrin dimer under identical conditions. The significance of this difference is not known but could reflect differences in the availability of phosphorylation sites in beta spectrin.

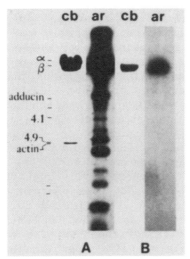

FIGURE 6   *Spectrin dimer contains additional phos-phoproteins: SDS PAGE analysis of A) spectrin dimer (30 ug) and B) beta spectrin (15 ug) isolated by HPLC ion exchange. Each was incubated with the addition of casein kinase (membrane) and ^{32}P-gamma ATP (640 cpm/pmol) at 37° C for 15 minutes. The reaction was stopped with the addition of 5X solubilizing buffer and analyzed by SDS PAGE and autoradiography.*

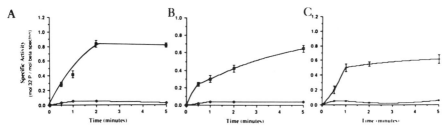

FIGURE 7   *Kinetics of in-vitro phosphorylation of purified beta spectrin by A) casein kinase (membrane), B) casein kinase (soluble), C) calcium-calmodulin dependent kinase ( ) and cAMP dependent kinase ( ). ( ) represent basal level of ^{32}P incorporated without the addition of kinase.   Beta spectrin was incubated with equal quantities of each kinase (50 units) and ^{32}P-gamma ATP (600 cpm/pmol). The reaction was stopped with the addition of 5X solubilizing buffer and analyzed by SDS PAGE. Each assay was done in triplicate. ^{32}P quantitation was measured as described in* METHODS.

The total level of phosphorylation achieved in spectrin dimer or purified beta spectrin was unchanged if the kinases were used in combination or alone. The ability of spectrin to be phosphorylated to the same extent under these conditions by each kinase suggests that either the sites phosphorylated are the same, or there are different sites which cannot be simultaneously phosphorylated. In contrast to in-vitro phosphorylation, in-vivo labeling studies with intact erythrocytes or erythrocyte ghost membranes show approximately four moles of phosphate incorporated per mole of spectrin dimer (Table 1). These values are in agreement with the reported values in the literature (18). The level of total endogenous phosphate in spectrin dimer as routinely purified is estimated to be 4.4 phosphates per mole of spectrin, as determined here by inorganic phosphate analysis. It is not known why the values for in-vitro and in-vivo levels of beta spectrin phosphorylation differ so substantially. One possibility is that spectrin may be a substrate for additional kinases in-vivo and/or phosphatases are not present in-vitro to allow all phosphorylation sites to be turned over. The in-vitro studies suggest either one phosphorylation site exchanged, or multiple sites turn over only partially to give a total of one phosphate incorporated.

	endogenous phosphate	in-vivo 32 P	in-vitro 32 P			
			mol phosphate / mol spectrin			
			CKI	CKII	Ca-CaM	cAMPd
spectrin dimer	4.4 ±0.6	4.3 ± 0.3	0.9 ± 0.2	1.1 ± 0.1	1.3 ± 0.1	0.35 ± 0.03
beta spectrin	ND	3.0 ±0.1	0.8 ± 0.1	0.7 ±0.02	0.65 ± 0.1	0.06 ± 0.02

TABLE 1 Summary of phosphate quantitation of spectrin dimer and isolated beta spectrin. Values determined are expressed as mol phosphate per mole of beta spectrin + S.E. ND:not determined.

DISCUSSION

The present study has examined the kinases present in the erythrocyte and their activity towards spectrin. As shown here, spectrin is multiply phosphorylated and is a substrate for a number of different protein kinases, suggesting that spectrin phosphorylation is regulated by multiple control mechanisms. In addition, spectrin itself is not a kinase, but is isolated from the erythrocyte membrane with a number of different kinases, the most predominant one being casein kinase.

Spectrin dimer purified by gel filtration co-purifies with cAMP independent (casein), dependent, and calcium-calmodulin dependent kinases. Casein kinase activity similar to that associated with spectrin has also been found to contaminate a number of other purified erythrocyte membrane skeletal proteins, including protein 4.1 (34), protein 2.1 (35), and adducin (unpub. observ.). The ability of casein kinase to tightly bind to specific substrates may be one mechanism by which protein phosphorylation is controlled in the erythrocyte membrane.

Purification of spectrin by HPLC ion exchange chromatography isolated the beta spectrin subunit which was completely free of kinase activity. Reassociation of alpha and beta to form heterodimer did not restore kinase activity, although other studies have established the fidelity of reassociated heterodimer spectrin with respect to other properties (36). These results, therefore, strongly indicate that spectrin has no intrinsic kinase activity, in contrast to previous studies that have suggested that spectrin undergoes "autophosphorylation" (1,17,37). Based on the results presented here, spectrin autophosphorylation is presumably due to endogenous and tightly bound casein kinase contaminating the spectrin preparations.

In-vitro and in-vivo spectrin phosphorylation studies were performed and the total amount of phosphate incorporated into spectrin ranged from one mole of phosphate per mole of spectrin dimer in-vitro to four moles of phosphate incorporated per mole in-vivo. These results are in agreement with earlier studies (2,5,14,18). With the exception of the cAMP dependent kinases, each kinase catalyzed the incorporation of approximately one mole of phosphate per mole

of beta spectrin. The values for incorporation are slightly
higher when spectrin dimer is used as a substrate, but the
values for spectrin dimer and isolated beta spectrin are
comparable.

Both type I and type II cAMP dependent kinases from
human erythrocytes have been described (2,3,7,8). Protein
2.1 (35,38), protein 4.1 (2,12,39) and protein 4.9 (12,40)
have been identified as substrates. The specificity of type
I or II has not been distinguished. In the present study,
two cAMP dependent kinases were isolated from the
erythrocyte and neither was able to incorporate ^{32}P into
spectrin dimer or beta spectrin. In addition, cAMP dependent kinase from rabbit skeletal muscle was tested and found
to be inactive towards spectrin dimer or isolated beta
spectrin. Previous studies of spectrin phosphorylation in
intact erythrocytes has shown an apparent cAMP dependent increase in spectrin phosphorylation (6,8,37,41,42). Since
protein 2.1 is a known substrate for cAMP dependent kinases
(35,38), and is often difficult to distinguish from beta
spectrin on one dimensional SDS PAGE, its contribution to
these results must be considered. In addition, the phosphorylation of alpha spectrin by cAMP dependent kinases has
been reported (37,42). The studies reported here find no
evidence of alpha spectrin phosphorylation, even after in
vivo stimulation by cAMP. The reason for this discrepancy
is not known. It may be due to differences in the cAMP concentrations used, as alpha spectrin phosphorylation has only
been observed at high cAMP concentrations (42).

Finally, calcium-calmodulin dependent kinase has been
identified in human ghost preparations (9). The results
presented here demonstrate that in-vitro, spectrin is a substrate for calmodulin dependent kinase. This phosphorylation may be important with regards to calcium-stimulated
phosphorylation in the erythrocyte.

The reason for the difference in phosphorylation
levels achieved in-vivo and in-vitro is not clear. It may
be that a critical phosphatase required for phosphate turnover has been lost or inactivated during spectrin preparation. It has been shown that most phosphatase activity in
the erythrocyte is found in the cytoplasm (43). Alternatively, conformational differences between in-vivo and in-
vitro states of spectrin may play a role. There is

precedence in the literature for differences in the level of ^{32}P incorporated in proteins labeled <u>in-vitro</u> or <u>in-vivo</u>. Neuron coated vesicle proteins show an increased incorporation <u>in-vivo</u> (44), and MAP2 protein contains up to thirty phosphates <u>in-vivo</u> and yet only ten phosphates per mole of protein can be incorporated <u>in-vitro</u> (45,46). Rather than postulating a loss of phosphatase, these differences have been attributed to tertiary and quaternary structural conformational changes which presumably regulate the accessibility of phosphorylation sites.

REFERENCES

1. Hosey, M.M. and Tao, M. (1976). An analysis of the autophosphorylation of rabbit and human erythrocyte membranes. Biochem. 15:1561.

2. Hosey, M.M. and Tao, M. (1977). Selective phosphoryla tion of erythrocyte membrane proteins by the solubil ized membrane protein kinases. Biochem. 16:4578.

3. Dreyfuss, G., Schwartz, K.J., and Blout, E.R. (1978). Compartmentalization of cyclic AMP-dependent protein kinases in human erythrocytes. Proc. Nat'l. Acad. Sci., U.S.A. 75:5926.

4. Simkowski, K.M. and Tao, M (1980). Studies on a soluble human erythrocyte protein kinase. J. Biol. Chem. 255:6456.

5. Tao, M., Conway, R., and Cheta, S. (1980). Purifica tion and characterization of a membrane-bond protein kinase from human erythrocytes. J. Biol. Chem. 255:2563.

6. Erusalimsky, J.D., Balas, N., and Milner, Y. (1983). Possible identity of a membrane-bound with a soluble cyclic AMP-dependent erythrocyte protein kinase that phosphorylates spectrin. Biochem. Biophys. Acta 756:171.

7. Rubin, C.S. (1979). Characterization and comparison of membrane-associated and cytosolic cAMP-dependent protein kinases. J.Biol. Chem. 254:12439.

8. Boivin, P., Garbarz, M., Dhermy, D., and Galand, C. (1981). In-vitro phosphorylation of the red blood cell cytoskeleton complex by cyclic AMP-dependent protein kinase from erythrocyte membrane. Biochim. Biophys. Acta 647:1.

9. Nelson, M.J., Daleke, D.L., and Huestis, W.H. (1982). Calmodulin-dependent spectrin kinase activity in resealed human erythrocyte ghosts. Biochim. Biophys. Acta 686:182.

10.   Palfrey H.C., and Waseem, A. (1985). Protein kinase C in the human erythrocyte. J. Biol. Chem. 260:16021.
11.   Cohen, C.M. and Foley, S.F. (1986). Phorbol ester and Ca^{2+}-dependent phosphorylation of human red cell membrane skeletal proteins. J. Biol. Chem. 261:7701.
12.   Horne, W.C., Leto. T.L., and Marchesi, V.T. (1985). Differential phosphorylation of multiple sites in protein 4.1 and protein 4.9 by phorbol ester-activated and cAMP dependent protein kinase. J. Biol. Chem. 260:9073.
13.   Faquin, W.C., Chahwala, S.B., Cantley, L.C., and Branton, D.(1986). Protein kinase C of human erythrocytes phosphorylates bands 4.1 and 4.9. Biochim. Biophys. Acta 887:142.
14.   Harris, W.H., and Lux, S.E. (1980). Structural characterization of the phosphorylation sites of human erythrocyte spectrin. J. Biol. Chem. 255:11512.
15.   Palmer, F.B., amd Verpoorte, J.(1971). The phosphorus components of solubilized erythrocyte membrane proteins. Can. J. Biochem. 49:337.
16.   Avruch, T. and Fairbanks, G. (1974). Phosphorylation of endogenous substrates by erythrocyte membrane protein kinases. Biochem. 13:5507.
17.   Imhof, B.A., Acha-Orbea, H.J., Libermann, T.D., Reber, B.F.X., Lutz, J.H., Winterhalter, K.H., and Birchmeier, W. (1980). Phosphorylation and dephosphorylation of spectrin from human erythrocyte ghosts under physiological conditions: autocatalysis rather than reaction with separate kinase and phosphatase. Proc. Nat'l. Acad. Sci., USA 77:3264.
18.   Harris, W.H., Levin, N., and Lux, S.E. (1980). Comparison of the phosphorylation of human erythrocyte spectrin in the intact red cell in various cell-free systems. J. Biol. Chem. 255:11521.
19.   Anderson, J.M. and Tyler, J.M. (1980). State of spectrin phosphorylation does not affect erythrocyte shape of spectrin binding to erythrocyte membranes. J. Biol. Chem. 255:1259.
20.   Birchmeier, W. and Singer, S.J. (1977). On the mechanism of ATP-induced shape changes in human erythrocytes. J. Cell Biol. 73:647.
21.   Sheetz, M.P. and Singer, S.J.(1977). On the mechanism of ATP-induced shape changes in the human erythrocyte membranes. I. The role of the spectrin complex. J. Cell. Biol. 73:638.

22.   Graham, C., Avruch, J., and Fairbanks, G.(1976).   Phos
       phoprotein phosphatase of the human erythrocyte.
       Biochem. Biophys. Res. Comm. 72:701.
23.   Usui, H., Imazu, M. Maeta, K., Tsukamoto, H., Azuma,
       K., and Takeda, M. (1988).   Three distinct forms of
       type 2A protein phosphatase in human erythrocyte
       cytosol.   J. Biol. Chem. 263:3752.
24.   Morrow, J.S. and Marchesi, V.T. (1981).   Self-assembly
       of spectrin oligomers in vitro: a basis for a dynamic
       skeleton.   J. Cell. Biol. 88:463.
25.   Morrow, J.S. Haigh, W. B., and Marchesi, V.T. (1981).
       Spectrin oligomers: a structural feature of the
       erythrocyte cytoskeleton.   J. Supra. Struct and Cell.
       Biochem. 17:275.
26.   Yoshino, H. and Marchesi, V.T. (1984). Isolation of
       spectrin subunits and reassociation in vitro. Analysis
       by fluorescence polarization.   J. Biol. Chem.
       259:4496.
27.   McGuinness, T.L., Lai, Y., and Greengard, P. (1985).
       Ca^{2+}/Calmodulin-dependent protein kinase II.   J. Biol.
       Chem. 260:1696.
28.   Cook, P.F., Neville, M.E., Vrana, K.E., Hart, F.T.,
       and Roskoski, R. Jr. (1982).   Adenosine cyclic 3',5'-
       monophosphate dependent protein kinase: kinetic
       mechanism for the skeletal muscle catalytic subunit.
       Biochem. 21:5794.
29.   Fenner, C., Traut, R.R., Mason, D.T., and Wikman-
       Coffelt, J. (1975).   Quantitation of Coomassie blue
       stained proteins in polyacrylamide gels based on
       analysis of eluted dye. Anal. Biochem. 63:595.
30.   Tishler, P. and Epstein, C.J. (1968).   A convenient
       method of preparing polyacrylamide gels for liquid
       scintillation spectrometry. Anal. Biochem. 22:89.
31.   Duck-Chong, C.G. (1979). A rapid sensitive method for
       detection of phospholipid phosphorus involving digest
       ion with magnesium nitrate.   Lipids 14:492.
32.   Laemmli, U.K. (1976).   Cleavage of structural proteins
       during the assembly of the head of bacteriophage T4.
       Nature 227:680.
33.   Morrow, J.S. and Haigh, W.B. (1983). Erythrocyte
       membrane proteins: detection of spectrin oligomers by
       gel electrophoresis.   Met. Enz. 96:298.
34.   Leto, T.L, Correas,E., Tobe, T., Anderson, R.A., and
       Horne, W.C., (1986). Structure and function of human
       erythrocyte cytoskeletal protein 4.1.   In Bennett, V.,
       Cohen, C.M., Lux, S., and Palek, J., (eds.) Membrane
       Skeletons and Cytoskeletal-Membrane Associations.
       Alan R. Liss, Inc., N.Y. pp 201.

35. Cianci, C.D., Georgi, M. and Morrow, J.S. (1988). Phos
     phorylation of ankyrin down-regulates its cooperative
     interaction with spectrin and protein 3. J. Cell
     Biochem. 37:301.
36. Coleman, T.R., Fishkind, D.J., Mooseker, M.S., and Mor
     row, J.S.(1989). Contributions of the Beta-subunit to
     spectrin structure and function. Cell Mot. in press.
37. Lutz, H.U.(1984). A cAMP dependent phosphorylation of
     spectrin dimer. FEBS 169:323.
38. Weaver, D.C. and Marchesi, V.T. (1984). The structural
     basis of ankyrin function. I identification of two
     structural domains. J. Biol. Chem. 259:6165.
39. Plut, D.A, Hosey, M.M., and Tao, M. (1978). Evidence
     for the participation of cytosolic protein kinases in
     membrane phosphorylation in intact erythrocytes. Eur.
     J. Biochem. 82:333.
40. Husain, A. Levin, A., and Branton, D. (1988). Aboli
     tion of actin-bundling by phosphorylation of human
     erythrocyte protein 4.9. Nature 334:718.
41. Beutler, E. Galand, C.(1981). In vitro phosphorylation
     of the red blood cell cytoskeleton complex by cAMPd
     protein kinase from red blood cell membrane. Biochem.
     Biophys. Acta 647:1.
42. Lutz, H., Stringaro-Wipf, G., and Maretzki, D. (1986).
     Red cell spectrin phosphorylation and cytoskeletal
     anchorage. J. Card. Pharm. 8 Suppl. s76.
43. Usui, H., Kinohara, N., Yoshikawa, K., Imazu, M., Im
     aoka, T., and Takeda, M. (1983). Phosphoprotein phos
     phatases in human erythrocyte cytosol. J. Biol. Chem.
     258:10455.
44. Keen, J.H. and Black, M.M. (1986). The phosphorylation
     of coated membrane proteins in intact neurons. J.
     Cell. Biol. 102:1325.
45. Tsuyama, S, Terayama, Y., and Matsuyama, S. (1987).
     Numerous phosphates of microtubule-associated protein
     2 in living rat brain. J. Biol. Chem. 262:10886.
46. Tsuyama, S., Bramblett, G.T., Huang, K.-P., and
     Flavin, M. (1986). Calcium/phospholipid-dependent
     kinase recognizes sites in microtubule-associated
     protein 2 which are phosphorylated in living brain and
     are not accessible to other kinases. J. Biol. Chem.
     261:4110.

Cellular and Molecular Biology of Normal
and Abnormal Erythroid Membranes, pages 131–144
© 1990 Alan R. Liss, Inc.

MODULATION OF ERYTHROPOIETIN RECEPTOR EXPRESSION ON ERYTHROPOIETIN RESPONSIVE AND UNRESPONSIVE CELL LINES[1]

Virginia C. Broudy, Nancy Lin, Betty Nakamoto
and Thalia Papayannopoulou

Department of Medicine, University of Washington
Seattle, Washington   98195

ABSTRACT   Erythropoietin exerts its effects
on erythropoiesis by binding to a specific
receptor. The erythropoietin receptor is
found on erythroid precursor cells,
megakaryocytes, and on a number of human and
murine cell lines, but the mechanisms that
govern its expression are not well
understood. We used 125 I-erythropoietin to
quantitate erythropoietin receptors on both
erythropoietin-responsive and unresponsive
cell line under conditions that modify their
differentiation or proliferation. The human
erythroleukemia cell line OCIM1 expresses
3000 receptors per cell with a binding
affinity of 280 pM. Induction of the
erythroid phenotype with δ-aminolevulinic
acid or its suppression with phorbol
myristate acetate resulted in a 1.5-fold
increase or a 70% decrease, respectively, in
the number of erythropoietin receptors per
cell. Murine GM979 cells display 1700
erythropoietin receptors per cell; treatment
of these cells with dimethylsulfoxide
resulted in a 4-fold increase in receptor

[1]This work was supported by National Institutes of
Health Grants DK31232 and DK30852.

display concomitant with increased cellular
hemoglobin content. The murine B6SUtA cell
line expresses approximately 150
erythropoietin receptors per cell with a
binding affinity of 400 pM, and responds to
erythropoietin with differentiation and
limited proliferation. Induction with
erythropoietin results in enhanced receptor
expression, without a change in binding
affinity. These data indicate that display
of the erythropoietin receptor is dynamic,
and that the early stages of erythroid
differentiation are accompanied by increased
erythropoietin receptor expression.

INTRODUCTION

Erythropoietin is a glycoprotein that
promotes the survival, proliferation, and
maturation of erythroid precursor cells. The
availability of large quantities of
erythropoietin, produced by recombinant DNA
technology, has facilitated investigation of its
mechanism of action (1). The biological effects
of erythropoietin are mediated via interaction
with a cell surface receptor. Receptors for
erythropoietin have been identified on erythroid
precursor cells (2-10) and on megakaryocytes (8,
11) but not on other normal hematopoietic cells.
Normal placental tissue expresses erythropoietin
receptors; these receptors may play a role in the
transplacental passage of erythropoietin during
gestation (12). Finally, a number of erythroid
and multipotent cell lines display the
erythropoietin receptor (8, 13-23), and these
provide a model in which to examine the regulation
of receptor expression.

Thus, information is available about the
cellular distribution of the erythropoietin
receptor, but less is known about the factors that
govern its expression. Exposure to erythropoietin
may rapidly down-modulate the receptor on the
erythropoietin-responsive cell lines TSA8 and TF-1
(14, 23) and on normal spleen cells (9).

Additionally, high concentrations of IL-3 may
down-modulate erythropoietin receptor display (9,
19). We examined erythropoietin receptor
expression on cell lines under conditions that
modify their differentiation and/or growth. The
results of these studies suggest a model in which
there is an initial increase in erythropoietin
receptor expression as early hematopoietic cells
begin to express the erythroid program, followed
by a decline in receptor numbers during terminal
erythroid maturation.

METHODS

Cell Culture

The murine erythroleukemia cell lines
Rauscher Red-1.5 (22, 24) and GM979 (25) were
cultured in RPMI 1640 supplemented with 10% fetal
calf serum. The B6SUtA murine cell line was
cultured as described (26). The OCIM1 human
erythroleukemia cell line was maintained in IMDM
supplemented with 10% fetal calf serum and 10^{-4}M β-
mercaptoethanol (27). To determine the effect of
induction on erythropoietin receptor expression,
1% dimethylsulfoxide (DMSO), 100 nM phorbol
myristate acetate (PMA), or 500 nM δ-
aminolevulinic acid (δ-ALA) were added to the
culture media for 1 to 4 days. In other
experiments, the cells were cultured in the
presence of 2.5 U/ml human recombinant
erythropoietin for varying periods of time. The
erythropoietin used for cell culture was expressed
in baby hamster kidney cells and partially
purified (biological activity 6000 U/mg) (28).

Quantitation of Receptors.

Erythropoietin receptor numbers and binding
affinities were measured as previously described
(17). Briefly, 1-2x 10^6 cells were incubated with
125 I-erythropoietin (300-900 Ci/mmol, Amgen) with
or without a 100 fold excess of unlabeled
erythropoietin (129,000 U/mg, Amgen) for 3 hours

at 15° C . Cell-associated 125 I-erythropoietin
was separated from free 125 I-erythropoietin by
sedimentation through phthalate oil. Both cell-
associated and free 125 I-erythropoietin were
measured in a Packard gamma counter, and equations
for one or two classes of receptors were fitted to
the data using the method of maximum likelihood
(29).
      Cells cultured in erythropoietin would have
partial saturation of their receptors, interfering
with accurate measurement of receptor numbers. To
circumvent this problem, the cells were washed
twice and suspended in erythropoietin-free medium
for 90 minutes to permit internalization and
degradation of surface-bound erythropoietin (2).

RESULTS

Time Course of Erythropoietin Binding

      To identify equilibrium binding conditions,
Rauscher Red 5-1.5 cells were incubated with 125
I-erythropoietin at 15°, 22° , or 37° C for 1 to 4
hours. In 3 experiments performed at 37° C,
binding of 125 I-erythropoietin was maximal at 60
minutes, and then progressively declined, probably
due to internalization and degradation of the
hormone (date not shown). At 22° C, binding
continued to increase up to 4 hours (Fig. 1).
Although the initial rate of binding at 15° C was
slower than at the higher temperature, binding
reached a plateau at 3 hours (Fig. 1). Binding of
125 I-erythropoietin to OCIM1 cells at 15° C also
reached a plateau at 3 hours (data not shown).
Binding at 15° C is a reversible process; addition
of a 100-fold molar excess of unlabeled
erythropoietin at 3 hours results in a progressive
decline in cell-associated 125 I-erythropoietin
(data not shown). Moreover, performing the
binding studies at 15° C inhibits significant
internalization and degradation of erythropoietin
(17). Consequently, a 3-hour incubation at 15° C
was used for all subsequent binding experiments.

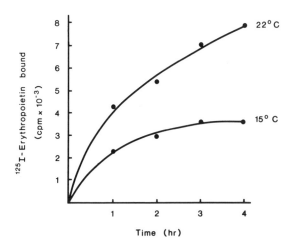

Time (hr)

Figure 1. Time and Temperature Dependence of Erythropoietin Binding. Rauscher Red 5-1.5 cells (10^6) were incubated with 0.3 nM 125 I-erythropoietin at 15° C or 22° C for 1 to 4 hours. Binding was calculated as the difference between total counts in the pellet and counts trapped in the presence of a 100-fold excess of unlabeled erythropoietin.

Erythropoietin Binding is Not Inhibited by Other Growth Factors.

Several other human growth factors were tested for their ability to compete with 125 I-erythropoietin for binding. Since certain of the hematopoietic growth factors such as granulocyte-macrophage colony-stimulating factor (GM-CSF) are species-specific, the human cell line OCIM1 was used for these experiments. OCIM1 cells were incubated with 0.15 nM 125 I-erythropoietin for 3 hours at 15° C with or without a 100 fold molar

excess of each of the following: unlabeled
erythropoietin, human erythroid potentiating
activity (EPA), insulin, human GM-CSF, or human
granulocyte colony-stimulating factor (G-CSF)
(Table 1).   In this experiment, the addition of
unlabeled erythropoietin resulted in 95% reduction
of binding of 125 I-erythropoietin.   None of the
other growth factors tested competed with 125 I-
erythropoietin for binding.   Similar results were
obtained with Raucher Red 5-1.5 cells.

TABLE 1
COMPETITION WITH 125 I-ERYTHROPOIETIN
FOR BINDING TO OCIM1 CELLS

Competitor	CPM Bound
0	821
Epo	38
EPA	738
Insulin	749
GM-CSF	834
G-CSF	762

Induction or Suppression of the Erythroid Program
Alters Erythropoietin Receptor Expression

To determine whether DMSO would affect the
display of the erythropoietin receptor, GM979
cells were cultured with 1% DMSO for 4 days and
receptor number and binding affinity were
quantitated.   Uninduced GM979 cells expressed
approximately 1700 receptors per cell with a
binding affinity of 540 pM.   Induction with DMSO
resulted in a four-fold increase in the number of
erythropoietin receptors per cell and increased
production of hemoglobin (Table 2).   These results
demonstrate that induction of erythroid
differentiation in GM979 cells is accompanied by
increased display of erythropoietin receptor.

TABLE 2

EFFECT OF DMSO ON ERYTHROPOIETIN RECEPTOR
EXPRESSION ON GM979 CELLS

Induction	Receptors/Cell	% Benzidine(+)
--	1660 ± 15*	0
1% DMSO x 4 days	6800#	34

*Mean ± SEM of 3 experiments.
#Average of 2 experiments. The fraction of cells
staining with benzidine was assessed in 1 of these
experiments.

The OCIM1 human erythroleukemia cell line
expresses about 3000 receptors per cell with a
binding affinity of 280 pM (17). Expression of
the erythroid phenotype in OCIM1 cells is enhanced
by δ-ALA (27) and abrogated by PMA (30).
Treatment OCIM1 cells with 500 nM δ-ALA for 2
days resulted in a 1.5-fold increase in
erythropoietin receptor display (one experiment).
In contrast to these results, treatment of the
cells with 100 nM PMA for 24 hours resulted in a
70% reduction in the number of erythropoietin
receptors per cell (mean of 4 experiments). The
binding affinity was not changed by either δ-ALA
or PMA treatment. These results show that
expression of the initial stages of the terminal
erythroid program or its suppression are
paralleled by erythropoietin receptor display.
B6SUtA is a multipotent murine cell line that
responds to erythropoietin with differentiation
and limited proliferation (26). These cells
express a single class of erythropoietin receptors
with a binding affinity of 400 pM (data not
shown). The B6SUtA cells were cultured with or
without erythropoietin and receptor number and
binding affinity were determined. Over a 6 day
period, receptor density increased 2-fold, and the
fraction of benzidine positive cells increased
from 0 to 40% (Table 3). There was no change in
binding affinity during this period. In time
course experiments, an increase in erythropoietin
receptor display was first identified 24 hours

after the addition of erythropoietin (data not shown).

Table 3
CORRELATION OF ERYTHROPOEITIN RECEPTOR EXPRESSION
AND HEMOGLOBIN INDUCTION IN B6SUtA CELLS

Culture Conditions	Receptors/Cell	% Benzidine(+)
IL-3	145	0
IL-3 + Erythropoietin x 3 days	191	10
IL-3 + Erythropoietin x 6 days	310	40

DISCUSSION

The binding affinity for the human cell line OCIM1 is 280 pM, similar to that described for the human erythroleukemia cell lines HEL and K562 (8, 17, 18). These cell lines express a single class of erythropoietin receptors, and do not respond to erythropoietin. The JK-1 human erythroleukemia cell line displays 2 classes of receptors with binding affinities of 60 and 280 pM; erythropoietin induces proliferation in this cell line (21). The properties of these human erythroleukemia cell lines suggest that the high affinity receptor may mediate responsiveness to erythropoietin. However, the human TF-1 cell line, which expresses a single class of low affinity receptors (400 pM), also proliferates in response to erythropoietin (23). Additionally, murine B6SUtA cells which express a single low affinity binding site (400 pM), can differentiate to early erythroblasts in the presence of erythropoietin, indicating that a second high affinity site is not an absolute requirement for cells to proliferate or differentiate in response to erythropoietin.

Chemical agents that augment or abrogate expression of the erythroid program modulate display of the erythropoietin receptor in concert with other erythroid markers. Treatment of GM979 cells with DMSO resulted in a 4-fold increase in receptor numbers, concomitant with increased cellular hemoglobin content, in accord with the results of other investigators (20). Exposure of OCIM1 cells to δ-ALA or TPA for 24 hours resulted in enhanced or diminished expression of the erythropoietin receptor, respectively. Changes in other erythroid markers paralleled the change in erythropoietin receptor expression on OCIM1 cells (27, 30). The results with OCIM1 cells demonstrate that erythropoietin receptor expression increases or decreases within a single cell line in conjunction with the erythroid phenotype.

These results were obtained in erythropoietin- unresponsive cell lines, and employed chemical agents as inducers. In view of recent data that gene regulation following chemical induction of erythroid differentiation may differ from that induced by erythropoietin (31), we explored the effect of erythropoietin itself on expression of its receptor. Erythropoietin-induced differentiation was accompanied by increased receptor expression in B6SUtA cells without a significant change in binding affinity. Thus induction of the erythroid program with either chemical agents or with erythropoietin results in enhanced receptor expression. These results may seem paradoxical in view of reports that late erythroid maturation is accompanied by a decline in receptor expression (6, 8, 10). Quantitation of erythropoietin binding to morphologically recognizable marrow erythroid precursor cells shows a decline in binding as cells mature from proerythroblasts to orthochromatic erythroblasts (8, 10), and erythropoietin receptor expression decreases as fetal mouse liver cells mature <u>in vitro</u> (6). The difference between these reports and our data may reflect the level of maturation of the cells selected for study. B6SUtA is a multipotent cell line that can form mixed colonies consisting of erythroid cells, neutrophils, and basophils (26); our results show that erythropoietin receptor numbers increase as these cells differentiate to early erythroblasts. The fetal mouse liver cells and the marrow erythroid precursor cells are a more mature population of cells, and receptor expression decreased during the late stages of terminal erythroid maturation. We speculate that we did not see a decline in receptor display because B6SUtA cells do not attain the level of erythroid maturation reached by normal erythroblasts or fetal liver cells.

As has been described for a number of other hermatopoietic growth factors (32), erythropoietin can down-modulate its receptor over a period of hours. TF-1 cells exposed to erythropoietin exhibited a rapid decline in erythropoietin receptor expression without a change in Kd (23). The maximal decrease in receptor numbers (to 50% of baseline values) was achieved by 3 hours, and was followed by a gradual return toward baseline numbers. In preliminary experiments, we have observed that erythropoietin treatment diminishes receptor expression on the human OCIM2 cell line (27). The kinetics and magnitude of erythropoietin-induced receptor down-modulation on OCIM2 cells resemble those on TF-1 cells.   High concentrations of erythropoietin (50 U/ml) down-modulate receptors on normal murine spleen cells within 2 hours (9). These observations suggest that erythropoietin can rapidly down-modulate the display of its receptor.

The available data suggest that erythropoietin receptor expression is regulated in a number of ways. There is a slow, progressive change in receptor display in association with expression of the erythroid gene program. This model features an initial increase in receptor numbers as early cells begin to express the erythroid program, followed by a decline in receptor display during terminal maturation of the cells. Additionally, erythropoietin itself can down-modulate the expression of its receptor over a period of hours. Whether down-modulation of the receptor is a prerequisite for erythropoietin biological effect awaits further investigation.

REFERENCES

1.   Lin F-K, Suggs S, Lin C-H, Browne JK,
      Smalling R, Egrie JC, Chen KK, Fox GM, Martin
      F, Stabinsky Z, Badrawi SM, Lai P-H,
      Goldwasser E (1985). Cloning and expression

of the human erythropoietin gene. Proc Natl
Acad Sci USA 82:7580

2. Sawyer ST, Krantz SB, Goldwasser E (1987).
    Binding and receptor-mediated endocytosis of
    erythropoietin in friend virus-infected
    erythroid cells. J Biol Chem 262:5554

3. Mufson RA, Gesner TG (1987). Binding and
    internalization of recombinant Human
    Erythropoietin in Murine Erythroid Precursor
    Cells. Blood 69:1485

4. Sawyer ST, Krantz SB, Luna J (1987).
    Identification of the receptor for
    erythropoietin by cross-linking to Friend
    virus-infected erythroid cells. Proc Natl
    Acad Sci USA 84:3690

5. Mayeux P, Billat C, Jacquot R (1987). The
    erythropoietin receptor of rat erythroid
    progenitor cells. J Biol Chem 262:13985

6. Fukamachi H, Saito T, Tojo A, Kitamura T,
    Urabe A, Takaku F (1987). Binding of
    erythropoietin to CFU-E derived from fetal
    mouse liver cells. Exp Hematol 15:833

7. Sawada K, Krantz SB, Sawyer ST, Civin CI
    (1988). Quantitation of specific binding of
    erythropoietin to human erythroid colony-
    forming cells. J Cell Physiol 137:337.

8. Fraser JK, Lin F-K, Berridge MV (1988).
    Expression of high affinity receptors for
    erythropoietin on human bone marrow cells and
    on the human erythroleukemic cell line, HEL.
    Exp Hematol 16:836.

9. Fraser JK, Nicholls J, Coffey C, Lin F-K,
    Berridge MV (1988). Down-modulation of high-
    affinity receptors for erythropoietin on
    murine erythroblasts by interleukin 3. Exp
    Hematol 16:769.

10. Akahane K, Tojo A, Fukamachi H, Kitamura T,
    Saito T, Urabe A, Takaku F (1989). Binding
    of iodinated erythropoietin to rat bone
    marrow cells under normal and anemic
    conditions. Exp Hematol 17:177.

11. Fraser JK, Tan AS, Lin F-K, Berridge MV
    (1989). Expression of specific high-affinity
    binding sites for erythropoietin on rat and
    mouse megakaryocytes. Exp Hematol 17:10.

12. Sawyer ST, Saunda K, Krantz SB (1987).
     Structure of the receptor for erythropoietin
     in murine and human erythroid cells and
     murine placenta.   Blood 70(Suppl 1):184a.
13. Todokoro D, Kanazawa S, Amanuma H, Ikawa Y
     (1987).   Specific binding of erythropoietin
     to its receptor on responsive mouse
     erythroleukemia cells.   Proc Natl Acad Sci
     USA 84:4126.
14. Fukamachi H, Tojo A, Saito T, Kitamura T,
     Nakata M, Urabe A, Takaku F (1987).
     Internalization of radioiodinated
     erythropoietin and the ligand-induced
     modulation of its receptor in murine
     erythroleukemia cells.   Intl J Cell Clon
     5:209.
15. Sakaguchi M, Koishihara Y, Tsuda H, Fujimoto
     K, Shibuya K, Kawakita M, Takatsuki K (1987).
     The expression of functional erythropoietin
     receptors on an interleukin-3 dependent cell
     line.   Biochem Biophys Res Commun 146:7.
16. Sasaki R, Yanagawa S, Hitomi K, Chiba H
     (1987).   Characterization of erythropoietin
     receptor of murine erythroid cells.   Eur J
     Biochem 168:43.
17. Broudy VC, Lin N, Egrie J, De Haen C, Weiss
     T, Papayannopoulou Th, Adamson JW (1988).
     Identification of the receptor for
     erythropoietin on human and murine
     erythroleukemia cells and modulation by
     phorbol ester and dimethyl sulfoxide.   Proc
     Natl Acad Sci USA 85:6513.
18. Fraser JK, Lin F-K, Berridge MV (1988).
     Expression and modulation of specific, high
     affinity binding sites for erythropoietin on
     the human erythroleukemic cell line K562.
     Blood 71:104.
19. Tsao C-J, Tojo A, Fukamachi H, Kitamura T,
     Saito T, Urabe A, Takaku F (1988).
     Expression of the functional erythropoietin
     receptors on interleukin 3-dependent murine
     cell lines.   J Immunol 140:89.

20. Tojo A, Fukamachi H, Saito T, Kasuga M, Urabe A, Takaku F (1988). Induction of the receptor for erythropoietin in murine erythroleukemia cells after dimethyl sulfoxide treatment. Cancer Res 48:1818.

21. Hitomi K, Fujita K, Sasaki R, Chiba H, Okuno Y, Ichiba S, Takahashi T, Imura H (1988). Erythropoietin receptor of a human leukemic cell line with erythroid characteristics. Biochem Biophys Res Commun 154:902.

22. Weiss TL, Barker ME, Selleck SE, Wintroub BU (1989). Erythropoietin binding and induced differentiation of rauscher erythroleukemia cell line red 5-1.5. J Biol Chem 264:1804.

23. Kitamura T, Tojo A, Kuwaki T, Chiba S, Miyazono K, Urabe A, Takaku F (1989). Identification and analysis of human erythropoietin receptors on a factor-dependent cell line, TF-1. Blood 73:375.

24. De Both NJ, Vermey M, Van't Hull E, Klootwijk-Van-Dijke E, Van Griensven LJLD, Mol JNM, Stoof TJ (1978). A new erythroid cell line induced by Rauscher murine leukaemia virus. Nature 272:626.

25. Brown BA, Padgett RW, Hardies SC, Hutchison III CA, Edgell MH (1982). β-Globin transcript found in induced murine erythroleukemia cells is homologous to the β hO and βh1 genes. Proc Natl Acad Sci USA 79:2753.

26. Greenberger JS, Sakakeeny MA, Humphries RK, Eaves CJ, Echner RJ (1983). Demonstration of permanent factor-dependent multipotential (erythroid/neutrophil/ basophil) hematopoietic progenitor cell lines. Proc Natl Acad Sci USA 80:2931.

27. Papayannopoulou Th, Nakamoto B, Kurachi S, Tweeddale M, Messner H (1988). Surface antigenic profile and globin phenotype of two new human erythroleukemia lines: Characterization and interpretations. Blood 72:1029.

28. Broudy VC, Tait JF, Powell JS (1988). Recombinant human erythropoietin: Purification and analysis of carbohydrate linkage. Arch Biochem Biophys 265:329.

29. Lipkin EW, Teller DC, de Haen C (1986). Equilibrium binding of insulin to rat white fat cells at 15°C. J Biol Chem 261:1694.
30. Papayannopoulou Th, Raines E, Collins S, Nakamoto B, Tweeddale M, Ross R (1987). Constitutive and inducible secretion of platelet-derived growth factor analogs by human leukemic cell lines coexpressing erythroid and megakaryocytic markers. J Clin Invest 79:859.
31. Todokoro K, Watson RJ, Higo H, Amanuma H, Kuramochi S, Yanagisawa H, Ikawa Y (1988). Down-regulation of c-myb gene expression is a prerequisite for erythropoietin-induced erythroid differentiation. Proc Natl Acad Sci USA 85:8900.
32. Walker F, Nicola NA, Metcalf D, Burgess AW (1985). Hierarchical down-modulation of hemopoietic growth factor receptors. Cell 43:269.

Cellular and Molecular Biology of Normal
and Abnormal Erythroid Membranes, pages 145–160
© 1990 Alan R. Liss, Inc.

THE BIOGENESIS OF MEMBRANE SKELETON IN MAMMALIAN RED CELLS

Manjit Hanspal, Jatinder S. Hanspal
and Jiri Palek

Department of Biomedical Research,
St. Elizabeth's Hospital of Boston,
Tufts University, School of Medicine,
Boston, MA   02135

ABSTRACT   Erythropoiesis involves a
sequence of events whereby a pluripotent
stem cell becomes committed to the
erythroid cell lineage and then progresses
through at least two replicative progenitor
stages, known as burst-forming
unit-erythroid (BFU-E) and colony-forming
unit-erythroid (CFU-E) stages, before
reaching the distinct erythroblast stages
of terminal differentiation. Part of the
terminal differentiation program of these
erythroid progenitor cells requires the
reorganization of the plasma membrane and
the biogenesis of the erythroid membrane
skeleton, a network of submembrane proteins
that confers mechanical stability to the
red cell membrane. The known temporal
sequence of the expression and assembly of
the constituent polypeptides suggest an
asynchronous synthesis with the synthesis
of α, β-spectrin, ankyrin and protein 4.1
occurring at the CFU-E stage and that of
band 3 at an early normoblast stage. The
synthesis and assembly of ankyrin and
protein 4.1 continues well after the
synthesis of other components of the
membrane skeleton has been down regulated.
Several defects in synthesis and assembly

of these proteins in abnormal red cells
(hereditary spherocytosis and hereditary
pyropoikilocytosis) are discussed with the
aim to learn from these defects about the
rate limiting steps involved in the
biogenesis of the mammalian erythroid
membrane skeleton.

INTRODUCTION

The erythrocyte membrane skeleton is a
two-dimensional network lying in apposition to
the cytoplasmic face of the plasma membrane.
This protein network is composed of a mainly
hexagonal lattice of fibers of spectrin
tetramers that are interconnected by junctional
complexes containing actin, with the aid of
proteins 4.1, adducin and, possibly, other
proteins like myosin, tropomyosin and protein
4.9 (1-4). The skeleton is attached to the
plasma membrane via the association of spectrin
with ankyrin and protein 4.1 which are, in turn,
bound to several integral membrane proteins.
The assembly of this membrane skeleton
complex which occurs during erythroid
development has been studied extensively in
avian erythroid cells (see 5 for review) and to
some extent in mammalian erythroid cells and
erythroleukemic cell lines. In both mammalian
and avian erythroid cells, the synthesis of
erythroid plasma and skeletal membrane proteins
is detectable at the early stages of erythroid
development. However, the synthesis is
asynchronous. For example, the synthesis of
spectrin and ankyrin is initiated well before
that of band 3 (6,7) and the synthesis and
assembly of ankyrin and protein 4.1 continues
well after the synthesis of other components of
the membrane skeleton has been down regulated
(8,9).
It has been shown that the development of
the mouse and chicken erythroblast to a mature
erythrocyte is accompanied by changes in the
composition and properties of the plasma

membranes of cells (10,11). In mouse, an
important stage of this development involves
enucleation of the late erythroblast to produce
the incipient reticulocyte, when all of the
spectrin of the former cell is sequestered to
the membrane of the reticulocyte (10). Thus, in
the mouse erythroid series, an essential stage
in concentrating spectrin occurs during
erythroblast enucleation. Since avian red cells
retain their nucleus, mammalian and avian
erythroid cell differentiation may therefore
involve different mechanisms to achieve the
appropriate accumulation and assembly of
spectrin in the terminal mature erythrocyte.

I.   SYNTHESIS AND ASSEMBLY OF MEMBRANE
     SKELETAL PROTEINS DURING MAMMALIAN
     ERYTHROPOIESIS

A.   Synthesis and Assembly of Spectrin

     Mammalian and Avian erythroid cells
synthesize both α and β subunits of spectrin
with α spectrin synthesis being 2-3 times more
than that of β spectrin. However, in the
membrane skeleton, α and β spectrins are
assembled in stoichiometric amounts (Fig. 1),
suggesting that the association of α spectrin
with the membrane skeleton may be rate-limited
at least in part by the amount of β spectrin
synthesized. Both subunits of spectrin are
synthesized in excess of the amounts that
assemble onto the membrane skeleton (8,12,13).
This pattern of expression is also observed in
AEV- and S-13 transformed avian cells and
FVA-transformed mammalian cells (6,7). In
contrast, murine erythroleukemia (MEL) cells
appear to synthesize an excess of β spectrin
over α spectrin (14,15), which may suggest an
alternate pattern of spectrin synthesis and
assembly in these cells. However, it has been
shown by Pfeffer et al. (15) that, in induced
MEL cells, spectrin is localized not only at the
plasma membrane but also near virus containing

vacuoles which co-purify with plasma membranes.

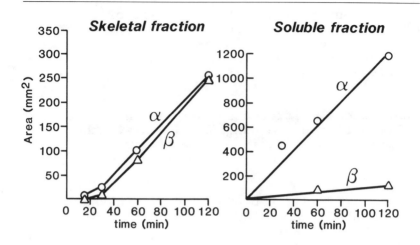

Figure 1.   Synthesis and assembly of α-and
β-spectrin in rat nucleated red cell precursors.
Nucleated red cell precursors from spleens of
phenylhydrazine anemic rats were labeled with
[^{35}S] methionine for different time periods
(15–120 min), lysed in a buffer containing
Triton X-100, and separated into a membrane
skeletal and a soluble fraction.   Aliquots of
each sample were immunoprecipitated with
affinity-purified anti-spectrin antibodies and
the immunoprecipitates were separated on 3.5–12%
polyacrylamide gradient gels.   The gels were
processed for fluorography and exposed to Kodak
XAR film.   The resulting autoradiograms were
scanned at 570 nm and the area under each peak
was integrated.   The area on the left-hand axis
represents the relative area.

Spectrin synthesis has been also studied in
early and late reticulocytes isolated from human
peripheral blood.   Early reticulocytes, like
nucleated red cell precursors, synthesize both α
and β subunits of spectrin with α spectrin

synthesis being 3 fold higher than that of β
spectrin. Likewise, in the membrane skeleton,
the two subunits are assembled in stoichiometric
amounts. Late reticulocytes, on the other hand,
do not synthesize α or β subunits of spectrin
(16).

After synthesis the subpopulation of
spectrin subunits that assemble rapidly with the
correct stoichiometry onto the membrane skeleton
is stable and is not degraded. In contrast, the
remaining unassembled subunits that fail to
assemble are rapidly catabolized (8,17,18). In
avian erythroid cells, this catabolism is highly
specific: β spectrin is degraded extremely
rapidly ($t_{1/2}$=15 min) by cytoplasmic
proteases, whereas α spectrin is turned over
more slowly ($t_{1/2} \approx$ 2 hr) by a lysosomal
route (19). During or immediately following
synthesis in avian erythroblasts, spectrin
monomers combine either as α β heterodimers,
which rapidly assemble onto the membrane
skeleton with high affinity, or as specific
homo-oligomers (β_4-spectrin or
α_2-spectrin). These latter forms are
apparently degraded rapidly. Although the
α_2 homo-oligomer cannot bind to the membrane
skeleton, the β_4 homo-oligomer is competent
to bind, but with a lower affinity than the
heterodimer (18).

The assembly of spectrin is also critically
determined by the available binding sites at the
membrane. For example, in nb/nb mutant mice,
which do not synthesize ankyrin, the red cells
accumulate only 50% of the normal amount of
spectrin (13) thus suggesting that the
ankyrin-band 3 association provides the primary
class of binding sites for the newly synthesized
spectrin at the membrane.

B. The Expression of Ankyrin and Protein 4.1

In both mammalian and avian erythropoiesis,
ankyrin and protein 4.1 are the last components
to be assembled on the membrane skeleton
(8,9,20). Like spectrin, ankyrin is synthesized

in excess of the amounts that assemble onto the membrane. A fraction of the newly synthesized ankyrin assembles rapidly on the membrane and is stable, while the remaining cytosolic ankyrin is degraded rapidly (17). The unassembled ankyrin that accumulates transiently in the soluble pool is unable to bind to β spectrin, suggesting that the excess soluble ankyrin must also exist in some modified form which cannot interact with β spectrin (18).

The fact that during development ankyrin synthesis continues after the spectrin synthesis has ceased (8,9), suggests that stable ankyrin assembly on the membrane can occur independently of spectrin. The presence of band 3 at the membrane is also not an essential prerequisite for ankyrin assembly since ankyrin can be deposited beneath the plasma membrane in the absence of band 3 during early CFUe stages of development (6,21). However, unlike the membrane skeleton of mature red cells, the membrane skeleton in the early erythroid precursors is very unstable with the skeletal proteins turning over very rapidly (6).

A difference in the morphogenesis of the membrane skeleton between avian and mammalian species is observed in the pattern of expression of protein 4.1. In avian erythroid cells, over 95% of the protein 4.1 synthesized rapidly assembles onto the membrane skeleton, irrespective of the stage in development (20). In mammalian erythroid cells, by contrast, large excess of newly synthesized protein 4.1 is found in the cytosol. Moreover, in rat nucleated red cell precursors and reticulocytes, two structurally related forms of protein 4.1 with MWs of 78 kd and 68 kd have been found. The ratios of the newly synthesized forms of protein 4.1 seems to be developmentally regulated as the 78 kd protein is predominantly synthesized at the nucleated red cell level and, as the cell matures into reticulocyte, the synthesis of 78 kd protein is down regulated while that of 68 kd protein continues (Hanspal and Palek, manuscript in preparation).

In avian erythroid cells, multiple variants
of protein 4.1 are found and are produced by a
combination of RNA processing and translational
control (22,23). This process is
developmentally regulated, and manifests itself
first in the expression of a set of lower MW
variants in early progenitor cells and late
polychromatophillic erythroblasts (24,25). As
the cells become postmitotic additional higher
MW variants are synthesized, resulting in the
accumulation of a set of early and late variants
in adult cells (23,24). The accumulation of
these variants may lead to the final
stabilization of the membrane skeleton.

C. The Assembly of Band 3 onto Preassembled
Membrane Skeleton

In avian erythroid cells, band 3 is the
last member of the membrane skeleton complex to
be synthesized. In FVA-transformed mammalian
cells, band 3 synthesis begins only after
induction with erythropoietin whereas spectrin
is synthesized even in the uninduced cells (7).
Previous in vivo pulse-labeling studies in mice
and rabbits (26,27) have also shown that band 3
synthesis is completed later than that of
spectrin and actin polypeptides.
In avian erythroid cells, the extent of
association of band 3 with the membrane skeleton
varies during chicken embryonic development.
Pulse-chase studies indicated that the band 3
polypeptides do not associate with the membrane
skeleton until they have been transported to the
plasma membrane. At this time, band 3
polypeptides are slowly recruited, over a period
of hours (as opposed to rapid assembly within
minutes of peripheral membrane proteins: α and
β spectrins, ankyrin and protein 4.1), onto a
preassembled membrane skeletal network and the
extent of this skeletal assembly is
developmentally regulated (9). During early
stages in development, the low levels of
membrane associated band 3 protein are most
likely due to the late onset of its synthesis.

However, once band 3 is inserted into the membrane, the stability of the membrane skeleton is dramatically increased and the skeletal proteins are no longer catabolized (6).

II.   MEMBRANE SKELETON OF ABNORMAL RED CELLS

A. Hereditary Spherocytosis (HS)

HS is a common, autosomal dominant disorder characterized by hemolytic anemia of varying severity and increased red cell osmotic fragility. Studies of the molecular basis of HS have localized the primary defect to one of the proteins of the red cell membrane skeleton.

Severe spectrin deficiency was first discovered in mice with a life-threatening spherocytic hemolytic anemia (28). Later, a similar deficiency was detected by Agre et al., (29) in a severe autosomal recessive HS. Subsequently, Agre et al., reported a partial spectrin deficiency in a majority of their HS patients (30,31). They found that the degree of spectrin deficiency was proportional to the increase in osmotic fragility and disease severity. It is unlikely that the spectrin deficiency represents the primary molecular defect in the majority of HS patients. In two recently studied patients with severe atypical HS, the underlying molecular defect causing spectrin deficiency involves the deficiency of ankyrin, the principal protein that anchors spectrin onto the membrane (32). The synthesis of spectrin is either normal (α spectrin) or incresed (β spectrin) but its incorporation into the membrane skeleton is diminished because of a marked deficiency of membrane associated ankyrin (33). The abnormal ankyrin is unstable and hence degraded in the cytosol prior to its assembly on the membrane (34). Partial ankyrin deficiency has been detected recently in some patients with the typical form of the autosomal dominant HS (35), and could represent the molecular basis of partial spectrin deficiency in these patients. Furthermore, HS has also been found to be linked with abnormalities involving chromosome 8 (36). In mice, chromosome 8 contains the gene for ankyrin (37). This protein is deficient in mice with severe spherocytic hemolytic anemia (nb/nb) which are also deficient in spectrin (13). Since ankyrin deficiency has been found in some patients with HS (32,38) and since recently, ankyrin gene in man is also mapped to chromosome 8 (Lambert et al., manuscript in preparation), it is possible that the ankyrin deficiency or dysfunction could underlie the deficiency of spectrin in a large subset of HS patients.

The severe autosomal recessive HS has been linked with polymorphism of α spectrin (39), the gene for which is located on chromosome 1 in both mouse and man (13,40). A subset of patients with autosomal dominant HS has a dysfunctional β spectrin (41,42), the gene for which is located on chromosome 14 (43).

B. Hereditary Pyropoikilocytosis (HPP)

HPP is a relatively rare, severe congenital hemolytic anemia characterized by striking micropoikilocytosis and microspherocytosis, autosomal recessive inheritance and a thermal instability of the red cells (44). The red cell membrane skeleton is markedly unstable in HPP subjects when subjected to shear stress (45). Two defects of the membrane skeleton have been identified in HPP. 1) The presence of mutant spectrin which is functionally expressed by defective spectrin dimer-dimer self-association, resulting in an increased amount of spectrin dimers as opposed to tetramers or oligomers in the skeleton (45). On a structural level, the 80 kd α I domain of spectrin, which represents the dimer-dimer self-association site, is altered in HPP subjects, as evidenced by limited tryptic digestion (46,47,48). On this structural basis, two most common variants of the α I domain of spectrin detected in HPP are Sp $\alpha^{I}/74$ and Sp $\alpha^{I}/46$; their tentative designation is based on the size of the abnormal tryptic peptide derived from the α I domain (46,47,49). 2) Second defect in the HPP red cell involves a partial deficiency of spectrin. This defect was originally described by Coetzer and Palek (50) and has been seen in all HPP patients studied so far in our laboratory.

The molecular basis of spectrin deficiency in HPP red cell membrane is presently unknown. Subjects with classical HPP may be compound heterozygotes for an α spectrin mutation (inherited from one parent) and for a defect in spectrin synthesis, inherited from the other parent (51,52). As noted above, α spectrin is synthesized in approximately three times the amount of β spectrin. On the membrane, however, the two polypeptides are assembled stoichiometrically, and their amount depends on the number of copies of membrane associated ankyrin (8,23). The unassembled α and β spectrions are rapidly catabolized in the cytosol. Because of this uneven α, β spectrin synthesis, a "thalassemia minor" like carrier of a synthetic defect of α spectrin is likely to be fully asymptomatic because the synthesis of α spectrin may still exceed that of β spectrin. It is possible, but remains to be proven, that this synthetic defect will lead to an increased quantitative expression of the α spectrin mutant and cause a concomitant partial spectrin deficiency.

In a recently studied HPP subject who is presumably a homozygote for mutant spectrin $\alpha^{I/46}$, the partial spectrin deficiency is due to increased susceptibiity of the mutant spectrin to degradation prior to its assembly on the membrane (53). The synthesis of α and β spectrins (as measured in reticulocyte cytosol) was normal but about 70% of α spectrin was degraded resulting in a diminished spectrin assembly on the membrane. These results are in agreement with the previous results of in vitro incubation experiments (50). In the latter, incubation of HPP spectrin with a lysate of nucleated erythroid precursor cells indicated

that HPP $\alpha^{I/46}$ spectrin, but not HPP
$\alpha^{I/74}$ spectrin, was more susceptible to
proteolytic degradation than a control, implying
that the decreased spectrin content of HPP is
not due to a single defect but that a more
complex mechanism is involved.

ACKNOWLEDGEMENTS

This work was supported by the National
Institutes of Health grant #PO1HL37462.

REFERENCES

1.   Branton D, Cohen CM, Tyler J (1981).
      Interaction of cytoskeletal proteins on the
      human erythrocyte membrane. Cell 24:24.
2.   Bennett V (1985). The membrane skeleton of
      human erythrocytes and its implications for
      more complex cells. Ann Rev Biochem
      54:273.
3.   Marchesi VT (1985). Stabilizing
      intrastructures of membranes. Ann Rev Cell
      Biol 1:531.
4.   Bennett V (1989). The spectrin-actin
      junction of erythrocyte membrane skeletons.
      Biochim Biophys Acta 988:107.
5.   Lazarides E (1987). From genes to
      structural morphogenesis: The genesis and
      epigenesis of a red blood cell.
      Cell 51:345.
6.   Woods CM, Boyer B, Vogt PK, Lazarides E
      (1986). Control of erythroid
      differentiation: asynchronous expression
      of the anion transporter and the peripheral
      components of the membrane skeleton in
      AEV-and S13-tranformed cells.
      J Cell Biol 103:1789.
7.   Koury MJ, Bondurant MC, Rana SS (1987).
      Changes in erythroid membrane proteins
      during erythropoietin-mediated terminal
      differentiation. J Cell Physiol 133:438.
8.   Hanspal M, Palek J (1987). Synthesis and

assembly of membrane skeletal proteins in
mammalian red cell precursors. J Cell Biol
105:1417.

9.   Cox JV, Stack JH, Lazarides E (1987).
Erythroid anion transporter assembly is
mediated by a developmentally-regulated
recruitment onto a preassembled membrane
cytoskeleton. J Cell Biol 105:1405.

10.   Geiduschek JB, SInger SJ (1979). Molecular
changes in the membranes of mouse erythroid
cells accompanying differentiation.
Cell 16:149.

11.   Chan L-NL (1977). Changes in the
composition of plasma membrane proteins
during differentiation of embryonic chick
erythroid cell. Proc Natl Acad Sci
USA 74:1062,

12.   Blikstad I, Nelson WJ, Moon RT, Lazarides E
(1983). Synthesis and assembly of spectrin
during avian erythropoiesis:
stoichiometric assembly but unequal
synthesis of α and β spectrin.
Cell 32:1081.

13.   Bodine DM, Birkenmeier CS, Barker JE
(1984). Spectrin deficient inherited
hemolytic anemias in the mouse:
characterization by spectrin synthesis and
mRNA activity in reticulocytes.
Cell 37:721.

14.   Lehnert ME, Lodish HF 91988). Unequal
synthesis and differential degradation of α
and β spectrin during murine erythroid
differentiation. J Cell Biol 107:413.

15.   Pfeffer SR, Huima T, Redman CM (1986).
Biosynthesis of spectrin and its assembly
into the cytoskeletal system Friend
erythroleukemia cells.
J Cell Biol 103:103.

16.   Hanspal M, Dainiak N, Palek J (1986).
Synthessis and assembly of spectrin in
human erythroblasts. Blood 68 Suppl 1:35a.

17.   Moon RT, Lazarides E (1984). Biogenesis
of the avian erythroid membrane skeleton:
receptor-mediated assembly and
stabilization of ankyrin (goblin) and

spectrin. J Cell Biol 98:1899.

18. Woods CM, Lazarides E (1986). Spectrin assembly in avian erythroid development is determined by competing reactions of homo-and hetero-oligomerization. Nature 321:85.

19. Woods CM, Lazarides E (1985). Degradation of unassembled α-andβ-spectrin by distinct intracellular pathways: regulation of spectrin topogenesis by β-spectrin degradation. Cell 40:959.

20. Staufenbiel M, Lazarides E (1986). Assembly of protein 4.1 during chicken erythroid differentiation. J Cell Biol 102:1157.

21. Koury MJ, Bondurant MC, Mueller TJ (1986). The role of erythropoietin in the production of principal erythrocyte proteins other than hemoglobin during terminal erythroid differentiation. J Cell Physiol 126:259.

22. Granger BL, Lazarides E (1984). Membrane skeletal protein 4.1 of avian erythrocytes is composed of multiple variants that exhibit tissue-specific expression. Cell 37:595.

23. Ngai J, Stack JH, Moon RT, Lazarides E (1987). Regulated expression of multipe chicken erythroid membrane skeletal protein 4.1 variants is governed by differential RNA processing and transational control. Proc Natl Acad Sci USA 84:4432.

24. Granger BL, Lazarides E (1985). Appearance of new variants of membrane skeletal protein 4.1 during terminal differentiation of avian erythroid and lenticular cells. Nature 313:238.

25. Yew NS, Choi HR, Gallarda JL, Engel JD (1987). Expression of cytoskeletal protein 4.1 during avian erythroid cellular maturation. Proc Natl Acad Sci USA 84:1035.

26. Chang H, Langer PJ, Lodish HF (1976). Asynchronous synthesis of erythrocyte membrane proteins. Proc Natl Acad Sci

USA 73:3206.

27. Koch PA, Gartrell JE, Gardner FH, Carter JR
(1975). Biogenesis of erythrocyte membrane
proteins in in vivo studies in anemic
rabbits. Biochim Biophys Acta 389:162.

28. Greenquist AC, Shohet SB, Bernstein SE
(1978). Marked reduction of spectrin in
hereditary spherocytosis in the common
house mouse. Blood 51:1149.

29. Agre P, Orringer EP, Bennett V (1982).
Deficient red cell spectrin in severe,
recessively inherited spherocytosis.
N Engl J Med 306:1155.

30. Agre P, Casella JF, Zinkham WH (1985).
Partial deficiency of erythrocyte spectrin
in hereditary spherocytosis.
Nature 314:380.

31. Agre P, Asimos A, Casella JF (1986).
Inheritance pattern and clinical response
to splenectomy as a reflection of
erythrocyte spectrin deficiency in
hereditary spherocytosis.
N Engl J Med 315:1579.

32. Coetzer TL, Lawler J, Liu SC, Prchal JT,
Gualtieri RJ, Brain MC, Dacie JV, Palek J
(1988). Partial ankyrin and spectrin
deficiency in severe atypical
hereditary spherocytosis.
N Engl J Med 318:230.

33. Hanspal M, Prchal JT, Hanspal J, Palek J
(1987). Synthesis and assembly of spectrin
and ankyrin in atypical hereditary
spherocytosis (HS) associated with
spectrin and ankyrin deficiency.
Blood 70 Suppl 1:53a.

34. Hanspal M, Hanspal J, Prchal JT, Palek J
(1988). Molecular basis of spectrin and
ankyrin deficiencies in atypical hereditary
spherocytosis (HS): Synthesis of unstable
ankyrin. Blood 72 Suppl 1:28a.

35. Palek J, Coetzer TL: Unpublished.

36. Chilcote RR, LeBean MM, Dampier C,
Pergament E, Verlinsky Y, Mohandas N,
Frischer H, Rowley JD (1987). Association
of red cell spherocytosis with deletion

of the short arm of chromosome 8.
Blood 69:156.

37. White R, Barker J (1987). Normoblastosis,
a mutant mouse with severe hemolytic
anemia. Blood 70 Suppl 1:57a.

38. Palek J, Lux SE (1983). Red cell membrane
skeletal defects in hereditary and acquired
hemolytic anemias. Sem Hemat 20:189.

39. Winkelmann JC, Marchesi SL, Watkins P
(1986). Recessive hereditary spherocytosis
is associated with an abnormal α spectrin
subunit. Clinical Research 34:474A.

40. Huebner K, Palumbo AP, Isobe M (1985). The
α-spectrin gene is on chromosome 1 in mouse
and man. Proc Natl Acad Sci USA 82:3790.

41. Wolfe LC, John KM, Falcone JC (1982). A
genetic defect in the binding of protein
4.1 to spectrin in a kindred with
hereditary spherocytosis.
N Engl J Med 307:1367.

42. Goodman SR, Shiffer KA, Casoria LA,
Eyster ME (1982). Identification of the
molecular defect in the erythrocyte
membrane skeleton of some kindreds
with hereditary spherocytosis.
Blood 60:772.

43. Prchal JT, Morley BJ, Yoon SH (1987).
Isolation and characterization of cDNA
clones for human erythrocyte β-spectrin.
Proc Natl Acad Sci USA 84:7468.

44. Zarkowsky, HS, Mohandas N, Speaker CB,
Shohet SB (1975). A congenital hemolytic
anemia with thermal sensitivity of the
erythrocyte membrane.
Br J Haematol 29:537.

45. Liu SC, Palek J, Prchal J, Castleberry RP
(1981). Altered spectrin dimer-dimer
association and instability of erythrocyte
membrane skeletons in hereditary
pyropoikilocytosis. J Clin Invest 68:597.

46. Lawler J, Liu SC, Palek J, Prchal J (1982).
Molecular defect of spectrin in hereditary
pyropoikilocytosis. Alterations in the
trypsin-resistant domain involved in
spectrin self-association.

J Clin Invest 70:1019.

47. Lawler J, Palek J, Liu SC, Prchal J,
Butler WM (1983). Molecular heterogeneity
of hereditary pyropoikilocytosis:
Identification of a second variant of
the spectrin α subunit. blood 62:1182.

48. Knowles WJ, Morrow JS, Speicher DW,
Zarkowsky HS, Mohandas N, Mentzer WC,
Shohet SB, Marchesi VT (1983). Molecular
and functional changes in spectrin from
patients with hereditary
pyropoikilocytosis. J Clin
Invest 71:1867.

49. Palek J (1985). Hereditary elliptocytosis
and related disorders. Clin Hematol 14:45.

50. Coetzer TL, Palek J (1986). Partial
spectrin deficiency in hereditary
pyropoikilocytosis. Blood 67:919.

51. Palek J (1987). Hereditary elliptocytosis,
spherocytosis and related disorder:
Consequences of a deficiency or a mutation
of membrane skeletal proteins.
Blood Reviews 1:147.

52. Palek J (1985). Hereditary elliptocytosis
and related disorders.
Clinics Haematol 14:45.

53. Hanspal M, Hanspal J, Palek J (1988).
Molecular basis of spectrin deficiency
in hereditary pyropoikilocytosis (HPP)
associated with mutant spectrin $\alpha^{I/46}$.
Blood 72 Suppl 1:43a.

**Cellular and Molecular Biology of Normal
and Abnormal Erythroid Membranes, pages 161–170**
© **1990 Alan R. Liss, Inc.**

TRANSPORT OF PHOSPHATIDYLSERINE ACROSS ERYTHROCYTE
MEMBRANES[1]

Jerome Connor and Alan J. Schroit

Department of Cell Biology, The University of Texas M. D.
Anderson Cancer Center, Houston, Texas 77030

A particularly interesting property of biologic
membranes is that many cells exhibit an asymmetric
distribution of phospholipids across the bilayer. Although
the origins of phospholipid asymmetry are unknown, recent
findings indicate that asymmetry is maintained by a
facilitative transport process involving specific lipid
transporters. In this article we summarize recent
observations on the transbilayer distribution of
phosphatidylserine (PS) in normal and pathologic red blood
cells (RBC). In addition, we discuss the mechanisms
responsible for maintaining PS exclusively in the inner
leaflet of normal cells and the events that may control its
"abnormal" expression in the outer leaflet of pathologic
RBC.

THE ERYTHROCYTE MEMBRANE

The erythrocyte membrane, the most extensively studied
mammalian plasma membrane, consists of a fluid lipid
bilayer in which the membrane proteins are embedded. The
membrane is attached to an intracellular cytoskeleton by
protein-protein and lipid-protein interactions that confers
on the erythrocyte its shape and stability (1-3).

---

[1] This work supported by National Institutes of Health
grant CA-47845.

One of the most interesting features of the cell membrane is the asymmetric distribution of membrane phospholipids between the two leaflets of the bilayer (4, 5). In RBC, the aminophospholipids reside preferentially in the inner leaflet, and the choline phospholipids are predominantly localized in the outer leaflet. Although most RBC membrane phospholipids show some preference for either leaflet, PS is the only major phospholipid that adopts a strict asymmetric distribution, being localized exclusively in the cell's inner leaflet (6, 7). This asymmetric organization is maintained through complex and at present, poorly understood interactions between specific membrane proteins. For example, certain proteins can anchor PS at specific sites within the bilayer whereas others specifically promote its movement between leaflets. Other lipid-related factors such as the degree of acyl chain unsaturation and charge may also be involved.

The physiological significance of phospholipid asymmetry is unclear. It has been suggested that defects in the normal asymmetric distribution of PS, for example PS exposure in the cells' outer leaflet which occurs in certain pathologic conditions (8-10), regulate homeostasis (11-13) by serving as a potent procoagulant surface and as a signal for triggering their elimination from the peripheral circulation by macrophages (14-17). These studies strongly suggest that the maintenance of PS asymmetry in human red cell membranes represents a homeostatic mechanism, the failure of which may lead to alterations in normal RBC function and ultimately to their elimination.

Despite the observations that PS is distributed asymmetrically within a bilayer membrane (18), the questions raised 15 years ago have only recently begun to be addressed. How is lipid asymmetry originated, maintained and regulated; what is its functional role, and, lastly, what are the pathologic consequences of breakdown of the regulatory processes that result in the exposure of PS in the cells' outer leaflet? While these fundamental questions have, for the most part, remained unanswered, recent evidence suggests that the preservation of PS in the cell's inner leaflet is of central importance in erythrocyte physiology.

CONTROL OF PHOSPHOLIPID ASYMMETRY IN RBC

The absence of PS in the outer leaflet of RBC and its rapid translocation from the outer to inner leaflet upon

the insertion of exogenously supplied lipids (see below),
clearly indicate the existence of mechanisms responsible
for the control and maintenance of the intrabilayer
distribution of PS. Two distinct mechanisms have been
proposed to be responsible for maintaining the asymmetric
distribution of PS in RBC: Direct interaction of PS with
the membrane skeleton (19-23) and a unidirectional ATP-
dependent translocation of PS from the outer to the inner
membrane leaflet (24-27).

Interaction of PS with the Cytoskeleton

    Experimental evidence in support of a direct membrane
skeleton-PS interaction have been obtained with both model
membrane systems and RBC. Studies with liposomes and
monolayer lipid films have demonstrated that spectrin (19)
and band 4.1 (28) specifically interact with PS. Similar
interactions between PS and spectrin in intact RBC were
demonstrated by Haest and colleagues (19-21). They showed
that oxidative cross-linking of spectrin by treatment of
RBC with diamide or tetrathionate resulted in enhanced PS
exposure in the cell's outer leaflet as determined by the
accessibility of PS to degradation by phospholipase A_2.
Recent evidence suggests, however, that band 4.1 may also
be partially responsible for maintaining PS in the inner
leaflet. Protein 4.1-deficient RBC were found to contain
significant amounts of outer leaflet PS (29). Further
support for the involvement of protein 4.1 has been
obtained from in vitro experiments which have shown that
purified band 4.1 avidly binds PS (30, 31). In contrast,
in vitro oxidation of protein 4.1 or protein 4.1 isolated
from sickle cells (32), which express PS in the outer
leaflet, bind significantly less PS. Thus it appears that
both protein 4.1 and spectrin may contribute to the
maintenance of red cell asymmetry by virtue of their
capacity to fix PS in the inner leaflet.
    Other studies suggested that Ca^{2+}-PS interactions might
also be responsible for immobilizing PS in the cell's inner
leaflet. Experiments on the effects of Ca^{2+}-phosphate
complexes on the ability of fluorescent PS analogs to
transfer between membranes indicated that PS does not
spontaneously translocate from one bilayer leaflet to
another, but can be immobilized in the leaflet in which it
resides (33). By relating these findings to the known
distributions of PS in RBC, one can speculate that PS might
be physically held in the inner leaflet via Ca^{2+}/phosphate

complexes, and that under appropriate conditions Ca^{2+} might be sequestered away from the inner leaflet thus allowing it to attain a partial equilibrium between leaflets. That Ca^{2+} may play a role in the maintenance of membrane asymmetry by immobilizing PS in the bilayer is supported by the observations of Lew et al. (34) who showed that irreversibly sickled cells (ISC) possess intracellular inside-out vesicles in which nearly all the measurable intracellular Ca^{2+} is in the form of precipitates with phosphate. Interestingly, ISC express appreciable amounts of endogenous PS in their outer leaflet (8, 9, 11, 15). Additional evidence for the participation of Ca^{2+} in this process comes from the recent results of Chandra et al. (35), who have shown that Ca^{2+} ionophore-mediated loading of Ca^{2+} into RBC results in a concomitant loss in PS asymmetry (possibly by dissolution of Ca^{2+}/phosphate complexes).

Transbilayer Movement of PS

Seigneuret and Devaux (36) first observed that exogenously inserted anionic phospholipids adopt an asymmetric distribution in intact RBC. When spin-labeled PS and PE (phosphatidylethanolamine) were added to RBC, a temperature and time-dependent decrease in the fraction of spin-labeled lipid which could be reduced by ascorbate was observed. Since ascorbate cannot penetrate membranes, these observations indicated that the analogs were transported to the inner monolayer from their initial site of insertion in the outer leaflet. Similar observations have been obtained using unlabeled and fluorescent or isotopically-labeled lipids in RBC (25-27) and nucleated cells (37). Since PS does not translocate between leaflets of artificially generated vesicles (33, 38), these findings indicate that lipid transport in cell membranes is mediated by a facilitated transport mechanism involving lipid-specific transporters (39, 40). Indeed, the translocation of PS from the outer to inner leaflet in RBC was shown to be ATP-dependent, since transport does not occur in ATP-depleted cells but could be reconstituted in RBC ghosts resealed in the presence of Mg-ATP (36). Additional evidence indicating that the transport of anionic phospholipids is dependent on lipid-specific protein transporters can be obtained from experiments which showed that transport is inhibited by agents that react with protein sulfhydryls (25-27, 36, 37).

EVIDENCE THAT A COMPONENT OF RBC BAND 7 IS THE PS-SPECIFIC
TRANSPORTER

Data generated in our laboratory indicate that a
component of RBC membrane band 7 may be the PS transporter.
This is based on experimental results using appropriately
synthesized probes that preferentially label the
transporter. Experiments employing a ^{125}I-labeled
photoactivatable PS analog in intact human RBC indicated
that a large fraction of PS initially inserted into the
cell's outer leaflet was specifically transported to the
inner leaflet by a 31kDa protein (41).
Because the intrabilayer transport of PS in RBC
requires that the transporters sulfhydryls be reduced, we
reasoned that it might be possible also to identify the
transporter with appropriately labeled inhibitors. For
these experiments we synthesized a series of sulfhydryl-
reactive reagents which bind reduced thiols by thiol-
disulfide exchange. An iodinated derivative of
pyridyldithioethylamine, which specifically inhibited the
transport of PS in RBC, also preferentially labeled the
31kDa protein (42). Thus, a translocating substrate (the
photoactivatable PS analog) and an inhibitor of the
transport activity seem to label the same RBC protein,
strongly suggesting that a component of RBC band 7 is
responsible for specifically transporting PS between
membrane leaflets.
Interestingly, other studies involving analysis of RBC
proteins from various pathologic cells have shown an
anomaly in the appearance of band 7. For example, some
band 7 components seem to be absent in RBC from patients
with hereditary stomatocytosis and cryohydrocytosis (43,
44). Similar results have been obtained from sickle RBC.
Although band 7 is apparently present in normal quantities
in sickle RBC, it may be functionally inactive as a result
of oxidation of its sulfhydryls (45), which must be reduced
in order to transport PS between membrane leaflets (42).

PATHOLOGIC CONSEQUENCES OF PS EXPOSURE IN THE CELL'S OUTER
LEAFLET

The translocation of PS from the inner to outer
leaflet has been implicated in several important biological
processes, suggesting that both the biogenesis and the
maintenance of PS asymmetry are important components of
homeostasis. It has been shown, for example, that the

translocation of PS from the inner to outer leaflet in
activated platelets (12) and sickle RBC (8, 9) is important
in clotting mechanisms (11) and in the pathogenesis of
sickle cell anemia (13, 15), respectively. In addition,
the abnormal exposure of PS in the cells' outer leaflet was
shown to result in their binding to macrophages. Both
sickle RBC and RBC containing an exogenously inserted
fluorescent PS analog are bound by monocytes and
macrophages (14) and are rapidly cleared by the
reticuloendothelial system in vivo (16).

CONCLUSIONS

The physiologic significance of phospholipid asymmetry
is still unclear. Defects in the normal asymmetric
distribution of PS, for example PS exposure in the cells'
outer leaflet in certain red cell pathologies, may result
in the expression of altered membrane surface properties,
some of which may have pathophysiologic consequences.
Indeed, artificial membranes and RBC that contain PS in
their outer leaflet were shown to display potent
procoagulant activity and enhanced binding to cells of the
reticuloendothelial system. These studies suggest that the
maintenance of PS asymmetry in RBC represents a homeostatic
mechanism, which, if it fails, results in the exposure of
PS, which then serves as a "non-self" signal for its
elimination. Its unique property of residing
preferentially on the inner membrane of normal RBC, in
conjunction with the pathologic consequences of its
exposure in the outer leaflet, implies that PS may be a
recognition moiety. Thus the maintenance of homeostasis may
be regulated by translocation of PS from the inner to the
outer bilayer leaflet. This internal system, if its
existence is proved, may represent a common mechanism by
which normal RBC function and, ultimately its lifespan is
determined.

REFERENCES

1.   Lux SE (1979). Spectrin-actin membrane skeleton of
     normal and abnormal red blood. Semin Hematol 16:21.
2.   Sheetz MP (1983). Membrane skeletal dynamics: role in
     modulation of red cell deformability, mobility of
     transmembrane proteins, and shape. Semin Hematol
     20:175.

3. Mohandas N, Chasis JA, Shohet SB (1983). The influence
    of membrane skeleton on red cell deformability,
    membrane material properties, and shape. Semin Hematol
    20:225.
4. Rothman JE, Lenard J (1977). Membrane asymmetry.
    Science 195:743.
5. Op den Kamp JAF (1979). Lipid asymmetry in membranes.
    Annu Rev Biochem 48:47.
6. Verkleij AJ, Zwaal RFA, Roelofsen B, Comfurius P,
    Kastelijn D, van Deenen LLM (1973). The asymmetric
    distribution of phospholipids in the human red blood
    cell membrane. Biochim Biophys Acta 323:178.
7. Gordesky SE, Marinetti GV, Love R (1975). The reaction
    of chemical probes with the erythrocyte membrane. J
    Membr Biol 20:111.
8. Chiu D, Lubin B, Shohet SB (1979). Erythrocyte membrane
    lipid reorganization during the sickling process. Brit
    J Haematol 41:223.
9. Lubin B, Chiu D, Bastacky J, Roelofsen B, van Deenen
    LLM (1981). Abnormalities in the membrane phospholipid
    organization in sickled erythrocytes. J Clin Invest
    67:1643.
10. Kumar A, Gupta CM (1983). Red cell membrane
    abnormalities in chronic myeloid leukaemia. Nature
    303:632.
11. Bevers EM, Comfurius P, van Rijn, JLML, Hemker HC,
    Zwaal RFA (1982). Generation of prothrombin-converting
    activity and the exposure of phosphatidylserine at the
    outer surface of platelets. Eur J Biochim 122:429.
12. Bevers EM, Comfurius P, Zwaal RFA (1983). Changes in
    membrane phospholipid distribution during platelet
    activation. Biochim Biophys Acta 736:57.
13. Franck PFH, Bevers EM, Lubin BH, Comfurius P, Chiu DT-
    Y, Op den Kamp JAF, Zwaal RFA, van Deenen, LLM,
    Roelofsen B (1985). Uncoupling of the membrane
    skeleton from the lipid bilayer: The cause of
    accelerated phospholipid flip-flop leading to enhanced
    procoagulant activity of sickle cells. J Clin Invest
    75:183.
14. Tanaka Y, Schroit AJ (1983). Insertion of fluorescent
    phosphatidylserine into the plasma membrane of red
    blood cells. Recognition by autologous macrophage. J
    Biol Chem 258:11335.
15. Schwartz RS, Tanaka Y, Fidler IJ, Chiu D, Lubin B,
    Schroit AJ (1985). Increased adherence of sickled and
    phosphatidylserine enriched human erythrocytes to
    cultured human peripheral blood monocytes. J Clin
    Invest 75:1965.

16. Schroit AJ, Madsen JM, Tanaka Y (1985). In vivo recognition and clearance of red blood cells containing phosphatidylserine in their plasma membrane. J Biol Chem 260:5131.
17. McEvoy L, Williamson P, Schlegel RA (1986). Membrane phospholipid asymmetry as a determinant of erythrocyte recognition by macrophages. Proc Natl Acad Sci USA 83:3311.
18. Bretscher MS (1972). Asymmetrical lipid bilayer structure for biological membranes. Nature 236:11.
19. Haest CWM (1982). Interactions between membrane skeleton proteins and the intrinsic domain of the erythrocyte. Biochim Biophys Acta 694:331.
20. Haest CWM, Deuticke B (1976). Possible relationship between membrane proteins and phospholipid asymmetry in the human erythrocyte Membrane. Biochim Biophys Acta 436:353.
21. Haest CWM, Plasa G, Kamp D, Deuticke B (1978). Spectrin as stabilizer of the phospholipid asymmetry in the erythrocyte membrane. Biochim Biophys Acta 509:21.
22. Williamson P, Bateman J, Kozarsky K, Mattocks K, Hermanowicz N, Choe HR, Schlegel RA (1982). Involvement of spectrin in the maintenance of phase-state asymmetry in the erythrocyte. Cell 30:725.
23. Dressler V, Haest CWM, Plasa G, Deuticke B, Erusalimsky JD (1984). Stabilizing factors of phospholipid asymmetry in the erythrocyte. membrane. Biochim Biophys Acta 775:189.
24. Calvez-Yves, Zachowski A, Herrmann A, Morrot G, Devaux PF (1988). Asymmetric distribution of phospholipids in spectrin-poor erythrocyte vesicles. Biochemistry 27:5666.
25. Daleke DL, Huestis WH (1985). Incorporation and translocation of aminophospholipids in human erythrocytes. Biochemistry 23:5406.
26. Tilley L, Cribier S, Roelofsen B, Op den Kamp JAF, van Deenen LLM (1986). ATP-dependent translocation of amino phospholipids across the human erythrocyte membrane. FEBS Lett 194:21.
27. Connor J, Schroit AJ (1987). Determination of lipid asymmetry in human red cells by resonance energy transfer. Biochemistry 26:5099.
28. Shiffer KA, Goerke J, Duzgunes N, Fedor J, Shohet SB (1988). Interaction of erythrocyte protein 4.1 with phospholipids. A monolayer and liposome study. Biochim Biophys Acta 937:269.

29. Schwartz RS, Chiu DTY, Lubin B (1985). Plasma membrane phospholipid organization in human erythrocytes. Current Topics in Hematology 5:63.
30. Sato S, Ohnishi S (1983). Interaction of a peripheral protein of the erythrocyte membrane, band 4.1, with phosphatidylserine-containing liposomes and erythrocytes. Eur J Biochem 130:19.
31. Cohen AM, Liu SC, Lawler J, Derick L, Palek J (1988). Identification of protein 4.1 binding site to phosphatidylserine vesicles. Biochemistry 27:614.
32. Schwartz RS, Rybicki AC, Heath RH, Lubin BH (1987). Protein 4.1 in sickle erythrocytes: Evidence for oxidative damage. J Biol Chem 262:15666.
33. Tanaka Y, Schroit AJ (1986). Calcium/phosphate induced immobilization of fluorescent phosphatidylserine in synthetic bilayer membranes: Inhibition of lipid transfer between vesicles. Biochemistry 25:2141.
34. Lew VL, Hockaday A, Sepulveda M-I, Somlyo AP, Oritz OE, Bookchin RM (1985). Compartmentalization of sickle-cell calcium in endocytotic inside-outside vesicles. Nature 315:586.
35. Chandra R, Joshi PC, Bajpai VK, Gupta CM (1987). Membrane phospholipid organization in calcium-loaded erythrocytes. Biochim Biophys Acta 902:253.
36. Seigneuret M, Devaux PF (1984). ATP-dependent asymmetric distribution of spin-labeled phospholipids in the erythrocyte membrane: Relation to shape changes. Proc Natl Acad Sci USA 81:3751.
37. Martin OC, Pagano RE (1987). Transbilayer movement of fluorescent analogs of phosphatidylserine and phosphatidylethanolamine at the plasma membrane of cultured cells. J Biol Chem 262:5890.
38. Denkins YM, Schroit AJ (1986). Phosphatidylserine decarboxylase: Generation of asymmetric vesicles and determination of the transbilayer distribution of fluorescent phosphatidylserine in model membrane systems. Biochim Biophys Acta 862:343.
39. Bishop WR, Bell RM (1985). Assembly of the endoplasmatic reticulum phospholipid bilayer: The phosphatidylcholine transporter. Cell 42:51.
40. Backer JM, Dawidowicz EA (1987). Reconstitution of a phospholipid flippase from rat liver microsomes. Nature 327:341.
41. Schroit AJ, Madsen J, Ruoho AE (1987). Radioiodinated, photoactivatable phosphatidylcholine and phosphatidylserine: Transfer properties and differential photoreactive interaction with human erythrocyte membrane proteins. Biochemistry 26:1812.

42. Connor J, Schroit AJ (1988). Transbilayer movement of phosphatidylserine in erythrocytes: Inhibition of transport and preferential labeling of a 31000 dalton protein by sulfhydryl reactive reagents. Biochemistry 27:848.
43. Lande WM, Thiemann VW, Mentzer WC (1982). Missing band 7 membrane protein in two patients with high Na, low K erythrocytes. J Clin Invest 70:1273.
44. Lande WM, Thiemann PVW, Fisher KA, Mentzer WC (1984). Two-dimensional electrophoretic analysis of human erythrocyte cylindrin. Biochim Biophys Acta 778:105.
45. Rank BH, Carlsson J, Hebbel RP (1985). Abnormal redox status of membrane-protein thiols in sickle erythrocytes. J Clin Invest 75:1531.

Cellular and Molecular Biology of Normal
and Abnormal Erythroid Membranes, pages 171–183
© 1990 Alan R. Liss, Inc.

MOLECULAR ANATOMY OF ERYTHROCYTE MEMBRANE SKELETON IN HEALTH AND DISEASE[1]

Shih-Chun Liu, Laura H. Derick and Jiri Palek

Departments of Biomedical Research and
Medicine, Division of Hematology/Oncology,
St. Elizabeth's Hospital of Boston,
Tufts University School of Medicine,
Boston, Massachusetts 02135

ABSTRACT. In this article, we review ultrastrutural data on the molecular anatomy of the normal and abnormal red cell membrane skeleton as well as aspects relevant for membrane stability and deformability. The normal membrane skeleton is primarily organized into a hexagonal lattice composed of junctional complexes of short F-actin filaments crosslinked by spectrin tetramers and medium-sized oligomers. When uniformly extended, spectrin filaments in the skeleton can be stretched end to end up to 200 nm which is about 2.8 x the estimated distance between adjacent junctional complexes in the intact membrane. This estimation of maximum extension of the skeletal network without rupturing the interconnecting spectrin filaments correlates well with the data on red cell deformation which was obtained at extremely high shear stress. Visualization of the skeletal network

[1]This work was supported by grants from
the National Institutes of Health
(HL37462, 27215 and 15157-7).

in hereditary spherocytosis (HS) associated
with a partial deficiency of spectrin and in
hereditary pyropoikilocytosis (HPP) associated
with defects in spectrin self-association as
well as partial spectrin deficiency reveals
striking differences in skeletal structure.
In cases of HS with mild spectrin deficiency,
the integrity of the hexagonal lattice is near
normal.   In contrast, HPP skeletons with a
comparable   degree   of   spectrin   deficiency
exhibit a marked disruption presumably due to
the   superimposed   defect   of   spectrin   self-
association. In the normal red cell membrane,
about 65% of the cytoplasmic surface is covered
by the skeletal structure.   In contrast, this
value is reduced in HS; in severe HS associated
with 50% deficiency of spectrin, it is as low
as 35%.   Without sufficient skeletal protein
support, HS membranes exhibit a lipid bilayer
instability and a markedly increased propensity
to vesiculate.

INTRODUCTION

The   inner   side   of   the   mammalian   red   cell
membrane is laminated by a protein network composed
of spectrin, actin, band 4.1 and other associated
proteins (see 1-3 for reviews).   This network
provides the stability to the membrane and is a
major   determinant   of   red   cell   shape   and
deformability.
Spectrin, the major protein constituent of
the membrane skeleton, accounts for   75% of the
skeletal   mass.   The   native   species   of   spectrin
extracted   from   the   normal   red   cell   membrane   are
tetramers and medium-sized oligomers (4) formed by
a head-to-head association of dimeric subunits ($\alpha\beta$,
100 nm in contour length).   The distal ends of the
spectrin molecules are associated with short actin
filaments.   This   spectrin-actin   association   is
stabilized by the formation of a ternary complex
with the protein 4.1.   The skeleton is linked to

the membrane proper primarily by the associations of spectrin-band 2.1-band 3 and band 4.1-glycophorin (5-8) as well as spectrin-lipid and band 4.1-lipid interactions (9-11).

MOLECULAR ANATOMY OF UNIFORMLY EXTENDED MEMBRANE SKELETON

Earlier electron microscopic studies (12-19) of the membrane skeleton which used various techniques of specimen preparation revealed a filamentous weblike structure containing a variety of poorly defined elements of various sizes. The complication of high protein density in the native skeleton was recently overcome by examinations of membrane skeletal fragments (20) and artifacturally extended membrane skeletons (21-23) to improve the structural resolution.

An example of the intact spread skeleton (Figure 1) shows clear images of a primarily hexagonal lattice of junctional complexes crosslinked by spectrin filaments resembling those of spectrin tetramers and medium-sized oligomers such as hexamers. These junctional complexes (9-16 nm thick, 38-50 nm long) presumably represent short F-actin and associated proteins. This regularly ordered network entends over the entire membrane skeleton. Some of the junctional complexes are arranged in the form of pentagons and septagons. In addition, globular structures (9-12 nm in diameter) are attached to the majority of the spectrin molecules approximately 80 nm from the distal ends of the spectrin that are inserted into the junctional complexes. Presumably, these globular structures represent ankyrin- or ankyrin/band 3-containing complexes, since they are located at the known binding site of ankyrin on the spectrin molecule and they are absent when ankyrin and residual band 3 are extracted from the skeleton under hypertonic conditions (23).

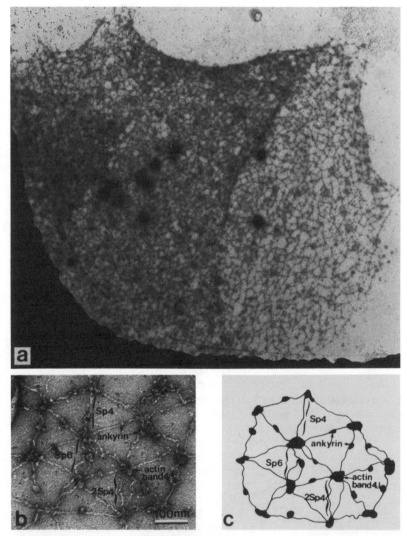

FIGURE 1. Spread membrane skeleton examined by negative-staining electron microscopy. (a) A large area of a spread network. (b) A higher magnification of the spread skeleton. (c) A tentative assignment of the structural elements in the schematic diagram. Sp4, spectrin tetramers; Sp6, spectrin hexamers; 2Sp4, double spectrin tetramers. Reproduced from Liu et al (23) with permission.

ULTRASTRUCTURAL BASIS OF MEMBRANE DEFORMATION

In order to explore the possible ultrastructural changes of the skeleton that accompany membrane deformation, we asked how the extended skeleton relates to the native skeleton in situ. We have focused on the following: (1) the density of the skeletal network as visualized by electron microscopy, (2) estimation of the surface area of the skeleton and (3) comparison of the skeletal deformation during unidirectional stretch as related to the cellular deformation of intact red cells.

The method we use to visualize the skeleton in situ first involves the fixation of ghosts with glutaraldehyde, then a brief sonication of the ghosts which produces small membrane openings ("windows") used to visualize the skeletal monolayer inside the ghosts by negative staining electron microscopy. The exposed skeletal network at the cytoplasmic surface of the membrane appears much denser than that of the extended skeleton, as previously observed with a slightly different method of specimen preparation (15-21). When we estimate the surface area of the fully extended skeleton, based on the known spectrin content (100,000 tetramers/cell), the estimated area covered by an extended hexagon (0.1 μm^2) and the number of spectrin tetramers required per hexagon (9 tetramers/hexagon), we can then calculate the total area of an extended skeleton (1,100 μm^2) which is about 8 times larger than the normal red cell surface area.

The maximum diameter of an uniformly extended skeleton is estimated to be 23 μm, which is about 2.8 x the red cell diameter. Based on this calculation with the spectrin tetramers fully extended (200 nm), the membrane skeleton can be stretched up to 2.8 x the red cell diameter. Further stretching will cause rupture of the skeletal network. A similar value for the maximum extension ratio of meshwork was also obtained by others (21,24,25). In addition, this estimation of maximum extension of the cell skeleton fits very well with the deformation data obtained previously by Sutera et al (26) which showed that red cells deformed under extremely high shear stress (2500 dynes/cm^2) in a ektacytometer. The long axis of these cells measured about 19 μm, which is about 2.2 x that of the red cell diameter. After cessation of the shear stress, these cells resume their normal discocyte shape. However, if the shear stress is increased to 4500 dynes/cm^2, one clearly sees both the cell fragments, and the dumbbell-shaped cells which are in the process of fragmentation, presumably due to the rupture of the membrane skeleton (27). The long axis of some of the stretched cells is about 2.8 x that of the resting red cell. Thus it appears that the maximum extension of the membrane skeleton without rupture is identical to an unidirectional extension of intact red cells. Figure 2 depicts a portion of the extended skeleton produced during specimen preparation. Note the presence of a dense region at the bottom where spectrin filaments run parallel along the horizontal direction. We speculate that the elongated red cell under high shear stress may have a similar type of skeletal rearrangement.

ULTRASTRUCTURAL ALTERATIONS IN HS AND HPP

To explore the possible skeletal alterations in hereditary spherocytosis (HS) and pyropoikilocytosis (HPP), we have studied the ultrastructure of the uniformly extended membrane skeletons in a subpopulation of HS patients with a partial spectrin deficiency ranging from 43-89% of normal spectrin levels and in patients with HPP who, in addition to a mild spectrin deficiency, carry a mutant spectrin that is dysfunctional with regard to its reduced ability to assemble from dimers into tetramers. We also evaluated the average number of crosslinking spectrin filaments associated with each junctional complex in large

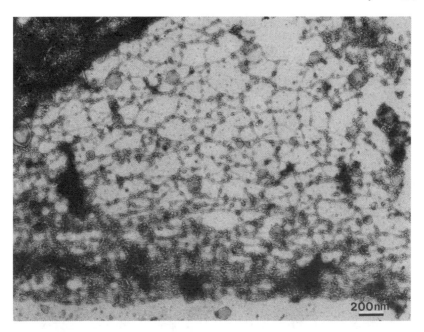

FIGURE 2. Asymmetric stretching of the membrane skeleton. The uneven spreading of the skeleton at the bottom region shows spectrin filaments running parallel along the horizontal direction.

areas of the skeleton (28). In most cases of HS, the hexagonal lattice was near normal or only minimally disrupted, with the exception of cases with severe spectrin deficiency (28), in which considerable skeletal disruption was noted.   In contrast to HS skeletons from cells with mild-to-moderate spectrin deficiency (e.g. 70% of normal), HPP skeletons with a comparable degree of spectrin deficiency exhibited a marked disruption of the skeletal lattice presumably due to a superimposed defect of spectrin dimers to form tetramers, that disrupted the two dimensional integrity of the skeletal network.

LIPID BILAYER-SKELETON UNCOUPLING:
POSSIBLE ROLE IN PATHOPHYSIOLOGY OF HS

The hallmark of the cellular lesion in HS is the membrane lipid loss leading to surface area deficiency as reflected by increased osmotic fragility (29). In addition, a release of spectrin-free vesicles has been demonstrated in vitro under various conditions. Possibly, a similar process may cause the loss of surface area in vivo. The principal molecular defect of the HS membrane skeleton is a partial deficiency of spectrin, resulting from either a primary defect of spectrin or a defect that is secondary to a deficiency or dysfunction of the spectrin binding protein, ankyrin (30). However, a direct link between the spectrin deficiency in HS and the membrane lipid loss has not been clearly established.

To address this problem, we studied ultrastructurally the separation of the lipid bilayer from the underlying membrane skeleton and the acceleration of membrane loss in HS. In addition, we measured the decrease of the surface area density of the monolayer skeleton in HS which might be related directly to its lipid loss.

The method we used to visualize separation of the lipid bilayer from the membrane skeleton involved the shape transformation of ghosts from discocytic to echinocytic shapes, produced by adding the physiological concentration of salt to hypotonically incubated ghosts. These echinocytic ghosts were then directly examined by negative staining electron microscopy (31).

Figure 3 shows some of the membrane spicules extended beyond the outer membrane rim of the flattened ghost allowing visualization of the surface contour of the spicule and its underlying structure. Striking ultrastructural alterations were detected in these membrane spicules. The continuity of the submembrane reticulum which extended into the spiny processes was interrupted

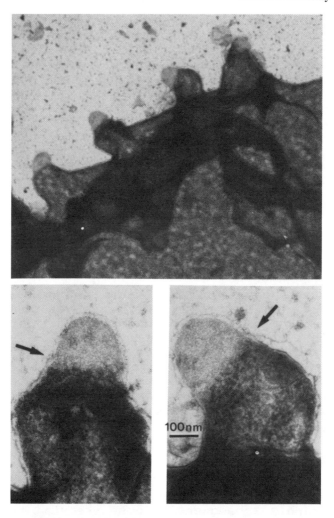

FIGURE 3. Negatively stained membrane spicules of echinocytic red cell ghosts. Echinocytic ghosts from normal red cells were produced by adding NaCl (150 mM) to normal white ghosts in 5 mM NaPi, pH 7.4 at 0°C and examined after 10 minute incubation. Arrows at the neck region of the spicule show the separation of the membrane lipid from the filamentous skeleton.

at the tips of the narrow projections, and a filamentous skeleton was separated from the lipid bilayer at the neck region of the projection. Some enclosed membrane microvesicles, which were lightly stained and did not contain any reticular structures typical of the membrane skeleton, were seen either attached to the tips of the processes or released from the echinocytic ghosts. It seems that the lipid bilayer, without the underlying skeletal support, is extremely unstable and thus prone to vesiculate from the membrane proper. The subsequent protein analysis of the isolated microvesicles indicated they retained band 3, band 7 and some band 4.1 as well as glycoproteins but contained very little spectrin or actin (< 5% of that in ghost membrane, 31).

In a preliminary study, we compared the vesiculation of normal ghosts to the ghosts from HS with severe (50%) spectrin deficiency by isotonic incubation. We found that HS ghosts released about three times more vesicles than normal (32). Since HS membranes are spectrin deficient, intuitively, one would suspect that the increased vesicle release in HS may be simply due to the fact that the amount of spectrin is insufficient to support the entire cytoplasmic surface of the lipid bilayer membrane. To directly evaluate the density of the skeletal protein network, we examined monolayer skeletons in the intact membrane in situ using the "window" technique described above. To obtain an estimate of the proportion of the surface area covered by the skeletal components in the membrane, we first traced the skeletal network of the electron micrograph. Subsequently these skeletal tracings were analyzed by a computer to obtain the percentage surface area covered by the tracings. Although this approach represents an imperfect, crude approximation, the preliminary data indicates that the proportion of the surface area covered by the tracing in the severe HS membrane (50% spectrin deficiency) is markedly reduced and measured only 36% as compared to 64% in the normal membrane (32).

It is very likely that this decrease in skeleton density underlies the destabilization of the lipid bilayer and the increased propensity of membrane loss in HS.

ACKNOWLEDGMENTS

We thank Patsy Bustos for manuscript preparation and Joan Joos for art work.

REFERENCES

1. Branton D, Cohen CM, Tyler J: Cell 24:24-32. 1981
2. Cohen CM: Semin Hematol 20:141-158, 1983
3. Marchesi VT: Annu Rev Cell Biol 1:531-561, 1985
4. Liu SC, Windish P, Kim S, Palek J: Cell 37:587-594, 1984
5. Bennet V, Stenbuck PJ: J Biol Chem 254:2533-2541, 1979
6. Bennet V, Stenbuck PJ: Nature 280:468-473, 1979

7. Havgreaves WR, Giedd KN, VerKleij A, Branton
    D: J Biol Chem 255:11965-11972, 1980
8. Anderson RA, Lovrien RE: Nature 307:655-658,
    1984
9. Cohen AM, Liu SC, Derick LH, Palek J: Blood
    68:920-926, 1986
10. Cohen AM, Liu SC, Lawler J, Derick LH, Palek
    J: Biochem 27:614-619, 1988
11. Rybicki A, Schwartz RS, Mueller T, Wang W,
    Chiu D, Lubin B: Blood 64:30a, 1984
12. Sheetz MP, Sawyer D: J Supramol Struct
    8:399-412, 1978
13. Timme AH: J Ultrastruct Res 77:199-209, 1981
14. Yu J, Fischman DA, Steck TL: J Supramol
    Struct 1:233-248, 1973
15. Tsukita S, Tsukita S, Ishikawa H: J Cell Biol
    85:567-576, 1980
16. Tsukita S, Tsukita S, Ishikawa H: J Cell Biol
    98:1102-1110, 1984
17. Nermut MV: Eur J Cell Biol 25:265-271, 1981
18. Espevik T, Elgsaeter A: J Micros (Oxf)
    122:159-163, 1981
19. Hainsfeld JF, Steck TL: J Supramol Struct
    6:301-311, 1977
20. Shen BW, Josephs R, Steck TL: J Cell Biol
    99:810-821, 1984
21. Byers TJ, Branton D: Proc Natl Acad Sci USA
    82:6153-6157, 1985
22. Shen BW, Josephs R, Steck TL: J Cell Biol
    102:997-1006, 1986
23. Liu SC, Derick LH, Palek J: J Cell Biol
    104:527-536, 1987
24. Waugh RE: Biophys J 39:273-278, 1982
25. Chasis JA, Mohandas N: J Cell Biol
    103:343-350, 1986

26. Sutera SP, Mehrjardi M, Mohandas N: Blood
     Cells 1:369-374, 1975
27. Sutera SP: Circulation Res 62:33-39, 1977
28. Liu SC, Derick LH, Agre PC, Palek J: Blood
     68:56a, 1986
29. Palek J: Blood Reviews 1:147, 1987
30. Coetzer TL, Lawler J, Liu SC, Prchal JT,
     Gualtieri RJ, Brain MC, Dacie JV, Palek J:
     New Engl J Med 318:230-234, 1988
31. Liu SC, Derick LH, Duquette MA, Palek J: Eur
     J Cell Biol, 1989
32. Liu SC, Derick LH, Palek J: Blood 72:31a,
     1988

Cellular and Molecular Biology of Normal
and Abnormal Erythroid Membranes, pages 185–199
© 1990 Alan R. Liss, Inc.

CONSEQUENCES OF STRUCTURAL ABNORMALITIES ON THE
MECHANICAL PROPERTIES OF RED BLOOD CELL MEMBRANE[1]

Richard E. Waugh and Sally L. Marchesi

Department of Biophysics
University of Rochester
School of Medicine and Dentistry
Rochester, NY 14642

and

Department of Pathology
Yale University School of Medicine
New Haven, CT 06510

ABSTRACT   The stability and deformability of
the red blood cell is governed by the
properties of its membrane. Abnormalities in
membrane mechanical function can result in
hemolytic anemia, and a number of structural
abnormalities in the membrane skeleton have
been identified in patients with inherited
hemolytic disorders. In an effort to
understand the connection between the
molecular lesion and its physiological
effect, we have studied the mechanical
properties of cells from patients having
inherited , biochemically identified,
molecular abnormalities of the membrane
skeleton. The abnormalities studied include
reductions in spectrin content, mutant
spectrins with reduced self-association, and
abnormal protein 4.1. Previously, a strong

[1]This work was supported by the Public Health
service under NIH grant nos. HL31524 (Waugh) and
DK 27932 (Marchesi).

correlation between the degree of spectrin
deficiency and the fractional reduction in
membrane shear rigidity has been observed,
regardless of the presence of other
abnormalities. In the present report we find
that membranes having abnormal spectrin self-
association exhibit higher shear rigidity
than normal. Cells from patients from three
kindreds, two with abnormal spectrin self-
association, exhibit increases in membrane
shear rigidity of 15-30 percent above normal.
This increase does not correlate with
quantitative reductions in spectrin dimer-
dimer interactions. The increase in rigidity
is associated with an apparent increase in
the resistance of the membrane skeleton to
isotropic deformations (local changes in
skeletal density). In contrast,
abnormalities in protein 4.1 structure have
no significant effect on the membrane shear
rigidity when small forces are applied to the
surface.

INTRODUCTION

The function of the membrane skeleton in the
red blood cell is mechanical. As described in
other entries in this volume, biochemical and
molecular-biological studies have provided much
information about the origins, structure, and
associations of the constituent molecules of the
skeleton. However, in assessing the function of
the skeleton it is appropriate to test its
mechanical behavior. Of particular interest is
the effect of specific structural abnormalities on
mechanical function of the intact membrane.
Understanding functional consequences of
abnormalities characterized at the molecular level
is essential for an accurate understanding of the
mechanisms underlying the pathological
consequences of the molecular abnormalities
identified in different hemolytic anemias.
The essential features of the mechanical
behavior of the red blood cell membrane have been
described [1,2]. Any membrane deformation can be

written in terms of three components: a change in surface area (isotropic deformation), an extension of the surface at constant area (shear deformation) and a change in curvature (bending) (Fig. 1). There are quantities that define the extent of deformation for each of these modes and quantities defining the "forces" that cause them to occur. (For details see [1].) The isotropic deformation is characterized by the fractional change in membrane area and driven by the isotropic force resultant (a force per unit length acting equally in all directions). Shear deformation is characterized by the extension ratio λ (the ratio of the deformed length of a material element to its resting length) and driven by the surface shear resultant. The bending of the membrane is given by the change in its radii of curvature, and driven by the bending moment resultant. In addition, for each of the modes there is a material coefficient that provides a measure of how strongly the membrane resists that type of deformation: the area expansivity modulus, the membrane shear modulus and the membrane bending stiffness. In addition to these elastic coefficients there also exist membrane viscosity coefficients that characterize the rate at which the membrane deforms in response to applied forces. In the present report we will limit our attention to elastic deformations of the surface.

The red cell membrane is a composite structure consisting of the lipid bilayer and the protein skeleton. In assessing the molecular basis of the mechanical behavior of the membrane, it is important to recognize which aspects of the mechanical behavior arise from the bilayer and which arise from the skeleton. The bilayer exhibits elastic character in area dilation and bending, but in shear deformation it behaves as a fluid. A pure lipid bilayer deforms readily in the plane of the surface (at constant area) and if placed in the circulation it would rapidly fragment until spherical particles were formed. The function of the membrane skeleton is to provide stability to the bilipid layer in shear deformation. Thus, measurement of the elastic

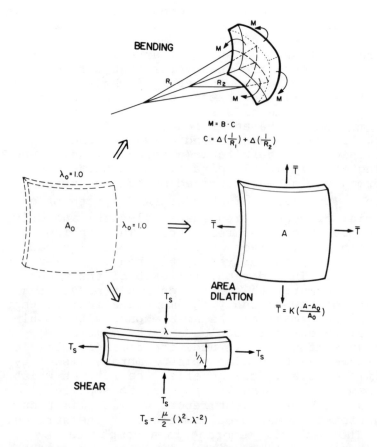

Figure 1.   Schematic of the different modes of deformation possible for membranes.   The change in membrane curvature (C) is driven by the bending moment resultant (M); the change in membrane area is driven by the isotropic force resultant $\bar{T}$; and the membrane extension (λ) is driven by the shear resultant T_S.   The membrane rigidity is characterized by the coefficients relating the forces to the deformations in each mode: the bending stiffness B, the area expansivity modulus K and the surface shear modulus μ.   Reprinted from [2] with permission.

shear modulus of the membrane provides a direct assessment of membrane skeletal function.

The structure and composition of the membrane skeleton have been reviewed extensively. (See [3], for example.) Briefly, the most abundant component of the skeleton is spectrin, a heterodimer which is capable of head-to-head association to form tetramers and higher oligomers. The ends of the heterodimer associate with the actin and protein 4.1 forming an extended hexagonal lattice-like structure [4]. The skeleton is attached to the bilayer via associations between spectrin, ankyrin and band 3 as well as via linkages between protein 4.1 and glycophorin C.

In a previous report, the effects of spectrin deficiency on shear elasticity of the membrane have been described [5]. Spectrin deficiency has been identified as an important feature of hereditary spherocytosis (HS) [6]. Blood samples from 17 patients from 10 kindreds with dominant or recessive HS and varying degrees of spectrin deficiency [5] were tested for abnormalities in the mechanical function of the membrane. In all cases the shear rigidity of the abnormal membranes was reduced, and the fractional reduction in the membrane shear modulus correlated strongly with the magnitude of the spectrin deficiency.

Two classes of underlying molecular defects have been identified in the disorder hereditary elliptocytosis (HE): abnormalities associated with protein 4.1 and mutant spectrins with reduced ability to self-associate. Chabanel *et al.* [7] have examined several cases of HE associated with abnormal spectrin in which membrane rigidity was increased. They postulated that the increased rigidity observed is due to an increase in the molar ratio of spectrin dimer to tetramer. In the present report, we examine three patients with mutant spectrin αI domains and abnormal spectrin self-association [8], one patient with a mutant spectrin αII domain (αIIa) and two patients with mutant forms of protein 4.1 [9].

METHODS

The apparatus and methods are described in detail elsewhere [5]. Briefly, samples drawn from patients and matched controls were shipped from a cooperating laboratory via overnight carrier. Cells were dispersed in a physiological buffer containing 4-5% autologous plasma. The dilute cell suspension was placed on the stage of an inverted microscope in a chamber formed between two coverglasses separated by a plastic spacer with a U-shaped cutout. A glass micropipette with an inside diameter of 1.0-1.2 μm was introduced into the open side of the "U". The pressure at the tip of the pipette was adjusted via a water-filled manometer positioned with a micrometer. Zero pressure was set within 0.5 mm H_2O (~50 dyn/cm^2) such that there was no flow of buffer into or out of the pipette tip. Cells were aspirated in the dimple region (Fig. 2) and the pressure was increased in increments of 0.5-1.0 mm H_2O. Experiments were recorded on video tape for subsequent analysis. The pressure was monitored with a pressure transducer and displayed and recorded in the video image. The length of the

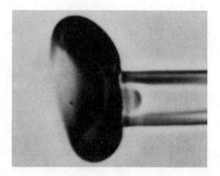

Figure 2. Photograph from a television monitor showing the aspiration of a red cell into a micropipette. The inside diameter of the pipette is ~1.2 μm. The length of the cell projection is measured as a function of the aspiration pressure.

cell projection in the pipette was measured from the recordings as a function of the aspiration pressure.

The membrane shear modulus, μ, was calculated from the length-pressure data pairs according to the theory of Evans [10]. The theoretical prediction is approximately linear, so in practice the modulus can be calculated by linear regression. The modulus is related to the slope of the length-pressure data pairs (dL/dP) by:

$$\mu = \left[\frac{2.45}{R_p^2} \frac{dL}{dP} \right]^{-1} ,$$

(1)

where R_p is the pipette radius.

Note that the determination of the modulus is independent of the intercept of the regression. This is an advantage because the change in the length of the projection can be measured much more accurately than its absolute magnitude. In fact, the measured intercept was always larger than the one predicted by the theory. This difference has always been attributed to measurement error, but results obtained in the present study suggest that the change in the intercept may reflect an important aspect of the membrane behavior that had not been considered in the original theoretical development. (See Discussion.)

RESULTS

In the present study, we have focused our attention on the disorder hereditary elliptocytosis (HE). Two types of molecular abnormality have been investigated. One class involves an abnormality in the structure of protein 4.1. The other involves several point mutations in the spectrin αI domain which result in reduced spectrin self-association, thought to result in an increased molar ratio of dimer to tetramer in the membrane.

TABLE 1
SUMMARY OF HE DEFECTS AND PROPERTIES

Defects	Dimer	μ/μ_o
Spectrin:		
αIT68, defic.	++	0.72
αIT50a	+++	1.13
αIT50b	+	1.20
αIIa	–	1.29
Protein 4.1:		
Shortened	–	0.94
Elongated	–	1.02

Examination of two families with abnormal protein 4.1 structure, one having an elongated form of the molecule and one having a shortened form, revealed no detectable abnormality in the elastic shear modulus for these membranes (Table 1). However, abnormalities were found in the elastic behavior of membranes with abnormal spectrin.

Cells from patients with four different types of spectrin variants were tested (Table 1). The characterization of the molecular defect is based on two-dimensional peptide maps [8,11]. The three spectrins with variant αI domains exhibit reduced self-association. This is evidenced by measurements of the mole fraction of dimer present in solution as a function of spectrin concentration (Fig. 3). In addition to reduced spectrin self-affinity, the αIT68 patient was spectrin-deficient [5].

The results of the mechanical tests for these four patients are shown in Figs. 4a-d. Membranes from three of the patients exhibited increased

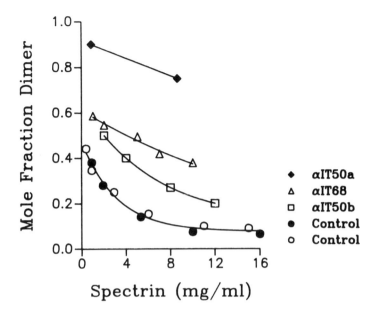

Figure 3. Mole fraction of dimer (relative to total spectrin) as a function of spectrin concentration in solution. Relative amounts of spectrin dimer and other oligomers were determined by dye elution from Coomassie Blue stained, non-denaturing acrylamide gels. (Data for controls and αIT68 replotted from [8]. Data for αIT50a from [11].)

rigidity compared to control values (shaded region in figures). This is evidenced by the decrease in the slope of the length, pressure data. The spectrin deficient membranes exhibited an increased slope (Fig. 4c), consistent with the decreased modulus observed for spectrin-deficient membranes [5]. The moduli calculated from the slopes of these data are listed in Table 1. In addition to a decrease in slope, the data for the abnormal membranes also have a reduced intercept, indicating that the deformation of the membrane at the initial aspiration pressure was smaller for these membranes. Note that neither the decrease

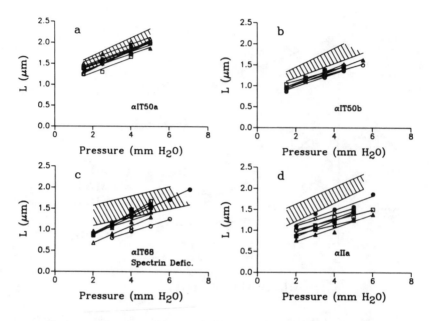

Figure 4a-d. Projection length (L) as a function of aspiration pressure for membranes having four different spectrin abnormalities. Shaded regions indicate the distribution of control data. In a, b and d, both the slope and intercept of the data for the abnormal membranes are reduced, although for "a" the change in intercept may not be significant. In c, the slope is increased, consistent with the spectrin deficiency, but the intercept is reduced.

in slope nor the decrease in intercept correlates with the reduction in spectrin self-affinity. In fact, the membranes with the lowest spectrin self-affinity (αIT50a) exhibited the least mechanical abnormality (Fig. 4a) and the membranes expected to have normal spectrin self-association (αIIa) show the greatest increase in membrane rigidity (Fig. 4d).
    The change in intercept observed for these abnormalities was unexpected. The theoretical

predictions of Evans [10] do not allow for this
possibility. To determine whether these
theoretical predictions were accurate for normal
membranes, measurements were performed on normal
membranes at high resolution (100X, oil immersion)
to obtain the most accurate absolute measure of
the membrane projection length. The results of
those measurements are shown in Fig. 5. Three
theoretical predictions are also shown. The solid
line is the theoretical prediction of Evans
[10,12] (neglecting membrane bending stiffness).
The lower dashed curve is Evans' prediction if the
bending stiffness of the membrane were five times
larger than has been measured [12]. The upper
dashed curve is based on the molecular theory of

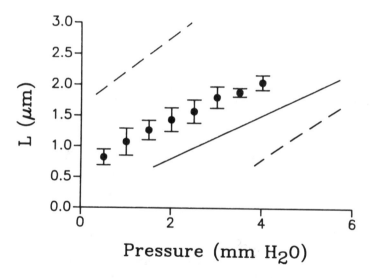

Figure 5. High resolution measurements of
projection length versus aspiration pressure for
normal membrane. Filled circles are means of
approximately 10 measurements, bars are plus or
minus one standard deviation. Solid curve is the
theoretical prediction of Evans [10] for an
incompressible skeleton. Lower dashed curve
accounts for a large membrane bending stiffness
[12]. Upper dashed curve is the prediction of
Markin and Kozlov [13] for a freely expandible
skeleton.

Markin and Kozlov [13]. Unlike the theory of
Evans, which constrains the membrane skeleton to
maintain constant area, Markin and Kozlov allow
the skeleton to change area locally, such that the
density of the skeleton is reduced in the region
near the pipet. The data clearly fall above the
original predictions of Evans. Error bars reflect
the uncertainty in the measurement of the
projection length. The addition of membrane
bending stiffness cannot account for the
disagreement between observation and Evans'
prediction. The data are shifted in the direction
predicted by Markin and Kozlov, suggesting that
local dilation of the membrane skeleton may
account for the larger-than-expected projections
that are observed.

DISCUSSION

The present study demonstrates that
abnormalities in spectrin may be associated with
an increase in membrane rigidity. This finding is
in agreement with a recent report by another
laboratory [7]. These findings contrast with a
previous study examining the effects of spectrin
deficiencies on membrane mechanical behavior, in
which only decreases in membrane rigidity were
observed [5].

The increase in rigidity observed in the
present study is manifested in two ways, by a
decrease in the slope of the length, pressure data
pairs and by a displacement of the data toward
smaller projection lengths at the same pressure
(decrease in apparent intercept). Although a
decrease in slope was expected for a more rigid
membrane, a change in the apparent intercept was
not. The theoretical prediction of Evans for an
incompressible membrane [10] contains only one
free parameter (the shear modulus), and changes in
the apparent intercept are not allowed. Thus, the
present results have prompted a re-evaluation of
the analysis used to interpret micropipet
experiments.

An alternative theoretical prediction has been
developed by Markin and Kozlov [13]. In that

analysis, the local area of the membrane skeleton
is allowed to change freely until the extensions
of the network reach 2.6, at which point the
spectrin molecules are fully extended and can
undergo no further deformation. Markin and
Kozlov's analysis for a freely expandible skeleton
predicts projection lengths that are appreciably
larger than those actually observed (Fig. 5).
However, Evans' analysis for an incompressible
skeleton predicts projection lengths that are too
small. Thus, the data indicate that local
dilation and compression of the membrane skeletal
area do occur, but that the resistance to such
dilation is finite. Furthermore, the displacement
of the apparent intercept of the length, pressure
data observed for some HE membranes suggests that
these membrane skeletons have an abnormally large
resistance to isotropic deformation (local changes
in skeletal area).

The mechanism responsible for the increased
rigidity of the membrane we have observed is not
known. Results obtained in another laboratory
indicated that there was a correlation between
increased membrane rigidity and an increase in the
ratio of dimer to tetramer in spectrin isolated
from the membrane, and it was suggested that the
increased rigidity they observed resulted from an
increase in the presence of dimer on the membrane
[7]. The results of the present study do not
support this conclusion. No correlation between
mole percent dimer and increased rigidity was
observed. In fact, membranes with an abnormality
that is not expected to affect dimer self-
association (αIIa) exhibited the greatest increase
in rigidity (Fig. 4d), whereas membranes having
the lowest spectrin self-affinity exhibited the
least mechanical dysfunction (Fig. 4a). Thus,
increased dimer to tetramer ratio does not appear
to be the direct cause of the increased rigidity.
Further biochemical and mechanical studies will be
needed to identify the mechanism responsible for
this increased rigidity.

In contrast to what was observed for the
spectrin abnormalities, abnormalities in the
structure of protein 4.1 had no effect on the

elastic rigidity of the membrane. Studies by
Takakuwa *et al.* [14] have shown that abnormal
protein 4.1 function results in decreased membrane
stability. This finding is consistent with
biochemical evidence that protein 4.1 stabilizes
the interaction between spectrin and actin. The
present results indicate that the increased
stability of the spectrin-actin association is not
essential for proper mechanical function when
forces on the membrane are small. Thus, while
protein 4.1 stabilizes the membrane skeleton
against fragmentation under conditions of high
stress, it contributes little to the membrane
response during "routine" deformations such as
those that occur normally in the microcirculation.

ACKNOWLEDGEMENTS

The authors thank Dr. Peter Agre for supplying
blood samples from the patients with αIT68 and
αIIa abnormalities and abnormalities in
protein 4.1.

REFERENCES

1. Evans EA, Skalak R (1979). Mechanics and
   thermodynamics of biomembrane. CRC Crit. Rev.
   Bioengr. 3:181.
2. Waugh RE, Hochmuth RM (1987). Forces shaping
   an erythrocyte. In Bereiter-Hahn J, Anderson
   OR, Reif W-E (eds): "Cytomechanics," Berlin:
   Springer-Verlag. pp. 249.
3. Bennett V (1985). The membrane skeleton of
   human erythrocytes and its implication for
   more complex cells. Ann. Rev. Biochem.
   54:273.
4. Liu S-C, Derick LH, Palek J (1987).
   Visualization of the hexagonal lattice in the
   erythrocyte membrane skeleton. J. Cell Biol.
   104:527.

5. Waugh RE, Agre P (1988). Reductions of erythrocyte membrane viscoelastic coefficients reflect spectrin deficiencies in hereditary spherocytosis. J. Clin. Invest. 81:133.

6. Agre P, Asimos A, Casella JF, McMillan C (1986). Inheritance pattern and clinical response to splenectomy as a reflection of erythrocyte spectrin deficiency in hereditary spherocytosis. N. Engl. J. Med. 315:1579.

7. Chabanel A, Sung K-LP, Rapiejko J, Prchal JT, Palek J, Liu SC, Chien S (1989). Viscoelastic properties of red cell membrane in hereditary elliptocytosis. Blood 73:592.

8. Marchesi SL, Letsinger JT, Speicher DW, Marchesi VT, Agre P, Hyun B, Gulati G (1987). Mutant forms of spectrin α subunits in hereditary elliptocytosis. J. Clin Invest. 80:191.

9. McGuire M, Smith BL, Agre P (1988). Distinct variants of erythrocyte protein 4.1 inherited in linkage with elliptocytosis and Rh type in three white families. Blood 72:287.

10. Evans EA (1973). New membrane concept applied to the analysis of fluid shear- and micropipette-deformed red blood cells. Biophys. J. 13:941.

11. Marchesi SL, Knowles WJ, Morrow JS, Bologna M, Marchesi VT (1986). Abnormal spectrin in hereditary elliptocytosis. Blood 67:141.

12. Evans EA (1980). Minimum energy analysis of membrane deformation applied to pipet aspiration and surface adhesion of red blood cells. Biophys. J. 30:265.

13. Markin VS, Kozlov MM (1988). Mechanical properties of the red cell membrane skeleton: analysis of axisymmetric deformations. J. Theor. Biol. 133:147.

14. Takakuwa Y, Tchernia G, Rossi M, Benabadji M, Mohandas N (1986). Restoration of normal membrane stability to unstable protein 4.1-deficient erythrocyte membranes by incorporation of purified protein 4.1. J. Clin. Invest. 78:80.

Cellular and Molecular Biology of Normal
and Abnormal Erythroid Membranes, pages 201–210
© 1990 Alan R. Liss, Inc.

USE OF THE POLYMERASE CHAIN REACTION FOR THE DETECTION AND CHARACTERIZATION OF MUTATIONS CAUSING HEREDITARY ELLIPTOCYTOSIS[1]

K.E. Sahr,[2] M. Garbarz,[3] D. Dhermy,[3] M.C. Lecomte,[3] P. Boivin,[3]
P. Agre,[4] K. Laughinghouse,[2] A. Scarpa,[2] T. Çoetzer,[5] J. Palek,[5]
S.L. Marchesi,[2] and B.G. Forget,[2]

[2]Yale University School of Medicine, New Haven, CT, 06510,
[3]Hopital Beaujon, 92118 Clichy Cedex, France, [4]Johns Hopkins
University School of Medicine, Baltimore, MD, 21205, and
[5]St. Elizabeth's Hospital, Tufts University School of Medicine,
Boston, MA, 02135.

ABSTRACT   We have determined the DNA sequence and exon/intron
organization of cloned genomic DNA encoding the αI domain of
human spectrin. This information was then used to synthesize
oligonucleotides for use in the polymerase chain reaction
technique to amplify specific exons of the α spectrin genes in
total cellular DNA of individuals with hereditary elliptocytosis and an associated abnormality (46-50kD or 65-68kD) of
the αI domain following partial tryptic digestion of spectrin.
Thirteen affected black individuals from 9 unrelated families
with the αI/68 kD anomaly were all found to carry the same
mutation, i.e. duplication of the codon for leucine residue
148: TTG-CTG to TTG-TTG-CTG. Thus the αI/68 kD protein
anomaly appears to be associated with a homogeneous genetic
defect at the DNA level. This approach was also applied to the
study of patients with the αI/50a kD and αI/50b kD anomalies
which are more heterogeneous at the amino acid sequence level.
The αI/50a defect resulted from a CTG (Leu) to CCG (Pro) base
change at residue 254 in two unrelated individuals or a TTC
(Ser) to CCC (Pro) base change at residue 255 in another
individual. In two other unrelated individuals with the αI/50a
polypeptide defect, the nucleotide sequence encoding residues
221 through 264 was normal. The αI/50b abnormality resulted
from a single base change of CAG (Glu) to CCG (Pro) encoding
residue 465 in two unrelated individuals. In a third
individual, the sequence of residues 445 through 490 was normal.

[1] The work was supported in part by grants from the National
Institutes of Health.

INTRODUCTION

Hereditary elliptocytosis (HE) is a heterogeneous disorder characterized by elliptical red cell shape. Several defects of the membrane skeleton have been identified in HE, including a number that have been localized to spectrin and are associated with peptide abnormalities detected by two dimensional fractionation of partial tryptic digests of spectrin (reviewed in references 1-3). Particularly frequent and well studied are abnormalities of the N-terminal or αI domain of spectrin which is functionally important for spectrin dimer self association. In many of these disorders, the normal 80 kD αI domain is susceptible to abnormal cleavage following partial tryptic digestion with the production of novel peptides 46-50 kD or 65-68 kD in size. Abnormal tryptic cleavages usually occur in the vicinity of amino acid changes (4). The abnormal 68 kD αI fragment has been shown to result from cleavage following arginine 131 and is associated with a leucine insertion between residues 148 and 150 of the α spectrin chain (4). The abnormal αI/50a peptide is the result of cleavage after arginine 250 and is associated with the substitution of proline for leucine at residue 254 or cleavage after lysine 252 associated with substitution of proline for serine at residue 255 (4). Similarly, the abnormal αI/50b peptide results from cleavage after arginine 462 associated with substitution of proline for glutamine at residue 465 of the α spectrin chain or cleavage after arginine 464 but without an amino acid substitution in the following 28 residues (4).

We have mapped and sequenced the exons in cloned genomic DNA encoding the normal αI domain of α spectrin (5). Twelve exons and their exon/intron boundaries were sequenced, a region encoding the first 526 amino acid residues of the αI domain peptide. Using the normal α spectrin gene sequence information, we designed three pairs of intronic oligonucleotide primers for use in the polymerase chain reaction (PCR) (6) to amplify and sequence the appropriate exons in DNA from individuals with the αI/68, αI/50a, and αI/50b kD variants of HE.

RESULTS

Exon/Intron Organization of the α Spectrin Gene.

Figure 1 shows the exon/intron organization that we have determined for cloned genomic DNA encoding most of the αI domain of spectrin. The DNA sequence of each exon and adjacent intronic regions was determined using the method of Sanger et al (7). The three exons encoding the regions associated with abnormalities in

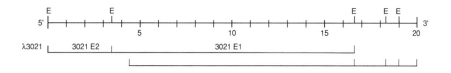

FIGURE 1. Exon/intron organization of the human α-spectrin gene. The EcoRI (E) sites in clone 3021(5) and another overlapping clone are shown.

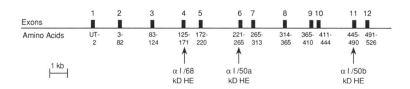

FIGURE 2. DNA sequence of exon 4 of the human α-spectrin gene showing the mutation associated with HE and the αI/68kD abnormality. Oligonucleotides corresponding to the underlined intronic sequences were used for PCR amplification.

A.

<u>ctcatctctgtataactcca</u>gtgttgttttccttcaacagGAAAACCATCCTGAC
　　　　　　　　　　　　　　　　　　　　221　GluAsnHisProAsp

CTACCCTTAATTCAGTCTAAGCAAAATGAGGTGAATGCTGCCTGGGAGCGCCTT
226 LeuProLeuIleGlnSerLysGlnAsnGluValAsnAlaAlaTrpGluArgLeu

　　　　　　　　　　　　　　　　　　　C C
CGTGGTTTGGCTCTCCAGAGACAGAAAGCTCTGTCCAATGCTGCAAACTTACAA
244 ArgGlyLeuAlaLeuGlnArgGlnLysAlaLeuSerAsnAlaAlaAsnLeuGln
　　　　　　　　　　　　　　　　　　↑ ↑
　　　　　　　　　　　　　　　　　ProPro

CGATTCAAAAGgtatggatctggccactgctttatagaaaactttgaagtgctt
262 ArgPheLysAr

tataaaaaccgt<u>gtctttgtattaggctct</u>

B.

<u>cttccatatacattatctcc</u>ttctttccaaagATGGAAATACTTGACAACAAC
　　　　　　　　　　　　　　　　　　445　MetGluIleLeuAspAsnAsn

　　　　　　　　　　　　　　　　　　　　　C
TGGACTGCCCTGCTGGAACTGTGGGACGAGCGTCATCGTCAGTATGAGCAGTGC
452 TrpThrAlaLeuLeuGluLeuTrpAspGluArgHisArgGlnTyrGluGlnCys
　　　　　　　　　　　　　　　　　　　　↑
　　　　　　　　　　　　　　　　　　　Pro

TTGGACTTTCATCTCTTCTACAGAGACAGTGAGCAAGTGGACAGTTGGATGAGT
470 LeuAspPheHisLeuPheTyrArgAspSerGluGlnValAspSerTrpMetSer

AGACAAGAGgtaacgggaggggtccataccatctctagaagtaatttctctcac
488 ArgGlnGlu

ccttcatttgccaccat<u>gactaccatgagttccctca</u>

FIGURE 3.　DNA sequence of exon 6 (A) and exon 11 (B) of the
human α-spectrin gene showing the mutations associated with HE and
the 50a kD (A) and 50b kD (B) abnormalities. Oligonucleotides
corresponding to the underlined intronic sequences were used for
PCR amplification.

HE are shown in Figure 1 and their DNA sequence is presented in Figures 2 and 3. From the nucleotide sequence information, we designed three pairs of intronic oligonucleotide primers (underlined in Figures 2 and 3) that were used in the PCR reaction (8) to amplify and sequence the relevant α spectrin exons in DNA from several individuals with HE or hereditary pyropoikilocytosis (HPP).

The αI/68 kD Abnormality.

The normal and mutant α spectrin exons of an individual heterozygous for the αI/68 kD peptide abnormality were amplified, subcloned into a double-stranded plasmid vector, and sequenced using the dideoxy chain termination method. In this individual, the index case (HP) described by Marchesi et al (4), there is a leucine insertion between residues 148 and 150 due to a duplication of leucine codon 148: TTG-CTG to TTG-TTG-CTG (Figure 2).

In order to determine if the αI/68 kD peptide abnormality is due to a single rather than multiple different defects, we studied the mutation in 13 affected black individuals from 9 unrelated families. PCR amplified DNAs were hybridized to labeled allele-specific oligonucleotide (ASO) probes complementary to either the normal or mutant DNA sequences (9), following transfer onto a nylon membrane (Figure 4). The amplified DNA of two unrelated normal individuals in lanes 1 and 2 hybridized only to the normal probe. Lane 3 contains amplified DNA from the heterozygous individual described above and it hybridized equally well to the normal and mutant probes. Lanes 4 through 6 and 8 through 12 contain DNA from individuals who were all shown to have the abnormal αI/68 kD tryptic fragment. The amplified DNA from each of these individuals hybridized to the mutation-specific probe. All but one were heterozygous for the mutation as evidenced by co-hybridization of the amplified DNA to the normal probe. The individual in lane 9 was homozygous for the polypeptide defect and was also homozygous for the TTG duplication as evidenced by lack of hybridization of the amplified DNA to the normal probe. The family member represented in lane 7 had normal spectrin. Amplified DNA from four other unrelated black individuals, three heterozygous and one homozygous for the αI/68 kD peptide abnormality, were similarly studied and all yielded similar results: positive hybridization to the mutant probe and, in the second homozygous individual, absence of hybridization to the normal probe (data not shown). The observation of the same TTG leucine codon duplication in all of the affected individuals studied suggests that HE associated with the αI/68 kD abnormality is due to a homogeneous genetic defect.

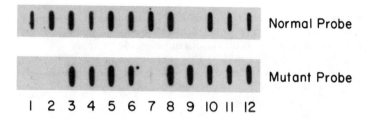

FIGURE 4. Slot blot hybridization to ASO probes of PCR amplified DNA of exon 4 from normal individuals and individuals with HE and the αI/68kD abnormality. See text for details.

The αI/50a kD Abnormality.

The αI/50a kD HE abnormality has been shown to be associated with separate proline substitutions involving either leucine 254 or serine 255 (4). These changes map to exon 6 (Figure 1). Using the oligonucleotide primers indicated in Figure 3A, we amplified total genomic DNA from one of the index cases of Afro-American ancestry (TS) studied by Marchesi et al (4). A single base change of CTG to CCG in the mutant allele results in the replacement of leucine 254 by proline (Figure 3A). The same mutation was identified in a second unrelated black individual from Togo with the αI/50a defect.

We also examined the mutation in the second individual (AR) with αI/50a HE that was studied by Marchesi et al (4). Using the same oligonucleotide primers, we amplified total genomic DNA. The PCR product was gel purified and reamplified asymmetrically as described by Gyllentsen et al (10) using a rate-limiting amount of the 5' primer. The total asymmetrically amplified DNA product was then directly sequenced using the rate-limiting primer and T7 DNA polymerase. This procedure results in the simultaneous sequencing of the amplified exon 6 from both normal and mutant alleles. In AR, a single base change of TCC to CCC in codon 255 of the mutant allele results in the replacement of serine by proline (Figure 3A).

We also studied genomic DNA from two other affected individuals, MA (11) and TN (12). Both of these unrelated black individuals have HPP associated with the αI/50a kD abnormality and total absence of the normal αI/80 kD peptide. DNA from both individuals was amplified and sequenced, either directly or after subcloning. No DNA sequence abnormalities were detected within exon 6 which encodes residues 221 through 264, i.e. 31 residues upstream and 12 residues downstream from the abnormal trypsin cleavage site identified in AR.

The αI/50b kD Abnormality.

The αI/50b kD abnormality is characterized by the presence of a 50 kD αI tryptic peptide and two smaller peptides of 17 and 19 kD not observed with the αI/50a kD defect. Sequence analysis of the 17 and 19 kD tryptic fragments from the index case (HB) revealed a substitution of proline for glutamine at position 465 (4). This change maps to α spectrin exon 11 (Figure 1). We amplified total genomic DNA from HB and a second unrelated affected black individual using the primers indicated in Figure 3B. The DNA products were subcloned and sequenced. In both individuals we detected a single base change of CAG (glutamine) to CCG (proline) in codon 465 of exon 11 of the mutant allele (Figure 3B).

In a third affected individual (DF) studied by Marchesi et al (4), the abnormal tryptic cleavage was shown to occur following residue 464, rather than residue 462 as in HB, but no amino acid substitution was identified in the 28 residues downstream from the cleavage site. Genomic DNA from DF was amplified, subcloned, and the entire exon 11 was sequenced. A total of 20 separate subclones were sequenced. A single subclone had an AAC (asparagine) to GAC (aspartate) change at position 450. In 19 additional subclones sequenced, however, this base change was not detected and the DNA sequence was completely normal. The base change noted in the single subclone is most likely due to an error introduced during amplification by the Taq polymerase. We conclude that the entire exon 11, encoding 19 amino acid residues upstream and 26 amino acid residues downstream from the abnormal trypsin cleavage site, is normal in both alleles of DF.

DISCUSSION

The present experiments confirm and extend our understanding of the amino acid changes associated with HE and the αI/50a, αI/50b and αI/68 kD abnormalities by demonstrating the specific nucleotide changes in the α spectrin genes of affected individuals. The αI/50a and αI/50b kD anomalies are heterogeneous at the molecular level. Two separate nucleotide changes resulting in two different amino acid replacements were observed in HE with the αI/50a kD abnormality. However, these mutations were absent in other unrelated affected individuals. At least two different defects are associated with HE and the αI/50b kD abnormality: a single nucleotide change resulting in the replacement of glutamine 465 by proline, and an as yet unidentified but different mutation.

In contrast, HE with the αI/68 abnormality appears to be the result of a single mutation. The same TTG codon duplication has been observed in 13 individuals from 9 unrelated black families as well as in 5 unrelated individuals of North African ancestry (13). The occurrence of the same mutation in all individuals studied is unlikely to be the result of multiple separate identical mutation events. Instead, it probably reflects a founder effect. It is tempting to speculate that the relatively high frequency of this defect is due to selection because of some type of beneficial effect in the heterozygous state, similar to the situation in sickle cell trait where individuals are protected against malaria. However, there is currently no direct evidence for this possibility.

The duplication of leucine codon 148 in all αI/68 kD HE individuals studied is probably the result of the phenomenon called frameshift mutagenesis (14) in which there is an intrachromosomal mispairing of sister chromatids during meiosis in regions of short directly repeated sequences. Such direct repeats, as short as two nucleotides, have been shown to be associated with both deletions and insertions in the human globin genes (15-17).

Most known mutations causing the various types of HE occur close to the site of abnormal tryptic cleavage in the αI domain. The mutations thus far identified that are located the furthest away from the abnormal tryptic cleavage site occur in HE with the αI/78 kD abnormality where the amino acid replacements are at residue 35 or 39 and the abnormal cleavage at residue 10; i.e., 25 and 29 residues proximal to the mutation (18,19). In three individuals studied, two with the αI/50a kD abnormality and one with the αI/50b kD abnormality, a gene mutation was not identified in the exon encoding the site of the abnormal tryptic cleavage. In the case of the αI/50a variant, the affected exon encodes 29 and 14 amino acid residues to either side of the cleavage site. In the αI/50b variant, the affected exon encodes 19 and 26 amino acid residues to either side of the presumed cleavage site. Thus, the mutations in these individuals may be located more distal (or proximal) to the abnormal tryptic cleavage site in neighboring exons of the α spectrin gene. Or, as recently suggested in a case of HE with the αI/74 kD abnormality (20), the aberrant αI tryptic cleavage may not be the result of a mutation in the α spectrin chain, but, rather, a mutation in the apposing β spectrin chain.

ACKNOWLEDGMENTS

We thank E. Coupal and K. Miceli for skilled technical assistance, K. Haggerty for preparation of the manuscript; Dr. J. Delaunay and colleagues for helpful discussions; and Drs. J.D. Bessman, and H. Zarkowsky for providing blood samples from patients.

REFERENCES

1. Marchesi SL (1989). The erythrocyte cytoskeleton in hereditary elliptocytosis and spherocytosis. In Agre P, Parker JC (eds): "Red Blood Cell Membrane: Structure, Function, Clinical Implications," New York: Marcel Dekker, p 77.
2. Palek J (1987). Hereditary elliptocytosis, spherocytosis and related disorders: Consequences of a deficiency or a mutation of membrane skeletal proteins. Blood Reviews 1:147.
3. Zail S (1986). Clinical disorders of the red cell membrane skeleton. CRC Crit Rev Oncol Hemat 5:397.
4. Marchesi SL, Letsinger JT, Marchesi VT, Agre P, Hyun B, Gulati G (1987). Mutant forms of spectrin α-subunits in hereditary elliptocytosis. J Clin Invest 80:191.
5. Linnenbach AJ, Speicher DW, Marchesi VT, Forget BG (1986). Cloning of a portion of the chromosomal gene for human erythrocyte α-spectrin by using a synthetic gene fragment. Proc Natl Acad Sci USA 83:2397.
6. Saiki RK, Scharf S, Faloona F, Mullis KB, Horn GT, Erlich HA, Arnheim N (1985). Enzymatic amplification of β-globin genomic sequences and restriction site analysis for diagnosis of sickle cell anemia. Science 230:1350.
7. Sanger F, Nicklen S, Coulson AR (1977). DNA sequencing with chain-terminating inhibitors. Proc Natl Acad Sci USA 74:5463.
8. Saiki RK, Gelfand DH, Stoffel S, Scharf SJ, Higuchi GT, Horn KB, Mullis HA, Erlich HA (1988). Primer-directed enzymatic amplification of DNA with a thermostable DNA polymerase. Science 239:487.
9. Saiki RK, Bugawan TL, Horn GT, Mullis KB, Erlich HA (1986). Analsysis of enzymatically amplified β-globin and HLA-DQα DNA with allele-specific oligonucleotide probes. Nature 324:163.
10. Gyllensten UB, Erlich HA (1988). Generation of single-stranded DNA by the polymerase chain reaction and its application to direct sequencing of the HLA-DQA locus. Proc Natl Acad Sci USA 85:7652.
11. Knowles WJ, Morrow JS, Speicher DW, Zarkowsky HS, Mohandas N, Mentzer WC, Shohet SB, Marchesi VT (1983). Molecular and functional changes in spectrin from patients with hereditary pyropoikilocytosis. J Clin Invest 71:1867.
12. Lawler J, Palek J, Liu SC, Prchal J, Butter WM (1983). Molecular heterogeneity of hereditary pyropoikilocytosis: Identification of a second variant of the spectrin α-subunit. Blood 62:1182.
13. Roux AF, Morle F, Guetarni D, Colonna P, Sahr K, Forget BG, Delaunay J, Godet J (1989). Molecular basis of Sp α$^{1/65}$ hereditary elliptocytosis in North Africa: Insertion of a TTG triplet between codons 147 and 149 in the α-spectrin gene from five unrelated families. Blood (in press).

14. Streisinger G, Okada Y, Emrich J, Newton J, Tsugita A, Terzaghi E, Inouye M (1966). Frame shift mutations and the genetic code. Cold Spring Harbor Symp Quant Biol 31:77.
15. Marotta CA, Wilson JT, Forget BG, Weissman SM (1977). Human β-globin messenger RNA. III. Nucleotide sequences derived from complementary DNA. J Biol Chem 252:5040.
16. Bunn HF, Forget BG (1986). "Hemoglobin: Molecular, Genetic and Clinical Aspects." Philadelphia: Saunders, p 412.
17. Efstratiadis A, Posakony JW, Maniatis T, Lawn RM, O'Connell C, Spritz RA, DeRiel JK, Forget BG, Weissman SM, Slightom JL, Blechl AE, Smithies O, Baralle FE, Shoulder CC, Proudfoot NJ (1980). The structure and evolution of the human β-globin gene family. Cell 21:653.
18. Morle L, Morle F, Roux AF, Godet J, Forget BG, Denoroy L, Garbarz M, Dhermy D, Kastally R, Delaunay J (1989). Spectrin Tunis (Sp$\alpha^{I/78}$), an elliptocytogenic variant, is due to the CGG -> TGG codon change (Arg -> Trp) at position 35 of the αI domain. Blood (in press).
19. Lecomte MC, Garbarz M, Grandchamp B, Feo C, Gautero H, Devaux I, Bournier O, Galand C, d'Auriol L, Galibert F, Sahr KE, Forget BG, Boivin P, Dhermy D (1989). Sp $\alpha^{I/78}$ kD: A mutation of the αI spectrin domain in a caucasian kindred with HE and HPP phenotypes. Blood (in press).
20. Garbarz M, Devaux I, Grandchamp B, Picat C, Dhermy D, Lecomte MC, Boivin P, Sahr KE, Forget, BG (1989). Search for the genetic abnormality in a case of hemolytic hereditary elliptocytosis with homozygosity for the spectrin alpha I/74 variant. C R Acad Sci (Paris) 308:43.

Cellular and Molecular Biology of Normal
and Abnormal Erythroid Membranes, pages 211–221
© 1990 Alan R. Liss, Inc.

MOLECULAR HETEROGENEITY OF α SPECTRIN
MUTANTS IN HEREDITARY ELLIPTOCYTOSIS/
PYROPOIKILOCYTOSIS

Theresa Coetzer[1], Jack Lawler[1],
Josef Prchal[2], Ken Sahr[3],
Bernard Forget[3], Jiri Palek[1]

1. Dept. of Biomedical Research, St. Elizabeth's
   Hospital of Boston, Tufts University School
   of Medicine, Boston, MA 02135
2. University of Alabama at Birmingham,
   Birmingham, AL 35294
3. Department of Internal Medicine, Yale
   University School of Medicne,
   New Haven, CT 06510

ABSTRACT The most common molecular defects
associated with hereditary elliptocytosis
(HE) and pyropoikilocytosis (HPP) involve
the N terminal α I domain of spectrin (Sp)
representing the Sp heterodimer (SpD) self-
association site. In this concise review,
we discuss these α I abnormalities and correlate the functional and structural
defects with the heterogeneous clinical
expression. Studies on homozygotes for the
three most common α Sp mutants (Sp αI/74,
Sp αI/46, Sp αI/65) indicate that the
Sp αI/74 defect is the most severely
affected both on a functional and clinical
level, followed by Sp αI/46 and finally
Sp αI/65 which is the mildest defect.
Amino acid analysis of the abnormal tryptic
peptides revealed the new α I cleavage
sites and, in some cases, the primary
structural defect. Sp αI/65 appears to
be due to a single mutation involving an
insertion of leu at residue 149, whereas
the Sp αI/46 abnormality is heterogeneous.
The Sp αI/74 mutation occurs in individuals
from diverse racial backgrounds and is thus
also likely to be heterogeneous.

Furthermore, RFLP studies on Sp αI/74
kindred using α and β Sp probes suggest
that, in some cases, the primary defect may
reside in the β chain which, in turn, could
influence the susceptibility of the α chain
cleavage site to proteolytic digestion.

INTRODUCTION

Spectrin (Sp), the major structural protein
of the red cell membrane skeleton, is a long
filamentous molecule consisting of an α and
β subunit which interact along their length
to form a Sp heterodimer (SpD) (1). In the head
region of the protein, two SpD self-associate to
form tetramers (SpT) and to some extent, higher
oligomers (2, 3). The SpT are arranged into a
hexagonal lattice; the distal ends of the
molecules are interconnected at each corner of
the hexagon by junctional complexes consisting
of actin oligomers, and protein 4.1 (4). The
skeleton is attached to the lipid bilayer
membrane via (a) an interaction of β Sp with
ankyrin which, in turn, binds to the cytoplasmic
domain of the major integral membrane protein,
band 3 (5), (b) an interaction of Sp with
protein 4.1 which binds to glycophorin (6), and
(c) Sp-lipid interactions (7). The structure of
Sp may be analyzed by limited tryptic digestion
which cleaves the molecule into distinct,
proteolytically resistant, functional domains,
α I-α V and β I-β IV (8).
Further structural characterization indicated
that Sp consists of a series of homologous
repeats of 106 amino acids each (9). The N
terminal α I domain and the C terminal
portion of β Sp are involved in the
self-association of SpD into SpT. This
self-association is governed by a thermodynamic
equilibrium which is immobilized when Sp is
extracted at near 0°C and thus the proportion of
SpD present in crude 0°C Sp extracts reflects
the functional state of Sp in the membrane (2).

This article will present a concise review
of the α I Sp defects in hereditary
elliptocytosis (HE) and pyropoikilocytosis
(HPP). We shall also discuss the functional
effects of the different structural Sp mutations
on the self-association of the Sp molecule and
correlate this with the clinical expression.

ABNORMALITIES OF α Sp IN HE AND HPP

HE and HPP are a group of hereditary
hemolytic anemias in which three major clinical
subtypes have been described (10). These are 1)
common HE, which is most prevalent and includes
clinical presentations ranging from an
asymptomatic carrier state to a severe hemolysis
as seen in a closely related disorder, HPP, 2)
spherocytic HE and 3) stomatocytic HE or south
east asian ovalocytosis. In common HE, the
molecular defects thus far reported involve
either a dysfunction of Sp, or deficiency of
protein 4.1 or glycophorin C (10, 11). In HPP,
two defects are present: an Sp mutation and a
partial Sp deficiency. Spectrin dysfunction,
manifesting by defective SpD self-association,
represents the most common abnormality and
involves the α I domain of Sp. On a
functional level, the impaired self-association
results in an increase in the amount of SpD
present in the membrane which is detected by
examining 0°C Sp extracts on nondenaturing
polyacrylamide gels (12). On a structural
level, the abnormalities have been localized to
the α I domain of Sp by limited tryptic
digestion followed by two dimensional
isoelectric focusing/sodium dodecyl sulfate
polyacrylamide gel electrophoresis (IEF/SDS
PAGE) and immunoblotting with polyclonal
antibodies against the α I domain. In
affected HE and HPP individuals, the normal
80,000 dalton α I domain is decreased and
there is a concomitant increase in one or more
lower molecular weight peptides. Several
different structural mutants have been described

both in our laboratory and by others (13-23).
The three most common mutants are designated Sp
$\alpha^{I/74}$, Sp $\alpha^{I/65}$ and Sp
$\alpha^{I/46}$ based on the molecular weight of
the abnormal peptide.

MOLECULAR DETERMINANTS OF CLINICAL EXPRESSION

One of the interesting features of these
disorders is that there is a marked
heterogeneity in their clinical expression which
ranges from an asymptomatic carrier state to
severe transfusion dependent hemolytic anemia
(see above, 9, 10). We have previously shown
that the disease severity is related to the
percentage of SpD present in the membrane and to
the total Sp content (Table 1, 24).
Consequently, the most severely affected
patients, manifesting as severe hemolytic HE or
HPP, have a marked increase in the amount of
unassembled SpD . In addition, HPP red cells
are also partially deficient in Sp, either
because of an instability of the mutant Sp or
another genetic defect that may involve
diminished Sp synthesis (24a). In contrast, HE
individuals and asymptomatic carriers,
respectively, have a moderate or mild increase
in SpD content and have normal amounts of Sp on
the membrane. The percentage of SpD also
correlates with the severity of hemolysis. The
proportion of SpD, in turn, are influenced by
the amount of mutant Sp and by the functional
severity of the self-association defect (Table
1, 24).

TABLE 1

<u>DETERMINANTS OF CLINICAL SEVERITY IN</u>
<u>HE WITH DEFECTIVE Sp SELF-ASSOCIATION</u>

1. SpD content of the membrane.
   - Functional capacity of mutant Sp
     to self-associate.
   - Amount of mutant Sp.

2. Total Sp content of the membrane.
   - Mutant Sp stability.
   - Interaction of a structural Sp
     defect and a defect in Sp
     synthesis.

CORRELATION BETWEEN MUTANT Sp FUNCTION
AND STRUCTURE

The majority of HE/HPP individuals are
heterozygotes who possess some normal Sp, and,
consequently, the functional abnormalities of
the mutant Sp cannot be accurately established.
Recently, we have identified subjects who are
either homozygotes or double heterozygotes for
mutant forms of Sp, and, consequently, have no
normal Sp in their cells. In these subjects, we
could therefore correlate the structural defect
with the functional severity. We determined the
percentage SpD present in the membrane and also
investigated the self-association of the mutant
SpD by in vitro experiments in solution and on
inside out vesicles (IOV). Our studies (25)
revealed a striking correlation between the type
of structural defect present and the functional
and clinical severity: Sp $\alpha^{I/74}$
homozygotes are the most severely affected; they
have a transfusion dependent hemolytic anemia
and their Sp is virtually incapable of
self-association, both in vivo (95% SpD in crude
0°C Sp extracts) and in in vitro experiments
where no SpT formation could be demonstrated
neither in solution nor on IOV. Sp
$\alpha^{I/46}$ homozygotes have a milder

hemolysis and have $\pm$ 50% SpD on the
membrane but the Sp $\alpha^{I/46}$ D are
incapable of forming SpT in vitro. In contrast,
Sp $\alpha^{I/65}$ homozygotes are clinically only
mildly affected and the Sp $\alpha^{I/65}$ D
partly retain the propensity to self-associate,
both on the membrane (26% SpD) and on IOV (50%
of the normal control level).

ELUCIDATION OF THE PRIMARY DEFECT

Amino acid sequence studies of the abnormal
tryptic peptides provide information regarding
the location of the cleavage site and, in some
cases, the primary structural defect (Figure 1).
Sp $\alpha^{I/65}$ is cleaved at arg 131 and there
is an insertion of leu at residue 149 as found
by several laboratories (23, 25, 26, 27). This
suggests that the Sp $\alpha^{I/65}$ defect is
homogeneous and is the result of a single
mutation. In the case of Sp $\alpha^{I/74}$ and

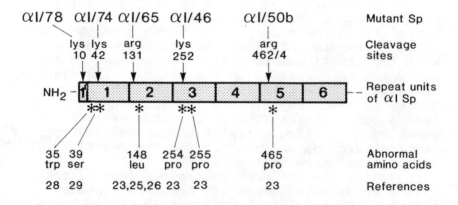

FIGURE 1. Cleavage site and primary
structural abnormalities of mutant α Sp.

Sp $\alpha^{I/46}$, respectively, the cleavage
sites were mappped to lys 42 (instead of the
normal arg 39) and lys 252 (Figure 1).
Sequencing of Sp $\alpha^{I/74}$ up to amino acid
60 revealed no abnormalities. Previous studies
(23) have revealed a pro substitution at
residues 254 or 255 in some Sp $\alpha^{I/46}$
individuals, whereas in patients studied in our
laboratory these residues were normal indicating
that the primary cause underlying this
structural defect is heterogeneous. Subjects
with Sp $\alpha^{I/78}$ (Sp Tunis) have an
abnormal cleavage site at lys 10 and two
different primary abnormalities have been
implicated: a trp substitution at residue 35
(28) or a ser substitution at residue 39 (29)
(Figure 1). The Sp $\alpha^{I/74}$ mutation is
also likely to be heterogeneous since it occurs
in individuals of diverse racial backgrounds
including caucasions, blacks, arabs and
melanesians. Furthermore, restriction fragment
length polymorphism (RFLP) studies using α
Sp (30) and β Sp (31) probes indicate that,
in some kindred, the primary defect may reside
in the β chain, which, in turn, could
influence the conformation of the apposing α
chain and, hence, the susceptibility of the
existing $\alpha^{I/74}$ cleavage site to
proteolytic digestion (25). With the
availability of genomic DNA sequences for α
and β Sp, our current attempts on
elucidating the primary structural defect of
these mutant spectrins involve amplification of
DNA from HE and HPP individuals by the
polymerase chain reaction (PCR) and subsequent
nucleotide sequencing.

ACKNOWLEDGEMENTS

    The authors wish to acknowledge the
cooperation of referring physicians Drs B Alter,
A Cao, C Dampier, R Gallanello, V Mankad, W
Wang.

REFERENCES

1. Cohen C (1983). The molecular organization
    of the red cell membrane skeleton. Semin
    Hematol 20:141.
2. Ungewickell E, Gratzer W (1987). Self-
    association of human spectrin. A thermo-
    dynamic and kinetic study. Eur J Biochem
    88:379.
3. Liu SC, Windisch P, Kim S, Palek J (1984).
    Oligomeric states of spectrin in normal
    erythrocyte membranes: biochemical and
    electron microscopic studies. Cell 37:587.
4. Liu SC, Derick L, Palek J (1987). Visual-
    ization of hexagonal lattice in the
    erythrocyte membrane skeleton. J Cell Biol
    104:527.
5. Bennett V (1982). The molecular basis for
    membrane-cytoskeleton association in human
    erythrocytes. J Cell Biochem 18:49.
6. Anderson RA, Lovrien RE (1984).
    Glycophorin is linked by band 4.1 protein
    to the human erythrocyte membrane skeleton.
    Nature 307:655.
7. Cohen AM, Liu SC, Derick LH, Palek J
    (1986). Ultrastructural studies of the
    interaction of spectrin with phosphatidyl-
    serine vesicles. Blood 68:920.
8. Morrow JS, Speicher DW, Knowles WJ, et al
    (1980). Identification of functional
    domains of human erythrocyte spectrin.
    Proc Natl Acad Sci USA 77:6592.
9. Speicher DW, Marchesi VT (1984).
    Erythrocyte spectrin is composed of many
    homologous triple helical segments. Nature
    311:177.
10. Palek J (1985). Hereditary elliptocytosis
    and related disorders. Clinics in
    Haematology 14:45.
11. Palek J (1987). Hereditary elliptocytosis,
    spherocytosis and related disorders:
    consequence of a deficiency or a mutation
    of membrane skeletal proteins. Blood
    Reviews 1:147.
12. Liu SC, Palek J, Prchal J, Castleberry RP

(1981). Altered spectrin dimer-dimer association and instability of erythrocyte membrane skeletons in hereditary pyropoikilocytosis. J Clin Invest 68:597.

13. Lawler J, Liu SC, Palek J, Prchal J (1982). Molecular defect of spectrin in hereditary pyropoikilocytosis: alterations in the trypsin-resistant domain involved in spectrin self-association. J Clin Invest 70:1019.

14. Lawler J, Palek J, Liu SC, et al (1983). Molecular heterogeneity of hereditary pyropoikilocytosis: identification of a second variant of the spectrin α-subunit. Blood 62:1182.

15. Knowles WJ, Morrow HS, Speicher DW, et al (1983). Molecular and functional changes in spectrin from patients with hereditary pyropoikilocytosis. J Clin Invest 72:1867.

16. Lawler J, Liu SC, Palek J, Prchal J (1984). Molecular defect of spectrin in a subgroup of patients with hereditary elliptocytosis: alterations in the α subunit domain involved in spectrin self-association. J Clin Invest 73:1688.

17. Lawler J, Coetzer TL, Palek J, et al (1985). Sp $\alpha^{I/65}$: a new variant of the α subunit of spectrin in hereditary elliptocytosis. Blood 66:706.

18. Lecomte MC, Dhermy D, Solis C, et al (1985). A new abnormal variant of spectrin in black patients with hereditary elliptocytosis. Blood 65:1208.

19. Lawler J, Coetzer T, Mankad VN, et al (1988). Spectrin $\alpha^{I/61}$: a new structural variant of α spectrin in a double heterozygous form of hereditary pyropoikilocytosis. Blood 72:1412.

20. Morle L, Alloisio N, Ducluzeau MT, et al (1988). Spectrin Tunis $\alpha^{I/78}$), a new α I variant that causes asymptomatic hereditary elliptocytosis in the heterozygous state. Blood 71:508.

21. Lambert S, Zail S (1987). A new variant of

the α subunit of spectrin in
hereditary elliptocytosis. Blood 69:473.

22. Marchesi S, Knowles WJ, Morrow JS, et al
(1986). Abnormal spectrin in hereditary
elliptocytosis. Blood 67:141.

23. Marchesi SL, Letsinger JT, Speicher DW,
(1987). Mutant forms of spectrin
α-subunits in hereditary
elliptocytosis. J Clin Invest 80:191.

24. Coetzer T, Lawler J, Prchal JT, Palek J
(1987). Molecular determinants of clinical
expression of hereditary elliptocytosis
and pyropoikilocytosis. Blood 70:766.

24a. Coetzer TL, Palek J (1986). Partial
spectrin deficiency in hereditary pyropoikilocytosis. Blood 67:919.

25. Coetzer T, Lawler J, Jarolim P, Palek J
(1988). Structural and functional heterogeneity of α spectrin mutants in
hereditary elliptocytosis/pyropoikilo-
cytosis. Blood 72, Suppl 1:38a.

26. Sahr KE, Garbarz M, Boivin P, et al (1988).
Use of the polymerase chain reaction (PCR)
for the detection of mutations causing
hereditary elliptocytosis (HE). Blood 72,
Suppl 1:34a.

27. Roux AF, Morle F, Guetarni D, et al (1988).
Molecular basis of Sp $\alpha^{I/65}$
hereditary elliptocytosis in North Africa:
insertion of a TTG triplet between codons
147 in the α-spectrin gene of five
unrelated families. Blood 72, Suppl 1:33a.

28. Morle L, Morle F, Alloisio N, et al (1989).
The diversity of hereditary elliptocytosis
in North Africa: protein aspects and
molecular genetics of Spectrin Tunis
(αI 35 Arg->Trp). J Cellular
Biochemistry, Suppl 13B:213.

29. Garbarz M, Lecomte MC, Devaux I, et al
(1988). The DNA's from HE and HPP
related patients with the spectrin
$\alpha^{I/78}$ kD variant contain a single
base substitution in EXON-3 of the
α spectrin gene. Blood 72,
Suppl 1:41a.

30. Linnebach AJ, Speicher DW, Marchesi VT,
     Forget BG (1986). Cloning of a portion
     of the chromosomal gene for human erythro-
     cyte α spectrin using a synthetic
     gene fragment. Proc Natl Acad Sci USA
     83:2397.
31. Prchal JT, Morley BT, Yoon SH et al (1987).
     Isolation and characterization of cDNA
     clones for human erythrocyte
     β spectrin. Proc Natl Acad Sci USA
     84:7468.

Cellular and Molecular Biology of Normal
and Abnormal Erythroid Membranes, pages 223–234
© 1990 Alan R. Liss, Inc.

THE DIVERSITY OF HEREDITARY ELLIPTOCYTOSIS IN NORTH AFRICA : PROTEIN ASPECTS AND MOLECULAR GENETICS

L.Morlé[a], A.-F.Roux[a,b], F.Morlé[a], N.Alloisio[a],
B.Pothier[a], K.E. Sahr[c], B.G.Forget[c], J.Godet[b], and
J.Delaunay[a]

a : CNRS URA 1171, Faculté de Médecine Grange-Blanche, 69373 Lyon Cedex 08, France
b : CNRS UMR 4, Université Claude-Bernard Lyon-I Villeurbanne Cedex, France
c : Department of Internal Medicine, Yale University School of Medicine, New Haven, CT 06510, USA

ABSTRACT. We provide a survey of the molecular alterations which underlie hereditary elliptocytosis in North Africa. In 12 families, we observed six elliptocytogenic variants, involving spectrin αI and αII domains, and protein 4.1. In addition, we found variants with no morphological change in the heterozygous state. $Sp\alpha^{I/65}$ hereditary elliptocytosis (six families) appeared clinically mild in the heterozygous state. It results from the insertion of a TTG triplet (Leu) at position 148 of spectrin αI domain (as is also the case in Black people). It is thought to have diffused northward from Subsaharian Africa. 4.1(-) hereditary elliptocytosis (2 families) is clinically mild in the heterozygous state and is

This work was supported by the Université Claude-Bernard Lyon-I, the Centre National de la Recherche Scientifique (URA 1171), and the Institut National de la Santé et de la Recherche Médicale (CRE 86 20 10).

due to the reduction of protein 4.1. Its
origin is unknown, however it was never
reported in Black people and occurs sporadi-
cally in Europeans. Spectrin Tunis (1 family)
yields a clinically silent elliptocytosis in
the heterozygous state. It is an example of a
unique variant, and is due to the CGG → TGG
codon change (Arg → Trp) at position 35 of
the αI domain.

INTRODUCTION

Hereditary elliptocytosis (HE) refers to a
group of conditions characterized by the presence
of red cells having an elliptic shape. Clinically,
elliptocytosis has a variable expression. At the
best, it is silent ; at the worst, it yields a
life-threatening hemolytic anemia. Between these
opposite situations, the entire spectrum of
severity is covered. Choosing ellipticity as the
primary criterion, elliptocytosis is transmitted
as a dominant or partially dominant character.
However, some morphologically recessive forms
exist. Over the last decade, it has been established that most cases of HE are due to mutations of
the red cell skeleton, the elegant collection of
which has been extensively reviewed (1). The
alterations involve mainly spectrin and protein
4.1. In addition, their nature and frequency vary
considerably according to ethnic groups. We had
the opportunity to investigate HE in North Africa.
North African populations display an extraordinary
genetic polymorphism that is accounted for by historical facts and that has already been documented concerning the abnormalities of hemoglobin. In
the present article, we will list the genetic
changes which we recorded as causing HE and
present some selected cases according to their
origin and/or recent data on their ultimate gene
alteration. We will also mention some variants
which remain morphologically silent in the heterozygous state.

NORTH AFRICA IS A CROSSROAD

North Africa, or Maghreb, designates a group of several countries, including Tunisia, Algeria and Morocco (from east to west). These countries lie between the western Mediterranean Sea in the north and the Sahara Desert in the south. Native North Africans are the Berbers who initially lived as nomads. From about the 12th century B.C., Phenicians came over from the Middle East (Lebanon, today). They founded Carthago (in Tunisia, today). The Romans took over shortly before the Christian era. Over the following centuries, North Africa underwent subsequent invasions, in particular by the Vandales (Northern Europe) and the Byzantines. From the 7th century on, the Arabs conquested the region, introducing the Moslem civilization which remained ever since. Still, other invasions took place, by the Turkish in particular. Admixtures from Black Africa occurred more continuously, either through the Sahara Desert or along coastal regions of West Atlantic Africa. Until recently, North African lowlands have been infested by malaria, a fact favoring the propagation of some red cell hereditary defects. The present - day genetics of North African people reflects the above historical perspectives. It is striking, for example, that hemoglobins S, C or G-Philadelphia, originating from Subsaharian Africa, coexist with hemoglobins O-Arab or Lepore, introduced from Europe or the Middle-East. In addition, relatively frequent consanguinity (especially in Algeria) favors homozygosity and allows the (usually dramatic) expression of variants that go undetected in the heterozygous state. Such genetic features fully apply to HE. In North Africa, we recently identified at the gene level the alterations responsible for $Sp\alpha^{I/65}$ HE and for HE due to spectrin Tunis [αI 35 Arg$\rightarrow$Trp]. Knowledge of the ultimate gene changes may help reconstitute the natural history of mutations, and locate there place and date of birth.

IN TWELVE NORTH AFRICAN FAMILIES, WE FOUND NINE DIFFERENT MUTATIONS

We will first list the elliptocytogenic mutations, as well as a few morphologically silent variants (in the heterozygous state), which we partially or completely identified in North Africa. Table 1 summarizes the data obtained in 12 North African families, some of which reside in France. In six families was $Sp\alpha^{I/65}$ HE recorded. In two families, we observed 4.1(-) HE (2). The Algerian 4.1(-) family has been first described by other authors and includes several homozygotes (3,4). Other cases corresponded to unique variants, some of which are not fully characterized as yet. We will describe below spectrin Tunis ($Sp\alpha^{I/78}$) in some detail. The $Sp\alpha^{I/74}$ abnormality was found by chance in one member of a $Sp\alpha^{I/65}$ HE family ; it occurred in the simple heterozygous state and remained morphologically silent. Spectrin Oran ($Sp\alpha^{II/21}$) (5) was remarkable in several respects : (i) it yielded disturbed peptide maps, following two-dimensional analysis of trypsin limit digests, that involved mostly the αII domain, but also the αIII and the βII domains ; (ii) in the absence of any detectable change of the αI domain and thereby probably related to the above changes, a defect of spectrin self-association was noted ; (iii) the variant was nearly undetectable in the heterozygous state (no clinical symptom, no morphological change, no alteration of the peptide maps ; only were some abnormal spots ascertained using anti αII domain antibodies), whereas homozygosity triggered a dramatic hemolytic anemia. Spectrin Tlemcen was an asymptomatic variant, clinically and morphologically, in the heterozygous state. It pertained to the 41 kDa fragment which contains the β-chain N-terminal region. The corresponding spots underwent sharp cathodic shifts with no detectable changes of their molecular weights. Finally, the other variants mentioned in Table 1 are still under investigation. We will now provide further detail on HE due to spectrin $\alpha^{I/65}$, spectrin Tunis ($\alpha^{I/78}$) and lack of protein 4.1.

Table 1   List of the mutations involving spectrin or protein 4.1 found in 12 North African families (February 1989).In most cases, elliptocytosis accompanied the variant in the heterozygous state, except for three cases (*), which remained morphologically silent in the heterozygous state. Δ: presence of homozygotes.

Type of HE, plus some asymptomatic variants in the heterozygous state.	Country of residence or origin	Number of families	References
$Sp\alpha^{I/78}$ (spectrin Tunis)	Tunisia	1	18,19
$Sp\alpha^{I/74}$*	Morocco	1[a]	8
$Sp\alpha^{I/65}$	Tunisia Algeria Morocco	1 4 1[a]	8,13, and unpubli- shed results
$Sp\alpha^{II/21}$ Δ (spectrin Oran)	Algeria	1[b]	5
$Sp\alpha^{II/...}$	Tunisia	1	Unpublished results
$Sp\alpha^{III/...}$*	Tunisia	1[c]	Unpublished results
Sp...	Tunisia	1[c]	Unpublished results
Spectrin Tlemcen (ßIV)*	Algeria	1[b]	Pothier *et al*, manuscript submitted
Absence of protein 4.1 Δ	Algeria Tunisia	1 1	2-4, and unpublished results

a, b et c : families harboring two mutations

THE $Sp\alpha^{I/65}$ ABNORMALITY

The $Sp\alpha^{I/65}$ abnormality was first discovered by Lecomte *et al* (6) in Blacks from several Subsaharian countries and from the French West Indies, and by Lawler *et al* (7) in American Blacks. Soon afterwards, Alloisio *et al* (8) found a similar variant in four North African families. At least in the North African cases did the condition-to whichever degree it was morphologically and biochemically expressed as we will see-, remained clinically asymptomatic. Although clinical manifestations were noted in some Black persons (6,7,9), the general trend for $Sp\alpha^{I/65}$ HE in Black people seems also to be that of mildness. $Sp\alpha^{I/65}$ homozygotes are moderately sick (10,11) and it is worth noting that hereditary pyropoikilocytosis, an aggravated manifestation of elliptocytosis, has never been seen in association with the $Sp\alpha^{I/65}$ abnormality. Probably, the overall mildness of the condition is accounted for by the retained propensity of the dimer to self-associate (8,11,12).

Despite the infraclinical status of $Sp\alpha^{I/65}$ HE in North Africa, which was confirmed in two other families since 1986 (13, and unpublished results), the morphological and biochemical expression remains strikingly variable, even in a given kindred. We found a significant correlation between the degree of elliptocytosis, the spectrin tetramer association constant and the percentage of the αI 65 kDa fragment (unpublished results). On the other hand, the percentage of the dimer in crude spectrin extracts (4°C) displayed a poor correlation, due to the residual ability of the dimer to self-associate (unpublished results). Contrasting with the absence of clinical signs in adults and in children, a transfusional history was recorded in two newborns in whom $Sp\alpha^{I/65}$ HE was found later on. Although we lack more precise indications, we note that the children who underwent these acute episodes are also those who have now the highest percentages of the αI 65 kDa fragment. Such variability in spectrin $\alpha^{I/65}$ expression is found in other variants of spectrin α-chain as well, but has not been explained thus far.

In two unrelated American Blacks with $Sp\alpha^{I/65}$ HE, Marchesi *et al* (9) found the insertion of a leucyl residue near position 150 of spectrin αI domain, using the methods of protein chemistry. Using a 13.5 kbp genomic α-spectrin probe (14) in five unrelated North African families, Roux *et al* (13) found that the ultimate lesion was a TTG insertion after codon 148, leading to the same leucine insertion in the polypeptide chain. Sahr *et al* (15) described the same change in a number of African and American Black families. At this point, it can be said that all families with $Sp\alpha^{I/65}$ HE are African or are of African origin, and that they all harbor the same mutation. It is not known whether the mutation has a monocentric or, as is the case for hemoglobin S, has a multicentric origin. It may be argued that a triplet insertion is much more improbable than the substitution of a single base and that, consequently, $Sp\alpha^{I/65}$ HE is likely to have occurred once rather than several times. Historical facts and the higher incidence of $Sp\alpha^{I/65}$ HE in Subsaharian Africa would suggest that the condition first arose in this part of Africa and later on diffused northward. A hypothetical protection against malaria would have favored its propagation. Noteworthy, $Sp\alpha^{I/65}$ HE has never been found thus far in ethnic groups not residing in or not originating from Africa.

4.1 (-) HEREDITARY ELLIPTOCYTOSIS

4.1 (-) HE generates a contrasting situation, although not strictly symmetrical. Conboy *et al* (16) showed that the above-mentioned Algerian 4.1 (-) HE (3,4) was associated with a DNA rearrangement upstream from the initiation codon for translation and with aberrant splicing of the 4.1 transcript. It is not yet known whether the Tunisian case of 4.1 (-) HE which we identified has the same alterations. On the other hand, Lambert *et al* (17) did not find this change in several South African families of European ascent, establishing therefore that 4.1 (-) HE is itself a heterogeneous disorder. How many different mutations are involved and how they spread remains to be established. We found nine families, which do not know to be related to each other, in one particular valley of the French Alps ; a distinct mutation may come into play, with a recent founding effect enhanced by sedentarity (unpublished results). It is puzzling that 4.1 (-) HE was never described among Black people, as a sporadic if not as an endemic mutation.

SPECTRIN TUNIS (αI 35 Arg $\to$ Trp)

Spectrin Tunis, first referred to as $Sp\alpha^{I/78}$, caused a clinically asymptomatic HE. On a morphological basis, the transmission was clearly dominant. There was a conspicuous defect of spectrin self-association (18). Upon one-dimensional analysis of spectrin limit digests, we found that the 78 kDa band, that is nearly indiscernible from the αI 80 kDa fragment (αI domain) under normal conditions, was increased. Kinetic analysis showed that the 78 kDa fragment developped at the reciprocal expense of the αI 80 kDa fragment.The 78 kDa band also reacted with anti αI domain antibodies kindly provided by Drs. J.Palek and J.Lawler.The αI 74 kDa fragment was not itself flanked with a shortened 72 kDa band. We assumed, therefore, that the sensitized cleavage point generating the αI 78 kDa fragment was near the α-chain N-terminus and, in any event, was upstream from the cleavage point that yields the 74 kDa fragment (since the latter was spared by the additional cleaving event). Indeed, aminoacid sequencing showed that abnormal proteolysis occurred after lysine 10 (19). It was infortunate that aminoacid sequencing was not able to reach the causal mutation which we anticipated to be nearby. Only could we establish that it did not involve the ten first positions (upstream from Lys 10). Using 20mer oligonucleotides complementary to genomic segments from introns 2 and 3, respectively, we thus carried out DNA amplification and sequencing. In two carriers of spectrin Tunis, we found the CGG→ TGG codon change (Arg→Trp) in position 35 (19).

Since Garbarz *et al* (20) found a variant with a similar protein phenotype in a French family, one could have wondered if the same allele was involved. This speculation was cut short, however, since they found that this other Spα$^{I/78}$ variant results from the AGG→AGT codon change (Arg→Ser) in position 39. Spectrin Tunis, therefore, appears as a unique variant at this point. It may be pointed out that the mutations yielding the Spα$^{I/78}$ phenotype, the mutation responsible for Spα$^{I/65}$ HE, and also the mutations causing Spα$^{I/50\ a\ or\ b}$ HE (9), are located in the *C* - terminal regions of helices 3 of the 106 aminoacid repeats described by Speicher and Marchesi (21). Although this remains speculative, these subdomains could be critical for appropriate "tension" of spectrin as a prerequisite for self-association.

CONCLUSIONS

The diversity of mutations causing HE in North Africa is superimposable to that observed as for hemoglobin abnormalities. It is largely accounted for by genetic admixtures which occurred at the occasion of known historical facts over the three past thousand years. The description of the ultimate genomic mutations causing Spα$^{I/65}$ HE and spectrin Tunis open new perspectives for the understanding of structure-function relationship near the spectrin self-association site.

ACKNOWLEDGEMENTS

We thank Drs. R. Kastally and S.Fattoum (Tunis), and Dr. P. Colonna (Algiers) for referring their patients' samples to us, Drs. J. Palek and J. Lawler for providing us with antibodies against spectrin αI domain, and Dr. M. Garbarz for his advise in DNA amplification.

REFERENCES

1. Palek J (1987). Hereditary elliptocytosis,
    spherocytosis and related disorders : conse-
    quences of a deficiency or a mutation of mem-
    brane skeletal proteins. Blood Reviews 1:147.

2. Alloisio N, Morlé L, Bachir D, Guetarni D,
    Colonna P., Delaunay J (1985). Red cell mem-
    brane sialoglycoprotein β in homozygous and
    heterozygous 4.1(-) hereditary elliptocytosis.
    Biochim Biophys Acta 816:57.

3. Féo C, Fischer S, Piau JP, Grange MG, Tchernia
    G (1980). Première observation de l'absence
    d'une protéine de la membrane érythrocytaire
    (bande 4.1) dans un cas d'anémie elliptocy-
    taire familiale.Nouv Rev Fr Hématol 22:315.

4. Tchernia G, Mohandas N, Shohet SB (1981)
    Deficiency of skeketal membrane protein band
    4.1 in homozygous hereditary elliptocytosis.
    Implications for erythrocyte membrane stabi-
    lity. J Clin Invest 68:454.

5. Alloisio N, Morlé L, Pothier B, Roux AF,
    Maréchal J, Ducluzeau MT, Benhadji-Zouaoui Z,
    Delaunay J (1988). Spectrin Oran ($\alpha^{II/21}$), a
    new spectrin variant concerning the αII domain
    and causing severe elliptocytosis in the homo-
    zygous state. Blood 71:1039.

6. Lecomte MC, Dhermy D, Solis C, Ester A, Féo C,
    Gautero H, Bournier O, Boivin P (1985). A new
    abnormal variant of spectrin in black patients
    with hereditary elliptocytosis. Blood 65:1208.

7. Lawler J, Coetzer TL, Palek J, Jacob HS, Luban
    N (1985). Sp$\alpha^{I/65}$: a new variant of the α sub-
    unit of spectrin in hereditary elliptocy-
    tosis. Blood 66:706.

8. Alloisio N, Guetarni D, Morlé L, Pothier B,
    Ducluzeau MT, Soun A, Colonna P, Clerc M,
    Philippe N, Delaunay J (1986).Sp$\alpha^{I/65}$ here-
    ditary elliptocytosis in North Africa. Am

J Hematol 23:113.

9. Marchesi SL, Letsinger JT, Speicher DW, Marchesi VT, Agre P, Hyun B, Gulati G (1987). Mutant forms of spectrin α-subunits in hereditary elliptocytosis. J Clin Invest 80: 191.

10. Garbarz M, Lecomte MC, Dhermy D, Féo C, Chaveroche I, Gautero H, Bournier O, Picat C, Goepp A, Boivin P (1986). Double inheritance of an $\alpha^{I/65}$ spectrin variant in a child with homozygous elliptocytosis. Blood 67:1661.

11. Coetzer T, Lawler J, Jarolim P, Palek J. (1988). Structural and functional heterogeneity of α spectrin mutants in hereditary elliptocytosis/pyropoikilocytosis. Blood 72 (Suppl 1):38a (Abstr).

12. Dhermy D, Garbarz M, Lecomte MC, Chaveroche I, Bournier O, Gautero H, Blot I, Boivin P (1986) Abnormal electrophoretic mobility of spectrin tetramers in hereditary elliptocytosis. Hum Genet 74:363.

13. Roux AF, Morlé F, Guetarni D, Colonna P, Sahr K, Forget BG, Delaunay J, Godet J (1989). Molecular basis of Sp$\alpha^{I/65}$ hereditary elliptocytosis in North Africa : insertion of a TTG triplet between codons 147 and 149 in the α-spectrin gene from five unrelated families.Blood (in press).

14. Linnenbach AJ, Speicher DW, Marchesi VT, Forget BG (1986). Cloning of a portion of the chromosomal gene for human erythrocyte α-spectrin by using a synthetic gene fragment. Proc Natl Acad Sci USA 83:2397.

15. Sahr KE, Garbarz M, Boivin P, Laughinghouse K, Marchesi SL, Forget BG (1988). Use of the polymerase chain reaction (PCR) for the detection of mutations causing hereditary elliptocytosis (HE). Blood 72 (Suppl 1):34a (Abstr).

16. Conboy J, Mohandas N, Tchernia G, Kan YW (1986). Molecular basis of hereditary elliptocytosis due to protein 4.1 deficiency. New Engl J Med 315:680.

17. Lambert S, Conboy J, Zail S (1988). A molecular study of heterozygous protein 4.1 deficiency in hereditary elliptocytosis. Blood 72 :1926.

18. Morlé L, Alloisio N, Ducluzeau MT, Pothier B, Blibech R, Kastally R, Delaunay J (1988). Spectrin Tunis ($\alpha^{I/78}$) : a new αI variant that causes asymptomatic hereditary elliptocytosis in the heterozygous state. Blood 71:508.

19. Morlé L, Morlé F, Roux AF, Godet J, Forget BG, Denoroy L, Garbarz M, Dhermy D, Kastally R, Delaunay J (1989). Spectrin Tunis (Sp$\alpha^{I/78}$), an elliptocytogenic variant, is due to the CGG-TTG codon change (Arg-->Trp) at position 35 of the αI domain. Blood (in press).

20. Garbarz M, Lecomte MC, Devaux I, Dhermy D, d'Auriol L, Boivin P, Grandchamp B (1988). The DNA's from HE and HPP related patients with the spectrin $\alpha^{I/78}$ kD variant contain a single base substitution in exon-3 of the α spectrin gene. Blood 72 (Suppl 1):41a (Abstr).

21. Speicher DW, Marchesi VT (1984). Erythrocyte spectrin is comprised of many homologous triple helical segments. Nature 311:177.

Cellular and Molecular Biology of Normal
and Abnormal Erythroid Membranes, pages 235–248

CLINICAL EXPRESSION OF SPECTRIN αI VARIANTS

P. Boivin, M.C. Lecomte. M. Garbarz. C. Féo[2],
O. Bournier. I. Devaux, C. Galand, H. Gautero,and D. Dhermy
INSERM U160 Hôpital Beaujon, 92118 Clichy France

ABSTRACT Variants of the αl domain of spectrin were
identified in 83 different subjects. 7 were carrying
the αI/78 variant, 14 the αI/74, 49 the αI/65 and 13
the αI/46. From these series of patients we tried to
define the relationship between the type and
functionnal consequence of the different variants and
the clinical status of patients.

INTRODUCTION

Many variants of spectrin have been observed in human
hereditary hemolytic disease. The most frequent concern the
α chain. often the αl domain, sometimes the α2 and may be
the α 4 domains. Other variants are due to the absence of a
peptide segment giving rise to a truncated chain. Variants
of αl domain are identified by limited tryptic digestion of
spectrin and recently by DNA analysis. In limited
proteolytic digestion the αl peptide of 80 kD is decreased,
replaced by a new peptide of lower molecular weight.

At the present day. we know at least eight different
well characterized variants of αl domain called αl/78 (5,
18), αl/74 (11, 12), αl/65 (10, 14). αI/61 (9), αl/50a
αl/50b (16 17), αl/46 (13) and αl/42-43 (8). All were
associated with an hereditary elliptocytosis which was
heterozygous in the great majority of cases and very seldon
homozygous.

Usually hereditary elliptocytosis (HE) is a benign
disease in heterozygote with two exceptions: the
pycnocytosis (or poïkilocytosis) in infancy (2) and the
pyropoïkilocytosis. Variants of spectrin αl domain were
identified in each clinical aspects of HE.

---

[1] This work was supported by INSERM Réseau Nord–Sud
   487NS1 and Association Claude Bernard
[2] INSERM U299. 94 Kremlin Bicêtre (France)

Some variants were observed as a single case; others were identified in several tenths of subjects. For these lasts it becomes possible to look for the relatioship between the variant type and the clinical status. Such a study could help in the knowledge of the functional role of the α1 domain segments were the mutations responsible of variants are localized.

In recent years, variants of the α1 domain of spectrin were identified and studied in our laboratory in 83 subjects with HE. Four types of variants were recognized: α1/74, α1/78. α1/65 and α1/46.

MATERIAL AND METHODS

60 of these 83 subjects were black. Fifty coming directly from western Africa: 6 from a single family had the α1/74 variant, 37 from 22 families the α1/65 variant and 7 from 7 families the α1/46 variant. Ten black subjects were native from the French West Indies, 1 had the α1/74 variant, 4 from 3 families the α1/65 variant and 5 from 2 families the α1/46. 14 subjects were caucasians and 9 were arabs from northern Africa. Among the former 7 from a single family had the α1/78 variant, 7 coming from 3 families had the α1/74 variant: among the arabs, 8 of 9 had the α1/65 variant from 5 families, 1 had the α1/46 variant.

Overall: 7 subjects had the α1/78 variant, 14 had the α1/74 variant, 49 the α1/65 variant and 13 the α1/46 variant. 46 subjects were adults, 29 were between 1.5 and 15 years old. 8 were less than 1.5 year old.

The prominence of the α1/65 variant in this series is explained on the one hand by the predominance in France of black immigrants from Mali where the α1/65 variant is the most frequent one, and on the other hand by results of a survey carried out in Western Africa by M.C. Lecomte and D. Dhermy. The results of this survey will be given elsewhere.

On the clinical point of view, we classified our 83 cases according to Palek (19). Classical hematological data were gathered as often as possible: however the frequent lack of accurate information, the frequence of associated diseases in African blacks (hemoglobinopathies, malnutrition iron deficiency) did'nt allow thorough analysis of the results.

Among the biological data which could reflect the disease severity: a study of erythrocyte deformability as a function of osmolality was carried out on most blood samples by one of us (Claude Féo) with an ektacytometer. Thermal sensitivity was evaluated 10 and 40 mn after exposure at 45 and 47°C either by microscopic examination or with the ektacytometer.

The variants were identified after limited tryptic digestion by one dimension electrophoresis and a combination of electrophoresis and isoelectric focusing according to O´Farrel with the technique of Speicher et al (22). For the one dimension electrophoretic we used a gradient 7-12 of polyacrylamide which allows a good separation of peptides. The percentage of the variant was measured by densitometry after one dimension electrophoresis and reported to the sums of variant and 80 kD peptide peaks.

The functional consequence resulting from the variant was evaluated from the % of spectrin dimers after membrane extraction at 4°C in a low ionic strength medium according to Liu et al (15). The various spectrin species extracted at 4°C were separated and measured either by sucrose gradient centrifugation or by non-denaturing gel electrophoresis and densitometry after staining.

The organizers of the present session whished it to be an exchange of ideas between clinicians and basic scientists; with this series of elliptocytosis as a basis we therefore tried to answer the following questions:

1. Does the type and/or the amount of the variant influence the clinical picture ?

2. Does the type and/or the amount of variant play a role in the spectrin functional alteration as seen at the tetramerization level ?

3. Is the intensity of the functional alteration correlated with the clinical picture ?

4. Is there a relationship between the type and amount of a variant and various hematological abnormalities such as erythrocyte deformability and thermal sensitivity ?

5. Are these abnormalities correlated with the intensity in the tetramerization dysfunction ?

CLINICAL AND HEMATOLOGICAL EXPRESSION

It is difficult to establish a relationship between the variant type and the clinical severity of elliptocytosis in heterozygotes because of the usual mildness of the disease.

Among 49 subjects with variant αI/65, 45 are practically asymptomatic: 2 cases correspond to new-born poïkilocytosis and 2 to the homozygous state: similar proportions of the various forms are seen with the 46 kD variant and it is noteworthy that among 62 subjects with αI/46 and αI/65 variants we did not see any HPP. Up until now we observed the αI/78 variant in 7 subjects from a single family with one case of HPP and one case of important hemolysis. Among the 14 subjects with the αI/74 variant, only 6 are asymptomatic but there are 2 cases of new-born poïkilocytosis and 4 cases of HPP in 3 different families.

From this overall clinical evaluation it appears that clinical manifestations are seen more often with the αI/74 than with the αI/65 and αI/46 variants.

If one looks in more details at the red cells morphological changes as a function of the variant and the different clinical forms no noticeable difference is seen.

BIOCHEMICAL DATA

If one considers the percentage of the abnormal component with respect to the type of variant, taking into account lot disparity, the percentages of the αI/65 variant are more dispersed than those of other variants and can be quite high, considering they are found in heterozygotes. In αI/65 homozygotes the amount is 100%. Among the αI/74 and αI/78 groups, the amounts of variant are higher in subjects with HPP than in simple heterozygotes. We saw above that the αI/65 variant was "clinically benign": therefore, apparently there is not any relationship between the amount of the variant and clinical expression in this particular group of subjects. It seems to be the same in the αI/46 group.

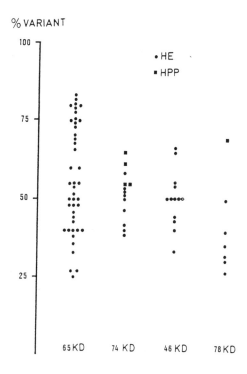

FIGURE 1. Percentage of variants after limited
tryptic digestion. The squares represent the cases of HPP

In Figure 2 showing the percentage of dimers in 4°C
extracts –this is supposed to represent the functional
alteration due to the variant –more important
discrepancies are obvious. This percentage is always
rather small in the αI/65 variant, even in homozygotes
were it was 40–50% respectively. Thus in the αI/65
variant, with the highest amount of the abnormal
component, the functional alteration is the weakest. These
results are in general agreement with those previously
reported by Th. Coetzer et al (3).

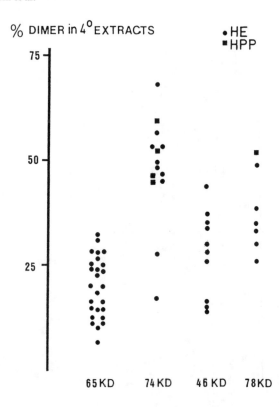

FIGURE 2. Percentage of spectrin dimers in 4°C extract. The squares represent the cases of HPP.

The amount of dimers is higher in αI/46 and αI/78 variants, but differences are more important with the αI/74 variant which often results in a considerable functional alteration. HPP with αI/74 and αI/78 variants have particularly high levels of dimers.

From the above it is obvious that there is no significant statistical relationship between the level of the αI/65 and the functional consequence as evaluated by the amount of dimers in the 4°C extract.

From Figure 3 there seems to be a weak relationship between the levels of variants and dimers in αI/46 variant, but a statistical significance is uncertain because of the small number of cases. On the contrary there is a clear correlation between the levels of αI/74 and αI/78 variant and dimers in 4°C extracts.

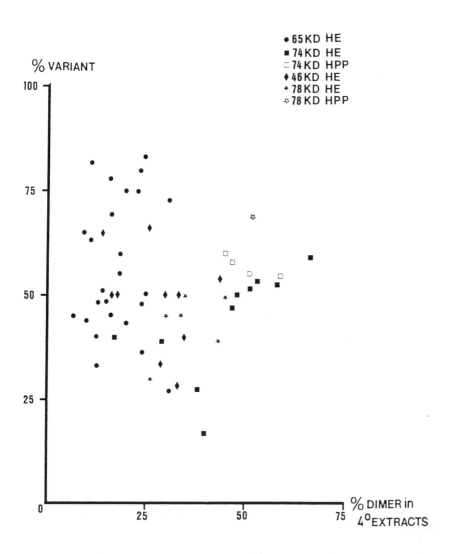

FIGURE 3. Relationship between the percentage of variant in tryptic digests and dimers in 4°C extracts.

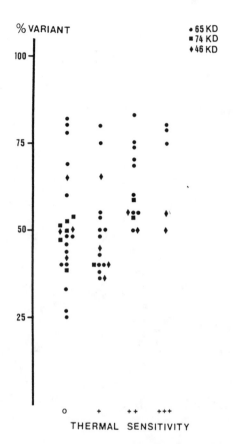

FIGURE 4. Thermal sensitivity at 45°C versus the percentage of variants in tryptic digests.

In the Figure 4 we represented the percentage of variant versus thermal sensitivity. This was appreciated after incubation of red cells at 45°C for 40 minutes by microscopic examination and counted as follows: 0, no morphological abnormality; +, less than 10% of red cells budding, ++ from 10 to 40% of red cells with deformation, +++ more than 40% of cells with morphological injuries. There is a moderate relationship between thermal sensitivity and variant level. The same type of diagram was used to look for a relationship between the percentage of dimer and thermal sensitivity. Such a relationship exist for the αI/78, αI/46 and αI/65 variants but not for the αI/74 variant (Figure 5).

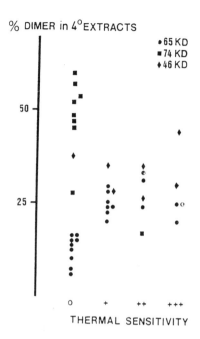

FIGURE 5: Thermal sensitivity at 45°C versus the percentage of dimers in 4°C extract.

Finally, there is a good statistical relationship between the percentage of αI/74, αI/78 and αI/65 variants on the ektacytometric index of deformability.

CONCLUSIONS

The present study allows to answer the above questions only partially and with caution because of the differences in the number of cases of each variant and the small number of variants:

1. In fact the type of variant does play a role in the clinical picture: the αI/65 variant is the mildest and the αI/74 the most severe. The effect of the variant percentage on the clinical picture cannot by really appreciate specially for the αI/65 variant.

2. The functional consequence of the variants as evaluated by the dimer levels in 4°C extract is the lowest for the αI/65 variant, the highest for the αI/74 and intermediate for the αI/46 and αI/78 variants. The dimer level is higher in HPP than in HE. Clinical severity correlates with dimer levels in αI/74 and αI/78 variant.

There is no relationship between the variant amount and the dimer level for the αI/65 variant (the highest variant level, the lowest dimer level); such a relationship exists for the αI/74 variant quite obviously and for the αI/78 variant. The αI/46 variant looks more like the αI/65.

3. Red cell deformability is negatively correlated with variant levels. Thermal sensitivity is correlated with dimer levels for the αI/65 and the αI/46 variants but not for the αI/74 variant. It also partially correlated with the variant percentage.

4. The number of observed cases allows to clearly define the clinical picture of the αI/65 variant. This variant is well defined on the biochemical point of view: it results from a clivage at the site 131 and the insertion of an extraleucine between the aminoacids 148 and 149 (17). The DNA mutation has been identified as a duplication of the codon for the residue 148 TTG-CTG to TTC-TTG-CTG (20, 21). The αI/65 variant is very probably an homogenous mutation specific to blacks. The presence in northern Africa (1) of cases known to be due to the same DNA mutation (20) probably reflects the likelyhood of populations migrations as does the presence of S and C hemoglobin in the same region.

In heterozygous subjects the αI/65 variant disease is a mild condition usually asymptomatic. The homozygous have a moderate hyperhemolysis much less severe than in HPP or αI/74 homozygotes despite of the fact that they have 100% of variant. Until now we did not observe double heterozygotes. But it is noteworthy that the patient reported by Iarocci et al (7) with two variants αI/65 and αI/50 seemed to have a less severe disease that the patient carrying the variants αI/74 and αI/61 recently reported by Lawler et al (9).

This clinical mildness is due to the weak consequence of the αI/65 variant on the tetramerization process even in homozygous which have about 40-50% of dimers in 4°C extracts.

5. The αI/74 variant stands out because of the following
- the relative severity of its clinical expression
- the importance of its functional consequence reflected by a high level of dimers in 4°C extracts
- a good correlation between the variant and dimer levels
- the absence of thermal sensitivity aside from HPP.

In most cases the αI/74 variant seems to be not due to an αI mutation. RFLP studies in kindreds with αI/74 homozygous suggested that the primary defect cannot be located on αl domain (4). Furthermore genomic DNA sequence of a homozygous patients with αI/74, responding to exons 2 and 3 encoding for the first 88 aminoacids of the spectrin αl domain did not show any abnormality (6). It was suggested that the primary defect resided in the β chain and that the presence of an abnormal β chain modified the αl domain conformation exposing the arginin 42 to proteolytic cleavage (as determined by microsequencing of the 74,000 peptide).

Cross-reconstitution of spectrin dimers with isolated α and β chains from controls and heterozygous patients with αI/74 variant furnishes very strong arguments for this hypothesis. We separated α and β chains by HPLC on anion exchanger mono Q, then reconstituted dimers and submitted them to limited tryptic digestion. Dimers reconstituted with controls α and β chain did not show 74 kD species. Dimer reconstituted with patient´s α chain and control β chain did not show 74 kD peptide. Dimer reconstituted with patients α and β chains obviously had the 74 kD peptide. Dimers reconstituted with control α chain and patient´s β chain displaid the 74 kD peptide. Indeed the αl/74 peptide was induced in normal α chain by the presence of the patient β chain.

6. It has been proposed that the functional importance of the various variants was related to the location of the trypsin cleavage site: the closer the site to the molecule NH2 terminal the more important the consequence. This hypothesis is contradicted by the description of the αI/78 variants; their cleavage site is at position 10; their dimer level is lower than for the αI/74 variant and the clinical picture is mild.

ACKNOWLEDGMENTS

We thanks N. Lemaire for preparing and typing this manuscript.

REFERENCES

1. Alloisio N, Guetarni D, Morlé L, Pothier B, Ducluzeau MT, Soun A, Colonna P, Clerc M, Philippe N, Delaunay J (1986). Spα1/65 hereditary elliptocytosis in North Africa. Am J Hematol 23:113-122.
2. Carpentier N, Gustavson LP, Haggard ME (1972). Pyknocytosis in a neonate: an unusual presentation of hereditary elliptocytosis. Clin Pediat 16:76-78.
3. Coetzer T, Lawler J, Prchal JT, Palek J (1987). Molecular determinants of clinical expression of hereditary elliptocytosis and pyropoikilocytosis. Blood 70:766-772.
4. Coetzer T, Lawler J, Jarolim P, Shar K, Forget B, Palek J (1989). Molecular heterogeneity of α spectrin mutants in hereditary elliptocytosis/pyropoikilocytosis. J Cell Biochem Suppl.13B:212.
5. Garbarz M, Lecomte MC, Devaux I, Dhermy D, d'Auriol L, Boivin P, Grandchamp B (1988). The DNA's from HE and HPP related patients with the spectrin α1/78 variant contain a single base substitution in Exon 3 of the α-spectrin gene. Blood 72 suppl.1:41a.
6. Garbarz M, Devaux I, Grandchamp B, Picat C, Dhermy D, Lecomte MC, Boivin P, Sahr K, Forget B (1989). Recherche de l'anomalie génétique dans une forme hémolytique d'elliptocytose hereditaire avec homozygotie pour le variant α1/74. C R Acad Sci (Paris) 308, Séries III:43-48.
7. Iarocci TA, Wagner GM, Mohandas N, Lane P, Mentzer WC (1988). Hereditary poikilocytosis anemia associated with the co-inheritance of two alpha spectrin abnormalities. Blood 71:1390-1396.
8. Lambert S, Zail S (1987). A new variant of the α subunit of spectrin in hereditary elliptocytosis. Blood 69:473-478.
9. Lawler J, Coetzer TL, Mankad Vn, Moore RB, Prchal JT, Palek J (1988). Spectrin-α1/61: a new structural variant of α-spectrin in a double-heterozygous form of hereditary pyropoikilocytosis. Blood 72: 1412-1415.
10. Lawler J, Coetzer TL, Palek J, Jacob HS, Luban N (1985). Spα1/65: a new variant of the α subunit of spectrin in hereditary elliptocytosis. Blood 66:706-709.

11. Lawler J, Liu SC, Palek J, Prchal J (1982). Molecular defect of spectrin in hereditary pyropoikilocytosis: alterations in the trypsin resistant domain involved in spectrin self-association. J Clin Invest 70:1019-1024.
12. Lawler J, Liu SC, Palek J, Prchal J (1984). A molecular defect of spectrin in a subset of patients with hereditary elliptocytosis. Alterations in the α-subunit domain involved in spectrin-self-association. J Clin Invest 73:1688-1695.
13. Lawler J, Palek J, Liu SC, Prchal J, Butler WM (1983). Molecular heterogeneity of hereditary pyropoikilocytosis: identification of a second variant of the spectrin α-subunit. Blood 62:1182-1189.
14. Lecomte MC, Dhermy D, Solis C, Ester A, Féo C, Gautero H, Bournier O, Boivin P (1985). A new abnormal variant of spectrin in black patients with hereditary elliptocytosis. Blood 65:1208-1217.
15. Liu SC, Palek J, Prchal JT (1982). Defective spectrin dimer-dimer association in hereditary elliptocytosis. Proc Natl Acad Sci USA 79:2072-2076.
16. Marchesi SL, Knowles WJ, Morrow JS, Bologna M, Marchesi VT (1986). Abnormal spectrin in hereditary elliptocytosis. Blood 67, 141-151.
17. Marchesi SL, Letsinger JT, Speicher DW, Marchesi VT, Agre P, Hyun B, Gulati G (1987). Mutant forms of spectrin α-subunit in hereditary elliptocytosis. J Clin Invest 80:191-198.
18. Morle L, Alloisio N, Ducluzeau MT, Pothier B, Blibech R, Kastally R, Delaunay J (1988). Spectrin Tunis (αI/78): a new αl variant that causes asymptomatic hereditary elliptocytosis in the heterozygous state. Blood 71:508-511.
19. Palek J (1985). Hereditary elliptocytosis and related disorders. Clin Haematol 14:45.
20. Roux AF, Morle F, Guetarni D, Colonna P, Sahr K, Forget BG, Delaunay J, Godet J (1988). Molecular basis of SpαI/65 hereditary elliptocytosis in North Africa: insertion of a TTC triplet between codons 147 and 149 in the α-spectrin gene of five unrelated families. Blood 72 suppl.1:33a.

21. Sahr KE, Garbarz M, Boivin P, Laughinghouse K,
    Marchesi SL, Forget B (1988). Use of the polymerase
    chain reaction (PCR) for the detection of mutations
    causing hereditary elliptocytosis. Blood 72
    suppl.1:34a.
22. Speicher DW, Morrow JS, Knowles WJ, Marchesi VT
    (1980). Identification of proteolytically resistant
    domains of human erythrocyte spectrin. Proc Natl Acad
    Sci (USA) 77:5673–5677.

Cellular and Molecular Biology of Normal
and Abnormal Erythroid Membranes, pages 249–265
© 1990 Alan R. Liss, Inc.

A NEW CYTOADHERENCE PROPERTY OF <u>PLASMODIUM</u>
<u>FALCIPARUM</u>-INFECTED ERYTHROCYTES:
ROSETTING WITH UNINFECTED ERYTHROCYTES

Shiroma M. Handunnetti, Aileen D. Gilladoga
and Russell J. Howard

Laboratory of Infectious Diseases
DNAX Research Institute
901 California Avenue
Palo Alto, California 94304-1104

ABSTRACT

Infection of human and <u>Aotus</u> monkey erythrocytes
with mature asexual stage parasites of the human
malaria <u>Plasmodium falciparum</u> induces the
appearance of a receptor for endothelial cells.
This receptor mediates attachment of infected
erythrocytes to endothelial cells lining small
blood vessels, leading to sequestration of mature
infected cells from the peripheral circulation.
The special pathology of acute cerebral malaria
in man is due to the blockage of blood flow by
attached infected erythrocytes in the small blood
vessels of the brain. We describe a second
specific receptor property acquired by the
surface of <u>P. falciparum</u>-infected erythrocytes:
attachment of uninfected erythrocytes around a
central infected erythrocyte containing a mature
asexual parasite. This phenomenon is called
'rosetting'. Methods for quantitation of
rosetting, <u>in vitro</u> selection of rosetting-
positive parasites, purification of rosettes and
recovery of pure infected cells from rosettes are
described. We show that some parasite strains
consistently form rosettes while others do not,
and, that the uninfected erythrocyte must also
bear specific receptor(s) to form a rosette. The
possible involvement of rosettes in affecting the

distribution of adherent infected cells in
different tissues is discussed, together with
other potential roles that rosettes could fulfil
to the parasite's advantage.

INTRODUCTION

The clinical symptoms of malaria infection are caused
exclusively by the proliferation of asexual bloodstages in
the blood. The parasite invades host red blood cells (RBC)
and differentiates through distinct morphological stages
(i.e., ring and trophozoite) before initiation of parasite
nuclear replication at the schizont stage. The parasite
cytoplasm divides subsequently to produce up to 20 RBC -
invasive daughter parasites which invade new RBC after
rupture of the original host cell. In the case of
Plasmodium falciparum malaria, the most lethal of the four
human malaria species, the cytoadherence properties of the
parasitized RBC (PRBC) have been linked to the special
pathology and virulence of this disease. P. falciparum
PRBC containing mature asexual parasites (trophozoites,
schizonts) are generally not detected in samples of
peripheral blood, unlike the ring-stage PRBC regularly seen
in light microscopy diagnosis. The mature PRBC are
'sequestered' in various tissues through adherence to the
endothelial cells lining the small blood vessel (1,2). In
small venules the adherent PRBC can markedly reduce blood
flow. In many acute cases of P. falciparum malaria an
especially dangerous syndrome of 'cerebral malaria' is
observed, in which the patient exhibits worsening nervous
dysfunction, coma and either resolution of the acute attack
or death (3). In cerebral malaria there is pronounced PRBC
sequestration in the brain, such that light and electron
microscopy of autopsy specimens reveal blood vessels
totally occluded by PRBC surrounded by necrotic brain
tissue (4). Adherence of P. falciparum PRBC to blood
vessel endothelial cells may afford the parasite two
advantages: mature PRBC require an environment of low pO_2
for optimal growth (5), and, mature PRBC are much less
deformable than ring-stage PRBC (6) so that mature PRBC are
rapidly cleared from the peripheral circulation (and
destroyed) by the filtering action of the spleen (7). This
acquired adherence property of P. falciparum PRBC has been
associated with the appearance of knob-like protrusions
(~100nm diameter) of the RBC membrane (1,8).

Two in vitro model systems have been developed to study the adherence properties of P. falciparum PRBC. Monolayers of human umbilical cord endothelial cells (primary cultures) bind mature PRBC but not immature PRBC or uninfected RBC (9). The C32 cell line of a human amelanotic melanoma (10) and other human cell lines (11) can also adhere P. falciparum PRBC and provides a convenient routine assay system.

A new cytoadherence property of mature asexual stages of P. falciparum has recently been identified - rosetting of uninfected RBC around a central intact PRBC (12). The phenomenon was first identified with P. fragile PRBC in the natural host the toque monkey (13), where appearance of PRBC rosetting during parasite development coincided with the disappearance of PRBC from the peripheral circulation. Comparison of several human and primate malarias for the presence of rosettes (12) subsequently revealed that parasites which sequester in vivo (e.g., P. falciparum and P. fragile) exhibit rosettes, whereas those which do not sequester (e.g., P. vivax and P. cynomolgi) also fail to rosette.

Here we use a quantitative assay for PRBC rosettes and simple methods for purification of intact rosettes, or the PRBC from disrupted rosettes, to define some fundamental properties of this cell-cell attachment phenomenon in P. falciparum malaria.

MATERIALS AND METHODS

Assay for Rosetting

The technique for counting rosettes was performed using a modification of the previously described method (13). Briefly, 10 ul of blood suspension was distributed evenly under a 22 x 22 mm coverslip and 100 consecutive PRBC examined under phase contrast optics. Alternately ethidium bromide was added to blood suspensions at 20 μg/ml and the specimen examined under ultraviolet light.

The number of PRBC that are not bound to RBC and those that are bound to one, two, or $\geq$ three RBC were counted. Triplicate counts were performed on each sample. Rosetting is expressed as the percentage of PRBC that are bound to $\geq$ three RBC.

Parasites

Four knob-positive (K+) C32 cell cytoadherence
positive (B+) strains of P. falciparum which have been
blood passaged in spleen-intact Aotus trivirgatus monkeys
were used: FMG strain (FMG) from Gambia; FVO strain from
Vietnam; Malayan Camp strain CHQ (MC) from Malaysia, St.
Lucia strain (SL) from El Salvador (14). Infected blood
containing 5-40% ring stage PRBC was cryopreserved (15) and
the animals cured with chloroquine. Prior to
cryopreservation heparinized infected blood was passed
through a column of CF11 cellulose to remove leucocytes
(16).
        Short term cultures of P. falciparum infected Aotus
blood was carried out as described previously (17).
Cryopreserved RBC from naive spleen-intact Aotus monkeys
were thawed and used for the rosetting assays.
        P. falciparum PRBC of Malayan Camp strain obtained
from Aotus monkeys were adapted to continuous in vitro
culture in human RBC. First, ring stage PRBC were cultured
for 24-36 h. and K+ trophozoite stage PRBC enriched with
0.5% gelatin/RPMI 1640. Second, K+ trophozoite stage PRBC
(collected from the supernatant) were selected for
cytoadherence-positive cells (18). The cells were added to
a monolayer of unfixed C32 melanoma cells (American Type
Culture Collection, Rockville, MD.) in 75cm^2 tissue culture
flasks and incubated for 1 h. at 37C° with gentle rocking
by hand every 10-15 min. The monolayer was washed with
RPMI 1640, pH 6.8 until all nonadherent cells were removed.
Fresh culture medium containing 15% fetal calf serum and
human O+ RBC (1% hematocrit) was added and the culture
incubated overnight. After the completion of schizogony
and rupture of the adherent PRBC, newly-invaded ring stage
PRBC were collected for continued culture.
        The progeny of the K+B+ parasites of the MC strain,
adapted to human RBC were assayed for rosetting. After the
first selection over C32 melanoma cells, 80-90% of PRBC
were in rosettes. This K+ rosetting-positive (R+)

phenotype was maintained by selection for R+ parasites using Percoll/sorbitol gradients (19). Rosetting parasites were collected from the 90% Percoll layer with RBC.

Purification of Non-Rosetting and Rosetting Parasites

Non-rosetting parasites from infected Aotus and human blood were purified by the Percoll/sorbitol density gradient method (19). The gradient was centrifuged at 10,000 r.p.m. (12,000 g) in an SS-34 (Sorvall Instruments Div. DuPont Co.) fixed angle rotor for 20 min at 20°C (Figure 4). Rosetting parasites (PRBC in rosettes) were purified using Percoll/sorbitol gradients centrifuged at 12,000 g for 5 min at 20°C.

Purification of PRBC from Rosettes

The K+R+ PRBC of MC strain were purified from PRBC/RBC rosettes by the following method: synchronized cultures containing trophozoite stage PRBC (5% parasitemia) were passed twice through a 25 G needle to disrupt rosettes. This RBC suspension was immediately layered over a Percoll/sorbitol gradient and centrifuged at 12,000 g for 20 min at 20°C. Trophozoite stage PRBC were collected from the interface between 60 and 70% Percoll (Figure 5).

RESULTS

Identification of Rosettes

In vitro cultures of P. falciparum asexual parasites in human RBC were examined by light microscopy for the presence of rosettes. In Figure 1 the appearance of PRBC without any attached uninfected RBC is shown, together with PRBC attached to 1, 2 or several uninfected RBC. Only PRBC containing trophozoites, schizonts or more mature intracellular parasites are seen with adherent uninfected RBC. In the same cultures cell-cell attachment of uninfected RBC alone was not observed. We have denoted any association of ≥ 3 uninfected cells with a PRBC as a 'rosette', however we always independently count the PRBC with 0, 1, 2 or ≥ 3 adherent RBC. We have consistently detected rosettes in some P. falciparum cultures of in vitro-adapted parasites and not in others (see below). Rosettes do not appear to represent an artifact of manipulation of the culture. Rosettes are observed if the culture flask is gently swirled to resuspend the settled cells and a droplet of blood placed directly, without other pipetation, onto a glass microscope slide. After gently placing a glass coverslip over the droplet the PRBC are examined. Rosettes identified by bright field microscopy, the mature PRBC recognized by the presence of an obvious parasite inclusion and parasite pigment. If ethidium bromide is added, fluorescence microscopy can be used to facilitate identification of any immature PRBC. Rosettes of <u>P. falciparum</u> PRBC have been seen with cultures in RBC of diverse blood group phenotypes (A+, B+, AB+, 0+) and with cultures containing 10–15% V/V of fetal calf serum, horse serum or human serum.

Rosetting of Uninfected Human RBC Around *P. falciparum* -Infected RBC

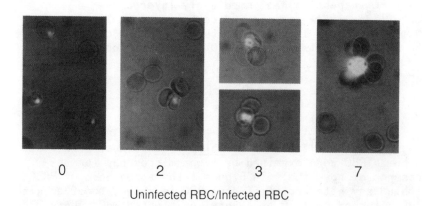

0   2   3   7

Uninfected RBC/Infected RBC

FIGURE 1. Rosettes identified by bright field light microscopy of ethidium bromide stained PRBC. The parasites in the panels with 0 or 2 uninfected RBC/PRBC were trophozoites, those in the panel with 3 uninfected RBC/PRBC were schizonts, while the extreme righthand panel shows a segmenter-infected PRBC.

The extent of rosetting of P. falciparum PRBC was determined with four parasite strains of diverse geographic origin in Aotus RBC (Figure 2). These parasites were derived from repeated infected blood passage in spleen-intact Aotus monkeys. Each strain exhibited sequestration of mature PRBC in Aotus monkeys, as well as adherence to human endothelial cells or C32 melanoma cells in vitro (14). Mature PRBC of these strains also express knob protrusions (i.e., K+ phenotype). For MC, FMG and FVO strains the analysis is shown for the same sample of cryopreserved infected blood thawed and cultured on two occasions to the late-trophozoite stage. None of these parasites in Aotus RBC rosetted more than 10% of PRBC with Aotus uninfected RBC (Figure 2). The very effective sequestration of Aotus PRBC in vivo, and their pronounced in vitro attachment to endothelial cells and C32 melanoma cells, do therefore not require the presence of PRBC rosettes.

Rosetting of *P. falciparum*-Infected RBC in *Aotus* Monkey Blood

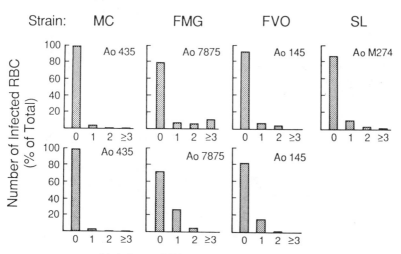

FIGURE 2. Comparison of four P. falciparum strains for rosetting in Aotus monkey blood. Results from repeated analysis of cryopreserved blood from individual infected animals (labeled Ao) are shown.

Parasites from three of the four strains adapted to growth in _Aotus_ monkey were successfully adapted to _in vitro_ growth in human RBC. During this _in vitro_ adaptation parasites were selected for the capacity of mature PRBC to float on gelatin (i.e., express knobs) and adhere to immobilized C32 melanoma cells. After several weeks of growth, when effectively all RBC present were human rather than _Aotus_, the extent of rosetting was re-examined (Figure 3). With SL and FMG strains of _P. falciparum_ in human RBC the extent of rosetting was < 10% of PRBC, as observed in _Aotus_ RBC. In contrast, ≥ 80% of MC-strain PRBC in human RBC formed rosettes with uninfected human RBC. These rosettes contained from 3 to 8 uninfected RBC around each central PRBC. This strain of parasites has since been cultured for several months _in vitro_, with once-weekly selection for adherence to C32 cells, or once-weekly selection for rosetting-positive cells (see Results below and Methods). The degree of rosetting for this MC strain varied from 60-90% of trophozoite-stage PRBC.

In order to maintain the rosetting phenotype of MC-strain _P. falciparum_ adapted to _in vitro_ growth in human RBC we devised a density gradient system to separate PRBC in rosettes from those not in rosettes (Figure 4). On a Percoll step gradient spun for 20 min., PRBC from non-rosetting strains of _P. falciparum_ band at the 60%/70% Percoll interface. Such PRBC contain < 5% uninfected RBC, and these RBC are not present in rosettes. With a rosette-positive parasite such as MC strain, and only 5 min. centrifugation, the PRBC band at this interface is a minor proportion of total mature-stage PRBC. Again, these PRBC are not in rosettes. The majority of PRBC are found at the 80%/90% interface, with > 70% of the PRBC in rosettes. The percentage parasitemia of this fraction is therefore lower, ranging from 10-30%. Uninfected RBC spin to the bottom of the tube at both centrifugation times. PRBC in rosettes can be collected from the 80%/90% Percoll interface and used to inoculate a new _in vitro_ culture, thereby propagating the desired phenotype.

Comparison of Rosetting in *Aotus* Monkey Blood
and in Human Blood from *In Vitro* Culture

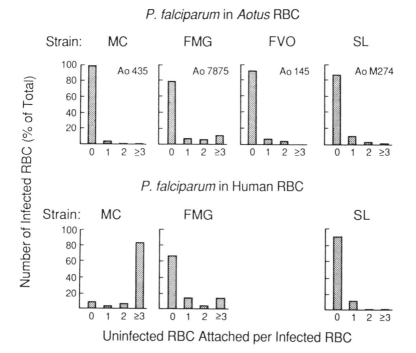

P. falciparum in *Aotus* RBC

FIGURE 3. Adaptation of P. falciparum parasites to in vitro culture in human RBC and analysis of rosetting.

PRBC in rosettes purified from such in vitro cultures are an ideal source of PRBC for detailed studies on surface antigens that might be responsible for rosette formation. To this end we devised a simple protocol to disrupt the purified PRBC rosettes and purify the PRBC. This protocol can also be utilized on the total infected blood (as shown in Figure 5), however in this case the purified PRBC will be derived from two potential populations: rosette-positive (R+) and rosette-negative (R-). Blood is passed through a 25 G needle to mechanically disrupt the rosettes then immediately layered on top of a Percoll step-density gradient and centrifuged. The PRBC then migrate exclusively to the 60%/70% Percoll interface from where they are collected at > 90% parasitemia. Such PRBC are no

longer rosetted. However, if these PRBC are mixed with
uninfected RBC they do reform rosettes (up to 80% PRBC in
rosettes compared to 76% PRBC in rosettes in the original
blood, Figure 5).

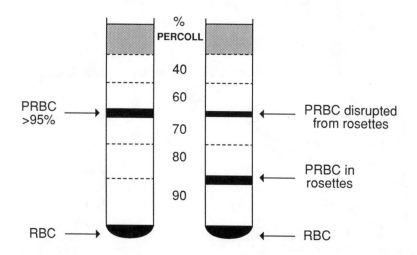

FIGURE 4. Purification of PRBC or PRBC in rosettes by
density gradient centrifugation: a schematic diagram
showing the final banding patterns. On the left, blood
from a R- parasite has been spun 12,000 g, 20 min. On the
right, blood from a R+ parasite has been spun at the same
force for only 5 min. When PRBC in rosettes are collected
they can be mechanically disrupted and rapidly spun again,
as shown on the left, to recover pure PRBC derived from
rosettes.

FIGURE 5.

Purification of PRBC from PRBC/RBC Rosettes

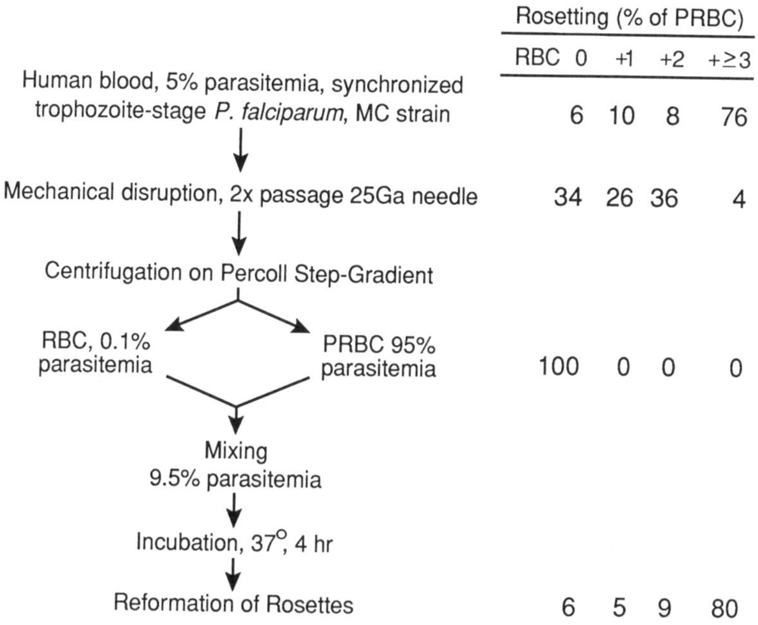

	Rosetting (% of PRBC)			
	RBC 0	+1	+2	+≥3
Human blood, 5% parasitemia, synchronized trophozoite-stage *P. falciparum*, MC strain	6	10	8	76
Mechanical disruption, 2x passage 25Ga needle	34	26	36	4
Centrifugation on Percoll Step-Gradient				
RBC, 0.1% parasitemia PRBC 95% parasitemia	100	0	0	0
Mixing 9.5% parasitemia				
Incubation, 37°, 4 hr				
Reformation of Rosettes	6	5	9	80

The striking difference in PRBC rosetting exhibited by MC strain parasites in Aotus versus human RBC could reflect a mutation which occurred during adaptation to in vitro culture (i.e., acquisition of the PRBC surface membrane rosetting receptor), or, a difference in the host RBC. Conceivably, mature stage parasites in Aotus RBC may express the rosetting receptor but some other parasite-induced change in Aotus RBC, which does not occur in human infected RBC, could prevent rosetting. It was also possible that uninfected Aotus RBC differed in their ability to form rosettes around PRBC compared with human uninfected RBC. To test these possibilities we purified Aotus monkey PRBC (trophozoite-stage, MC strain) to > 90% parasitemia by density gradient centrifugation then added either uninfected Aotus RBC or uninfected human RBC (Table 1). As anticipated from the low-level of PRBC rosetting observed with Aotus-infected blood, addition of Aotus uninfected RBC yielded only 2-18% rosettes. In contrast, human RBC added to Aotus PRBC yielded 44% and 62%

of PRBC in rosettes. It appears that the low level of PRBC rosetting in <u>Aotus</u> blood is not due to failure of the PRBC to express a surface receptor for uninfected RBC, but instead failure of <u>Aotus</u> uninfected RBC to form the rosette.

TABLE 1
ROSETTING OF <u>P. FALCIPARUM</u>-INFECTED <u>AOTUS</u>
MONKEY RBC* WITH HUMAN AND <u>AOTUS</u> RBC.

Source of RBC added to purified PRBC		Rosetting % of PRBC with RBC			
		0	+1	+2	+ ≥3
<u>Aotus</u>	435	94	4	0	2
	132	62	10	10	18
	9026	66	4	14	16
Human	1	19	18	19	44
	9	3	15	20	62

* MC strain, K+, cytoadherence-positive PRBC cryopreserved at ring-stage in <u>Aotus</u> blood then cultured < 36 hr. after thaw.

DISCUSSION

We have previously shown that rosetting of uninfected RBC around PRBC occurs in two natural host-parasite associations, <u>P. falciparum</u> infections in man and <u>P. fragile</u> infections in the toque monkey (12,13) in both of which the mature parasite stages are sequestered <u>in vivo</u>. In two other malaria parasites which do not show parasite sequestration, <u>P. vivax</u> infections in man and <u>P. cynomolgi</u> in the toque monkey, the mature parasite forms fail to rosette (12). In <u>P. fragile</u> infections rosetting and <u>in vivo</u> sequestration occur simultaneously within an erythrocytic cycle. Rosetting of PRBC in human <u>P. falciparum</u> isolates appears at the trophozoite stage, the stage at which parasites are sequestered <u>in vivo</u> and bind to C32 melanoma cells <u>in vitro</u>. These results suggested that the two cytoadherence properties of PRBC, adherence to endothelial cells and to uninfected RBC in rosettes, are closely related.

In the present study we have examined four strains of
P. falciparum from diverse geographic origins for
rosetting. These parasite strains have been blood passaged
in spleen-intact Aotus monkeys, show marked sequestration
in vivo and adhere strongly to C32 melanoma cells in vitro
(14). However, when ring-infected Aotus blood
(cryopreserved and thawed) was cultured for 36 h. and
assayed for rosetting at the mature trophozoite/schizont
stage, rosetting occured at a very low level (<10%) in all
four strains. Repeated rosetting assays of the different
strains (Figure 2) and preparations of a particular strain
from different monkeys (SMH, data not shown) showed
consistently low levels of PRBC rosetting. These results
suggest that the PRBC receptor for adherence to C32
melanoma cells and the PRBC receptor for rosetting with
uninfected RBC are different. The results could also
reflect failure of Aotus PRBC or RBC to express the
appropriate rosetting receptor(s). In order to address
this second question we investigated the ability of Aotus
PRBC to form rosettes with human and Aotus RBC. When
purified Aotus PRBC (>95% PRBC) are mixed with human RBC,
44-62% of PRBC formed rosettes whereas only 2-18% of PRBC
formed rosettes with Aotus RBC (Table 1). This result
indicates that the Aotus PRBC express the receptor for
rosetting and that the failure to form rosettes is due
either to lack of receptor(s) on uninfected RBC or the
presence of receptor molecules at a very low density.
Similar results were obtained with P. fragile infected
rhesus RBC: rhesus PRBC do not form rosettes with rhesus
uninfected RBC (0-9% PRBC in rosettes), whereas 33-49% of
PRBC form rosettes with toque monkey uninfected RBC (SMH,
data not shown). Thus, although rhesus PRBC express the
rosetting receptor, the rosetting receptor(s) are absent on
rhesus uninfected RBC. These results lead us to conclude
that PRBC/RBC rosetting requires two types of receptors,
one on the PRBC surface membrane and the other on the
uninfected RBC surface membrane. The molecular nature of
these receptor molecule(s) is unknown.
    When the Aotus isolates were adapted to human RBC and
C32-binding positive cells selected in vitro, rosetting of
PRBC varied in different parasite strains. In three
strains, FMG, FVO and SL, rosetting of PRBC was very low
(<10% of PRBC in rosettes) while in MC strain >80% of PRBC
were in rosettes.
    Rosetting appears to inhibit/interfere with the
binding of PRBC to C32 melanoma cells. The non-rosetting

parasite FMG, in human RBC, did adhere to C32 melanoma cells, and can be described as a R-B+ phenotype. In contrast, the rosetting positive parasites of MC strain in human RBC gave very low adherence to C32 cells and initially appeared to be R+B-. Rosettes of uninfected RBC formed around MC strain trophozoite-PRBC in vitro at the precise stage when adherence to C32 cells would normally be anticipated. Since uninfected RBC in rosettes could effectively block any interaction of the PRBC with the C32 cell monolayer, we mechanically disrupted purified rosettes of PRBC/RBC, purified the PRBC (Figure 4) and tested their adherence to C32 cells. The PRBC then bound strongly to C32 cells (SMH, data not shown). Thus, in vitro under the standard assay conditions, this parasite appears to have the R+B- phenotype, but in vivo where uninfected RBC are subjected to high shear forces in blood flow, the rosettes may be disrupted to reveal PRBC of R+B+ phenotype. In vitro with MC strain we observe PRBC in rosettes and a minority free of bound uninfected RBC. Only the latter will bind to C32 cells in the standard assay and selection protocol for C32 cell adherence.

Our findings support the following speculation of the functional significance of rosetting in vivo. Since rosetting competes with PRBC binding to C32 cells in vitro, it is very likely that rosetting would compete with PRBC binding to endothelial cells in vivo due to the obstruction of the endothelial cell receptor on PRBC by the uninfected RBC. However, rosetting may actually enhance the possibility of PRBC adherence to endothelial cells in vivo. If rosettes are formed in the peripheral circulation, PRBC in rosettes could then be selected for adherence in particular tissues by "clogging" of capillaries (Figure 6 "A"). Subsequent disruption by shear forces could then expose the PRBC receptor(s) for endothelial cell adherence (Figure 6 "B, C"). PRBC may therefore attach to small blood vessels in different tissues to non-rosetted PRBC. Non-rosetted PRBC will flow differently through narrow vessels and interact differently with the capillary wall compared to rosetted PRBC. Rosetting could therefore be an additional parasite survival mechanism that prevents destruction of PRBC in the spleen.

Schematic Diagram of the Possible Relationship
Between Infected-Erythrocyte Adherence to
Uninfected Erythrocytes (Rosetting) and Adherence
to Endothelial Cells Lining Blood Vessels

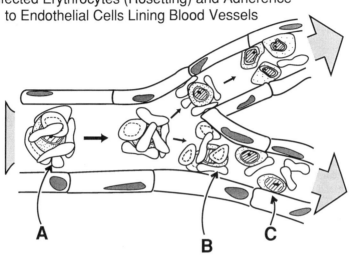

A   B   C

FIGURE 6.   Hypothetical role of P. falciparum rosettes
in vivo to promote PRBC attachment to endothelial cells in
vessels where the rosette, but not free PRBC, is occluded.

Rosetting in vivo could have other functional roles
such as, (a) protection of PRBC from recognition by
monocytes and other cells of the host immune system; (b)
facilitation of exchange of metabolites, lipids and
proteins between PRBC and uninfected RBC; (c) increased
parasite proliferation through more efficient merozoite
invasion.   Merozoites released from ruptured PRBC may
immediately invade adjacent uninfected RBC in rosettes and
thereby minimize their accessibility to host antibodies.
      Our continuing studies aim to identify the molecular
nature of the rosetting and endothelial cell receptors on
the surface of PRBC and explore their tolerance to the
pathology of P. falciparum malaria in natural infections.

ACKNOWLEDGEMENTS

      We are grateful to other members of our laboratory for
their assistance and critical comments. These studies

are supported by a WHO/TDR Training Fellowship and a Rockefeller Foundation Training Grant to SMH, by grants from the United States Agency for International Development (Grant#DPE-0453-G-SS-8049-00) and TDR/IMMAL component of WHO (Grant#TDR-880122), and by the direct support of DNAX Research Institute.

REFERENCES

1. Miller LH, Fremount HN, Luse SA (1971). Deep vascular schizogony of Plasmodium knowlesi in macaca mulatta. Am J Trop Med Hyg 20:816.
2. McPherson GG, Warrell MJ, White Nj, Looreesuwan S, Warrell DJ (1985). Human cerebral malaria: A quantitative ultrastructural analysis of erythrocyte sequestration. Am J Pathol 119:385.
3. Spitz, S (1946). The pathology of acute falciparum malaria. Military Surgeon _:555.
4. Aikawa M, Suzuki M, Gutierrez Y (1980). "Pathology of Malaria." New York: Academic Press, vol 2, p 47.
5. Scheibel LW, Ashton SH, Trager W (1979). Reduced oxygen tension provides a better environment for the in vitro parasite development. Exp Parasitol 47:410.
6. Miller LH, Usami S, Chien S (1971). Alteration in the rheologic properties of Plasmodium knowlesi-infected red cells. A possible mechanism for capillary obstruction. J Clin Investig 50:1451.
7. Wyler DJ, Oster CN, Quinn TC (1978). The role of the spleen in malaria infections. In "Role of the spleen in the immunology and parasitic diseases", Trop Dis Res Ser 1, Schwabe & Co, Basle, p 183.
8. Trager W, Rudzinska MA, Bradbury PC (1966). The fine structure of Plasmodium falciparum and its host erythrocytes in natural malarial infections in man. Bulletin, WHO 35:883.
9. Udeinya IJ, Schmidt JA, Aikawa M, Miller LH, Green I (1981). Falciparum malaria-infected erythrocytes specifically bind cultured human endothelial cells. Science 213:555.
10. Schmidt JA, Udeniya IJ, Leech JH, Hay RJ, Aikawa M, Barnwell J, Green I, Miller LH (1982). Plasmodium falciparum malaria. An amelanotic melanoma cell line bears receptors for the know ligand of infected erythrocytes. J Clin Invest 70:379.

11. Panton LJ, Leech JH, Miller LH, Howard RJ (1988).
     Cytoadherence of Plasmodium falciparum-infected
     erythrocytes to human melanoma cell lines correlates
     with surface OKM5 antigen. Infection and Immunity
     55:2754.
12. Handunnetti SM, Davie PH, Perera KLRL, Mendis KN
     (1989). Uninfected erythrocytes form rosettes around
     Plasmodium falciparum infected erythrocytes. Am J
     Trop Med Hyg 40:117.
13. David PH, Handunnetti SM, Leech JH, Gamage CP, Mendis
     KN (1988). Rosetting: A new cytoadherence property
     of malaria infected erythrocytes. Am J Trop Med Hyg
     38:289.
14. Howard JH, Barnwell JW, Rock EP, Neequaye J, Ofori-
     Adjei D, Maloy WL, Lyon JA, Saul AJ (1988). Two ~300
     kDa Plasmodium falciparum proteins at the surface
     membrane of infected erythrocytes. Mol Biochem
     Parasitol 27:207.
15. Meryman HT, Hornblower M (1972). A method for
     freezing and washing red blood cells using a high
     glycerol concentration. Transfusion 12:145.
16. Homewood CA, Neame KD (1976). A comparison of methods
     used for removal of white cells from malaria infected
     blood. Ann of Trop Med Parasitol 70:249.
17. Trager W, Jensen JB (1976). Human malaria parasites
     in continuous culture. Science 193:673.
18. Magoman C, Wollish W, Anderson L, Leech J (1988).
     Cytoadherence by Plasmodium falciparum-infected
     erythrocyte is correlated with the expression of a
     family of variable proteins on infected erythrocytes.
     J Exp Med 168:1307.
19. Aley SB, Sherwood JA, Marsh R, Eidelman O, Howard RJ
     (1986). Identification of isolate-specific proteins
     on sorbitol-enriched Plasmodium falciparum infected
     erythrocytes from Gambian patients. Parasitol 92:511.

**Cellular and Molecular Biology of Normal
and Abnormal Erythroid Membranes, pages 267–281**
© **1990 Alan R. Liss, Inc.**

DISCRETE SITES OF PERMEATION INDUCED IN THE HUMAN
RED CELL MEMBRANE BY MALARIA PARASITES[1]

Z.Ioav Cabantchik, Josefine Silfen
and Hava Glickstein

Department of Biological Chemistry, Institute of Life
Sciences, Hebrew University, Jerusalem, Israel 91904

ABSTRACT   So as to meet the increasing demand for
import of nutrients and export of waste products, the
intracellular malaria parasites produce profound
changes in the permeability properties of the host
(erythrocyte) membrane. Approximately 6 hours after
Plasmodium falciparum invades the human red cell, and
a few hours before any structural changes are detected
in the red cell membrane, the latter becomes permeable
to molecular species, which are otherwise impermeant
or very poorly permeant to uninfected cells. These
include polyols such as sorbitol and myoinositol,
amino acids such as gln and his , a variety of organic
acids and trace metal ions. The extent of permeation
of these agents increases gradually with intracellular
parasite development, depends on de novo protein
synthesis and is blocked differentially by a series of
bioflavonoid glycosides which also markedly decrease
parasite growth. Most of the water soluble permeants
gain access into the parasitized cell by a pore-like
pathway (anionic channel by patch clamp) while the
more hydrophobic ones would favor partitioning into
the parasite modified membrane. The pores are
irreversibly blocked by covalent binding analogs of
bioflavonoid-glycosides, the sites of binding are
endofacial, and they amount to a few hundred per cell.
The new sites of permeation can serve both as routes
for specific delivery of toxic agents into parasitized
cells and as specific targets whose inactivation leads
to arrest of parasite growth.

---

[1]Supported in part by grants NIH AI-20342 and AID
CDR C7-171.

INTRODUCTION

The red cell membrane is endowed with a battery of transport systems which can be classified according to their physiological role as supporters of cellular functions (e.g. glucose carrier, lactate carrier, nucleobase carriers, glutathione carrier, some amino acid carriers, Na-pump, Ca-pump), or as subservers of essential systemic functions (e.g. $Cl-HCO_3$ exchanger, urea carrier, adenosine carrier).

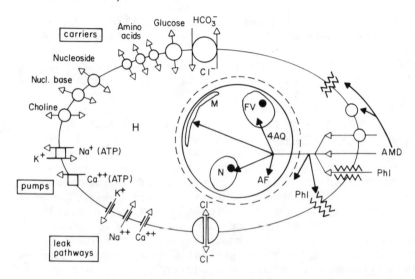

Figure 1. The major transport sytems of the red cell membrane which remain operative in a malaria parasitized cell are depicted on the left half while new pathways induced by the parasite appear on the right half. These pathways allow permeation (empty arrows) of substrates as well as of some antimalarial drugs (AMD) into the host cell cytosol (H), from where they can reach the inhibitory target (filled arrow) either of the host or of the parasite. Components of the parasite nucleus (N), mitochondria (M), food vacuole (FV) or parasite cytosol can serve as targets for drugs such as 4-aminoquinolines (4AQ), antifolates (AF), etc. Phlorizin (phl), which is selectively permeant to infected cells, inhibits parasite growth by a pleiotropic mechanism, affecting both host and parasite components.

Additional transport sytems which are present in the red cell membrane play only minor physiological roles and are merely remnants of a once metabolically active cell (e.g. various amino acid transporters, choline carrier, ion leak pathways (channels)) (Fig. 1).

In general, the traffic of solute across the red cell membrane is dominated by the electroneutral exchange of anions, which subserves the systemic removal of CO_2 from tissues to lungs (1) and constitutes the most specialized system of that membrane . Second in activity is glucose, whose carrier-mediated transport fuels the metabolic machinery (i.e. glycolysis) of human red cells (2). Upon parasite invasion of the red cell and the ensuing rise of metabolic activity (3) generated by the rapid growth and replication of the intracellular parasite, there is a commensurate increase in traffic of metabolites and catabolites across the red cell membrane (4,5). Much of this traffic is carried out by the constitutive transport mechanisms of the red cell, which, apparently, undergo only minor modifications during the life span of the intracellular parasite (5) (Fig. 2).

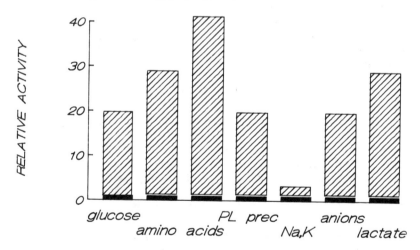

Figure 2. Nutrient traffic across the red cell membrane of a Plasmodium falciparum infected human red blood cell (trophozoite stage) is given in values relative to those obtained in uninfected cells for the respective substrate (PL prec the denotes phospholipid precursor-choline; Na,K refer to the leaks of those cations; anions refer to both inorganic and organic anions).

However, in order to meet the above metabolic demands, the parasite also induces permeability changes in the host cell membrane for a variety of substrates (5,6), which are either poorly permeant or impermeant to uninfected cells (notably gln and myoinositol). In principle, an increase in permeation of a discrete number of substrates can be accomplished by the constituents of the host membrane , provided their native activity in the uninfected cell or even their modified activity in the parasitized cell, have an intrinsically high capacity for carrying out enhanced fluxes. This is probably the case for glucose and nucleobases, whose increased traffic represents merely an increase in substrate concentration with minor changes in kinetic parameters (5). However, for some substrates for which the red cell membrane is either poorly permeable (e.g. amino acids such as gln, or phospholipid precursors such as myoinositol, ref. 6) or is limitingly permeable (e.g. lactate, ref. 7), new permeation pathways would have to be provided by the parasites either by de novo synthesis or by modification of the native red cell membrane constituents. In this work we describe various biophysical and biochemical properties of the new pathways, their use as targets for pharmacological agents with potential antimalarial activity and their use as vehicles for selective targeting of cytotoxic agents to malaria parasitized cells.

METHODS

All the methods quoted in the text were described in detail in various publications (7-11). Unless specified otherwise, all studies were conducted with the ItG2G1 (brazilian) cloned strain of P. falciparum. Other strains used were FCR_3 (Gambia), W2 (Indochina) and D6 (12).

Measurements and evaluation of transport

The measurement of transport across the parasitized red cell depends to a large extent on the ability to monitor the movement of solute across the red cell membrane, the outermost boundary of a highly compartmentalized cell. Although the available techniques for measuring transport have provided a wealth of kinetic data, it is not always clear that the information pertained the red cell membrane per se, rather than intracellular membranes, such as the parasite plasma membrane (Fig. 3).

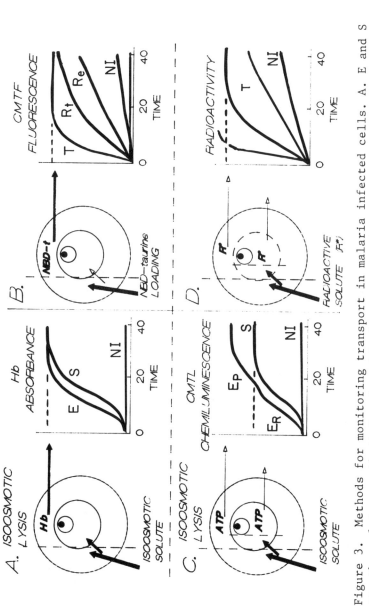

Figure 3. Methods for monitoring transport in malaria infected cells. A. E and S are the solutes erythritol and sorbitol, respectively; NI : uninfected cells. B. CMTF is the method of continuous monitoring of transport by fluorescence; Rt and Re are late and early rings and T are trophozoites. C. Same as B but luminescence replaces fluorescence; E and S represent the solutes erythritol and sorbitol and the subscripts R and P represent the erythrocyte and parasite-associated ATP. D. as in B.

Using isoosmotic solutions of various permeant solutes, one can follow the kinetics of hemolysis caused by solute (and water) ingress. This is done by measuring release of either hemoglobin (8) or ATP (10) from the host compartment into the medium. Differences in rate of hemolysis induced by solutes, usually represent differences in transport rates through the red cell membrane, provided the solutes are impermeant to parasites. However, for solutes which also permeate the parasite at rates comparable or faster than into the red cell, their different volume of distribution in the infected cell could affect the measurement of transport rate by up to a factor of two, at the most. Entry of solute into the parasite can also be followed by continuous mesurement of the released ATP by solute-induced hemolysis(10). Using tracers such as radioactively labeled (11) or fluorescent labeled (9) substances, one can also follow either their influx or efflux properties and obtain the transport kinetic parameters of the respective system(s). However, as some substances might be also permeant to the parasite, and some might even be modified by them chemically, it would need to be shown for each individual substance, that the actual rate determining step measured is associated with transport across the red cell membrane.

An additional problem often encountered with in vitro parasitized red cells, is the presence of various developmental stages, even in synchronized cultures. Since the relative activities of different solutes can also change with intracellular parasite development, it is therefore difficult to do quantitative comparisons of permeation data which are obtained with different cultures.

RESULTS and DISCUSSION

Biophysical properties of the new permeation pathways

Increased transport across the host cell membrane of parasitized cells was observed for a variety of solutes which range from polyols, inorganic and organic acids to a variety of amino acids (14). Attempts have been made to elucidate whether a single pathway or multiple pathways are involved in the permeabilization of the host cell membrane. On the basis of earlier studies of isoosmotic hemolysis using polyols, it was suggested that pores with an equivalent radius of 7 A° could accomodate the permeation of most solutes tested (14). Support for the pore-like mechanism was obtained from patch clamp studies of parasitized cells which indicated the presence of large conductance channels which were specific for anions (Stutzin and Cabantchik, unpublished observations) and from transport studies conducted with anionic probes (9,15). These studies also indicated that the pore-like structures were detectable about 6 hours after invasion of the red cell by Plasmodium falciparum, and that their number increased with intracellular development from a value of a few dozens per cell at the ring stage to a few hundred per cell at the trophozoite stage. The discriminatory capacity of these pathways for anions versus cations and for polyols of up to a given size, indicated that permeabilization was of a specific nature. As these pathways were blocked by amino reactive reagents, it was suggested that they beared positively charged groups which could confer the above discriminatory properties between anions and cations (15). The sites of action of the amino acid blocker was found to be on the cytoplasmic surface of the cell, thus requiring permeation of the blocker for inhibitory action.

However, more recent biophysical analysis of the pathways based on data obtained with the same methodology, but encompassing a considerably larger number of solutes, including amino acids, indicated that all the available permeation data could not be fitted to a single pore-like mechanism (17)(Figure 4). This conclusion is probably correct, despite the fact that the analysis was based entirely on data obtained with the isoosmotic lysis technique, which, as indicated above , provides only a semiquantitative measure for solute transport across the red cell membrane of the infected cell. Moreover, the solutes which showed anomalous behavior in terms of the pore model were all zitterionic amino acids (Figure 4). This would indicate either that the model is incorrect, thus requiring adoption of an alternative model or that the data obtained with amino acids might not be strictly comparable with those of polyols because of differences in charges between the two classes of substrates, in physicochemical properties of the isoosmotic solutions of both types of substrates and in the radii of the permeating forms of the solutes. A rather more appropiate model which could accomodate the data obtained with all the above solutes (17), but not organic acids (Silfen and Cabantchik, unpublished observations), was based on solute permeation which is determined by partitioning into an area of the

membrane which bears a character of a protein-lipid
mesophase (17).

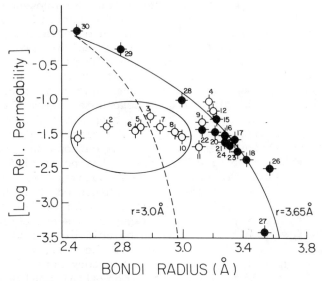

Figure 4. Fitting of transport data to the Renkin
model of diffusion through pores (16). Data adapted from
refs. 14 and 17 are given in terms of permeability
constants relative to 30-thiourea, the numbers denoting the
values for the solutes used. Amino acids (empty circles):1-
gly; 2-ala; 3-val; 4-ileu; 5-cys; 5-se; 7-thr; 8-asp; 9-
glu; 10-asn; 11-gln; 12-his. Polyols (filled circles): 135
arabitol; 16-xylitol; 17-sorbitol; 18-dulcitol; 19-ribose;
20-deoxyglucose; 21-rhamnose; 22-arabinose; 23-mannitol;
24-D-glucose; 26-sedoheptulose; 27-myoinositol; 28-
erythritol; 29-glycerol.

This was assumed to be conferred by parasite-derived
proteins interacting with red cell lipids . A third model
which could also fit all the transport data available
assumes both, specific pores induced by parasites and some
less-pecific diffusion pathways in the membrane, which
could result from changes in protein or lipid domains
generated either directly by parasite components or caused
indirectly by destabilization of the red cell cytoskeleton.
While the pore would allow passage of a variety of
hydrophilic substances, the other could also accomodate
most hydrophobic solutes. Selective inhibition of the
pore-activity by bioflavonoid-glycosides are among the

pieces of evidence which support that model.

Biochemical properties of the pores

In order to study the expression of the new pathways as a result of de novo protein synthesis, cycloheximide was added to a synchronous culture of rings (ca. 12 hrs after invasion) and the activity of the pores studied as a function of incubation time in culture conditions. Data shown in Figure 5 shows that cycloheximide blocked the appearence of the pores, commensurate with the arrest of protein synthesis. They suggest that the generation of the pathways was not a result of a catalytic modification of preexisting membrane entities, but most probably was a result of deposition of new membrane polypeptides. This study also indicates that the level of expression attained before addition of the protein synthesis inhibitor, was mantained throughout the period of incubation in which cycloheximide was present in the medium.

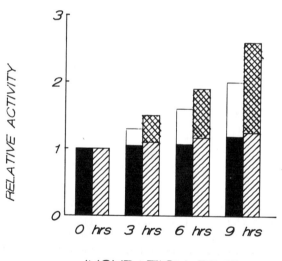

Figure 5.   Rings (10% parasitemia) obtained from synchronized cultures (12 hrs. after invasion) were exposed to cycloheximide (5 μg/ml) at zero time and tested either for transport (isoosmotic sorbitol) (filled and empty bars) or [^{3}H]ileu incorporation into TCA precipitable material (slashed and crossed bars). Data are given in terms of activities relative to those of controls at time zero.

Attempts to reveal the chemical identity of the pores relied on derivatives of phlorizin (Figure 6), an agent which has previously been shown to block the pathways and arrest parasite growth with similar efficacy (18)[1].

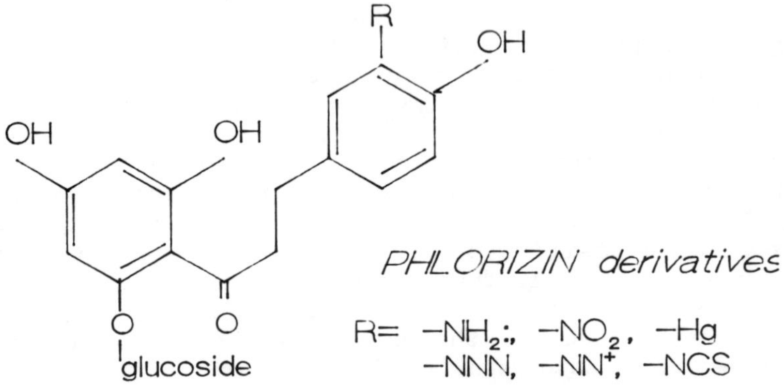

PHLORIZIN derivatives

R= $-NH_2$:, $-NO_2$, $-Hg$
$-NNN$, $-NN^+$, $-NCS$

Figure 6. Structure of phlorizin and various derivatized analogs.

Phlorizin analogs tested for their transport blocking capacity were analyzed in terms of structure-activity relationship (SAR) schemes (8). It was found , that the electron withdrawing capacity of the substituting group (Hammett's constant) was a determining factor for inhibitory action of these agents (Figure 7).

The most potent analog which also had an electrophilic group with covalent binding capacity, was the NCS derivative (ITC-phlorizin). When cells were exposed to the reagent first in a salt balanced medium supplemented with glucose and subsequently transferred to growth medium, this agent inhibited parasite growth with IC_{50} of 8 μM and the transport pathways (sorbitol) with an IC_{50} of 3 μM .

[1] The "antimalarial action" of phlorizin quoted in the Merck Index (1968/ 8th Edition or ealier) was credited to the discoverer of phlorizin for the notion that " because of its bitter-like properties", phlorizin is likely to be useful as many other antimalarial remedies".

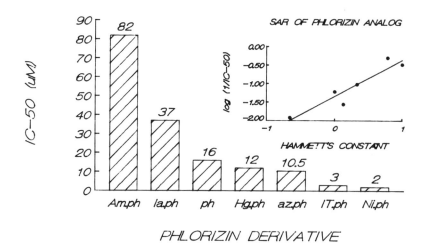

PHLORIZIN DERIVATIVE

Figure 7. The IC$_{50}$ (µM) of various phlorizin analogs on sorbitol-mediated hemolysis are given on the top of each column and SAR is given in the inset (8). ph refers to phlorizin and others are referred as: Am=amino; Ia=acetamido;IT=isothiocyano; az=azido; Ni=nitro and Hg.

When the agent was reacted first with trophozoites for 20 min. at 37°C and subsequently washed off, the respective IC$_{50}$'s obtained for growth and transport were between 5-10 fold higher than those obtained in the presence of the drug. Phlorizin, in those conditions, was more than 90% reversible as a blocker of the pathway and as an antimalarial.

Phlorizin derivatives were also used to discern between multiple transport systems induced by the parasites. As demonstrated in Figure 8, the IC$_{50}$ values for different substrates span more than two orders of magnitude: for cys, the values were higher than 500 µM, while for the hydrophobic amino acids they were in the 40-70 µM range and for the hydrophilic amino acids and polyols they were in the lower µM range. When present in solution during the flux measurement, the NCS derivative was 2-5 fold more inhibitory to transport of all the hydrophilic solutes than phlorizin itself, while for the more hydrophobic solutes , differences in potency between the two derivatives were between 1.2-1.5 fold.

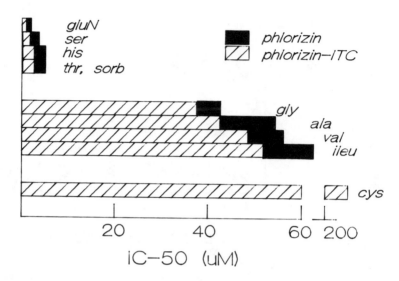

Figure 8. The inhibitory potency of phlorizin and its isothiocyano (ITC) derivative on solute-induced hemolysis. gluN refers to glutamine and sorb to sorbitol.

This clearly demonstrates that the different substrates utilize different routes of entry into parasitized cells , rather than they all utilize the same pathways but are affected differentially by the inhibitors. Although the latter possibility can not be completely excluded, several pieces of information support the former explanation. First, the inhibitory effect of either phlorizin or ITC-phlorizin appear to be non-competitive inasmuch as similar inhibitory effects were obtained after an initial exposure of the agent in the absence or presence of substrate (not shown). Second, the inhibition of the transport of hydrophilic solutes is associated with a maximum of 1,000 phlorizin binding sites per cell, all probably endofacial as revealed with radioactively labeled phlorizin (8,18). At this level of binding there is almost no effect on the transport of the hydrophobic solutes, cys or organic acids. Only at higher concentrations of phlorizin, there are detectable levels of inhibition of hydrophobic solute transport.

At present, the <u>modus operandii</u> of the phlorizins on the permeation pathways is not clear, except that the aspects of the pores which are blocked by them are endofacial and that the putative amino acid residues tagged by the reagent are lysines, due to the specificity of the NCS moiety for that group and in analogy with previous results obtained with NCS derivatives of disulfonic stilbenes (15). Because of the scarcety of binding sites per infected cell which precludes the use of radioactively labeled phlorizin or ITC-phlorizin for identification purposes, we have developed efficient anti-phlorizin antibodies using ITC-phlorizin derivatized thyroglobulin as macrmolecular carrier. Present aims are directed at the identification of the ITC-phlorizin putative targets in the membrane of the malaria infected cell which are chemically modified by the reagent.

Pharmacological properties of the pores

The possibility was considered of using the pores either as targets for pharmacological agents or as routes for specific delivery of drugs into malaria infected cells. Desferral, a typical antimalarial agent which affects parasite growth by chelating intracellular iron, gains access into infected cells but not into normal cells (19). Phlorizin and phlorizin-like agents showed relatively high efficacy as inhibitors of parasite development and specificity for malaria infected cells in in vitro cultures of erythrocytes. Their antimalarial action is apparently of a bimodal nature, affecting both componentes in the host membrane and in the parasite as well. Because of the glycosidic moiety, phlorizin is impermeant to normal red cells as well as to a variety of other cells (20). However, the agents are demonstrable permeant to infected cells, probably through the same pores they eventually block, that is after reaching inhibitory concentrations within the infected cell (Figure 1, ref. 8). In order to test the hypothesis of phlorizin inhibition at the parasite level, the agent was added to trophozoites whose host cell membrane were permeabilized with Sendai virus, but whose protein synthetic capacity was largely retained (8). Phlorizin inhibited protein synthesis in permeabilized cells, although with 1/3 to 1/2 the efficiency observed in intact infected cells. Similar differences in inhibitory potency on intact as compared to permeabilized cells, were also observed with desferral and with chloroquine (to be published). The studies strongly suggest that the inhibitory effect of phlorizin in intact cells can be attributed to interference with vital functions associated with the host cell membrane, i.e. transport. However, if sufficient agent can gain access to the host cytosol ,

additional effects on the parasite might ensue.   The
alternative hypothesis , that the agents affect directly
host cell cytosolic components but indirectly affect the
parasite, can not be discarded at the present stage.
      Finally, phlorizin is known to be toxic to mammals
due to blockage of Na/glucose cotransport mechanisms in
kidney and gut (20). However, other structural congeners of
this agent, like cosmetin and nitrophlorizin, have
substantially lower "side-effects" on these transport
mechanisms, but retain both their antimalarial and pore
blocking activity (8). This raises the prospects of using
these "permselective drugs" and blockers of parasite-
induced transport sytems as potential antimalarial agents.

REFERENCES

1.   Passow H (1988) Molecular apects of band 3 protein-
     mediated anion transport across the red blood cell
     membrane. Rev Physiol Biochem Pharamcol 103:62.
2.   Stein WD (1985) "Transport and diffusion across cell
     membranes". London, New York: Academic Press.
3.   Sherman IW (1984). Metabolism. In Peters W, Richard
     WHG (eds): " Handbook of Experimental Pharmacology",
     Berlin-Heidelberg: Springer-Verlag, p31..
4.   Sherman IW. (1985). Membrane structure and function of
     malaria parasites and the infected ertyrocyte.
     Parasitology 91:609.
5.   Sherman IW (1988). Mechanisms of molecular trafficing
     in malaria. Parasitology 96:557.
6.   Ginsburg M, Stein WD (1987). New permeability pathways
     induced by the malarial parasite in the membrane of
     its host erythrocyte: potential routes for targeting
     drugs into infected cells. Biosc Rep 7:455.
7.   Cabantchik, ZI, Kutner S, Krugliak M, Ginsburg H
     (1982). Anion transport inhibitors as supressors of P.
     falciparum growth in in vitro cultures. Mol Pharmacol
     23:92.
8.   Silfen J, Yanai P, Cabantchik ZI (1988). Bioflavonoid
     effects on in vitro cultures of P. falciparum:
     inhibition of permeation pathways induced in the host
     cell membrane by the intraerthrocytic parasite.
     Biochem Pharmacol 37: 4269.
9.   Kutner S, Brener WV, Ginsburg H, Alex SB, Cabantchik
     ZI (1985). Characterization of permeation pathways in
     the plasma membrane of human erythrocytes infected
     with early stages of P. falciparum. Association with

parasite development. J Cell Physiol 125:521.

10. Kanaani J, Ginsburg H (1988). Compartment analysis of ATP in malaria-infected erythrocytes. Biochem Intern 17:451.

11. Elford BC, Haynes JD, Chulay JD, Wilson RJM (1985). Selective shape-specific changes in the permeability to small hydrophilic solutes of human erythrocytes infected with P. falciparum. Molec Biochem Parasitol 16:43.

12. Bitouti AJ, Sjoes-dsma A, McCann PP, Kyle DE, Oduola AMJ, Rossan RN, Milhous WK, Davidson, DE Jr (1988). Reversal of chloroquine resistance in malaria parasite P. falciparum by Desipramine. Science 242:1301.

13. Gero AM, Bugledich EMA, Paterson ARP, Jamieson GP (1988). Stage specific alteration of nucleoside membrane permeability and nitrobenzylthioinosine insensitivity in P. falciparum infected erythrocytes. Molec Biochem Parasitol 27:159.

14. Ginsburg H, Kutner S, Zangwil M, Cabantchik ZI (1986b). Selectivity properties of pores induced in host erthrocyte membrane by P. falciparum. Effect of parasite maturation. Biochim Biophys Acta 861:194.

15. Breuer WV, Kutner S, Silfer J, Ginsburg H, Cabantchik ZI (1987). Covalent modification of the permeability pathways induced in the human ertyrocyte membranes by the malarial parasite P. falciparum. J Cell Physiol 133:55.

16. Renkin EM (1954). Filtration, diffusion and molecular seiving through porous cellulose membranes. J Gen Physiol 38:225.

17. Ginsburg H, Stein WD (1987). Biophysical analysis of novel transport pathways induced in red blood cell membranes. J. Membr Biol 96:1.

18. Kutner S, Breuer WV, Ginsburg H, Cabantchik ZI (1987). On the mode of action of phlorizin as an antimalarial agent in in vitro cultures of P. falciparum. Biochem Pharmacol 36:123.

19. Fritsch G, Jung A (1986). ^{14}C-desferrioxamine B: Uptake into erythrocytes infected with P. falciparum. Z Parasitenk 72:709.

20. Semenza G, Kessler M, Hosang M, Weber J, Schmidt U (1984). Biochemistry of the Na^+,D-glucose cotransporter of the small intestinal brush - border membrane. The state of the art in 1984. Biochim Biophys Acta 779:343.

**Cellular and Molecular Biology of Normal
and Abnormal Erythroid Membranes, pages 283–299
© 1990 Alan R. Liss, Inc.**

A MODIFIED BAND 3 PROTEIN, EXPRESSED ON THE SURFACE OF ERYTHROCYTES INFECTED WITH A KNOBBY LINE OF PLASMODIUM FALCIPARUM (HUMAN MALARIA), IS INVOLVED IN CYTOADHERENCE

I. W. Sherman, E. Winograd

Department of Biology, University of California
Riverside, California 92521

ABSTRACT Infections with the human malaria Plasmodium falciparum are characterized by the retention of parasitized erythrocytes in tissue capillaries and venules. Erythrocytes containing trophozoites and schizonts attach to the endothelial cells which line these vessels by means of ultrastructurally identifiable excrescences present on the surface of the infected cell. Such excrescences, commonly called knobs, are visible by means of scanning or transmission electron-microscopy. The biochemical mechanisms responsible for erythrocyte adherence to the endothelial cell are still undefined. In an attempt to identify the cytoadhesive molecule on the surface of the infected red cell we have prepared monoclonal antibodies to knob-bearing erythrocytes. One of these, monoclonal antibody 4A3, is an IgM that reacts (by means of immunofluorescence) with the surface of erythrocytes bearing mature parasites of a knobby line, and does not react with a knobless line. By immunoelectronmicroscopy 4A3 was localized to the knob region; in an in vitro cytoadherence assay the antibody blocked binding of knob-bearing cells to formalin-fixed amelanotic melanoma cells. 4A3 was used to immunoprecipitate a protein from extracts of knobby erythrocytes which had been previously surface iodinated. The antigen recognized by 4A3 had an Mr of 85 kDa. Peptide mapping suggests the 85 kDa antigen is homologous to band 3.

INTRODUCTION

As early as 1890 Bignami and Bastianelli (1) observed that during a P. falciparum infection only erythrocytes containing ring forms were present in the peripheral circulation, and trophozoite and schizont-infected red cells were conspicuously absent from the peripheral blood. Autopsy examination of fatal cases of P. falciparum malaria demonstrated the presence of trophozoite and schizont-infected red cells in the post-capillary venules of various body organs. Thus, the absence of the more mature stages of P. falciparum in the blood is due to the attachment of red cells bearing these stages to the venular endothelium, a phenomenon called sequestration. Animal studies have shown that the major deep tissue sites favored by P. falciparum for completion of asexual development are the heart, spleen, and skeletal muscles, and in humans the placenta of primigravada and the cerebral blood vessels (especially in acute infections) are also affected.

Erythrocytes containing trophozoites and schizonts attach to the post-capillary venular endothelium by means of excrescences present on the surface of infected erythrocytes (2,3,4). These excrescences, commonly called 'knobs', are visible by means of scanning (5,6) and transmission electron microscopy (7,3), and consist of an electron dense plaque underlying an elevation of the plasma membrane of the red cell. It has been suggested (8,9) that through the phenomenon of sequestration the intraerythrocytic parasite is able to evade destruction by spleen filtering mechanisms, and in this way the schizont can release merozoites to initiate another erythrocytic cycle of development. Since parasitized erythrocytes sequester in organs where the oxygen tension is lowest, and in vitro studies have indicated that low oxygen tensions favor parasite development (10), it is possible that this withdrawal from the blood is of benefit to the developing malarial parasite. Speculation aside, the attachment of P. falciparum-infected erythrocytes to the post-capillary venular endothelium undoubtedly impedes blood flow in those organs where sequestration takes place, and in the brain capillaries occlusion and endothelial cell damage are surely contributing factors to the pathogenesis of cerebral malaria (11,12). Indeed, Raventos-Suarez et al. (13) showed (using an ex vivo rat microcirculatory preparation) that knobs were indispensable for generating the circulatory obstruction, and that adherence was confined to endothelial cells lining the venule surface. It was their view that although knobs are sufficient for adherence, there is reason to believe that attachment also involves specific endothelial binding sites, and that splenic and plasma factors could modulate the interaction.

In addition to the phenomenon of sequestration of red cells infected with mature asexual parasites gametocyte-bearing red cells also undergo a portion of their development in the deep tissues. Mature gametocytes present in erythrocytes circulate freely, but the smaller growing gametocyte withdraws from the peripheral blood (14). The knoblike protrusions present on the surface of a red cell bearing a trophozoite or a schizont cannot explain the sequestration of an erythrocyte containing an immature gametocyte since knobs are completely absent from both immature and mature gametocytes. The presence of knobs in and of itself is also insufficient to define a functional binding site for sequestration since in some malarias i.e. P. malariae and P. brasilianum, the infected erythrocytes have knobs but in these species the infected cells do not sequester.

Several laboratories have correlated the presence of a parasite-synthesized high molecular weight protein with knobby cytoadherent lines of P. falciparum (15). This parasite-encoded protein, called Plasmodium falciparum erythrocyte membrane protein 1 (PfEMP1), has neither been isolated nor has its function been unequivocally demonstrated. There are also indications that the intraerythrocytic malaria parasite is able to alter the surface of the red cell by modifying existing host cell proteins. For example, Winograd et al. (16) showed that during the development of knobs there was a significant increase in the binding of IgG, and that the immunoglobulin was preferentially bound to the elevated region of the knob. The antigen recognized by the IgG appeared to be related to band 3, the anion transporter of the erythrocyte, since naturally occurring autoantibody to band 3 was found to bind to knobby red cells which had previously been stripped of their autologous IgG.

Evidence for modifications of band 3 in a knobby line of P. falciparum was also found in freeze fracture, immunocytochemical and lectin binding studies. Allred et al. (17) showed that in the protoplasmic leaflet of the membrane there was no increase in the number of intramembranous particles in the erythrocyte during knob formation, but specific and characteristic rearrangements of such particles did take place. Moreover, during parasite maturation from trophozoite to schizont there was a tendency for the distribution of IMP sizes in the region of the knob to be shifted toward smaller sized particles relative to that of the uninfected red cell. Sherman and Greenan (18) reported that in distinct contrast to the uniform distribution of ferritin particles seen on the surface of knobby infected red cells with ricin, wheat germ agglutinin and Limax flavus lectins, were clusters of ferritin-concanavalin A (Con-A). Typically, only 10-15% of the knobs showed such ferritin-Con A clusters. (Band 3 protein is the primary constituent of the intramembranous particle and also contains the binding site for con A.) Using immunoelectronmicroscopy we found that band 3 (as well as glycophorin and spectrin) were aggregated in the area of the knob, whereas the remainder of the red cell showed no such clustering (19).

The present work builds on these earlier findings and suggests that modifications of band 3, in the region of the knob, may play a role in cytoadherence.

MATERIALS AND METHODS

The FCR-3 strain (African) of P. falciparum was cultured according to the methods of Trager and Jensen (20).

Monoclonal antibodies were produced against live infected cells, and screened by immunofluorescence (21).

The methods of iodination of red cells and immunoprecipitation have been described earlier (21).

Band 3 was isolated following the methods of Drickamer (22) and the cytoplasmic domain (TR-41) and the chymotryptic fragments (CH-17 and CH-35) were prepared as described by Appel and Low (23) and Fukuda et al. (24) respectively. Two dimensional iodopeptide maps of isolated proteins were made according to Elder et al. (25) and Markowitz and Marchesi (26).

RESULTS

A detailed analysis of knobs on the surface of P. falciparum-infected erythrocytes by scanning electron microscopy (6) showed that when infected cells contained trophozoites knobs were sparse and the diameter of the knob

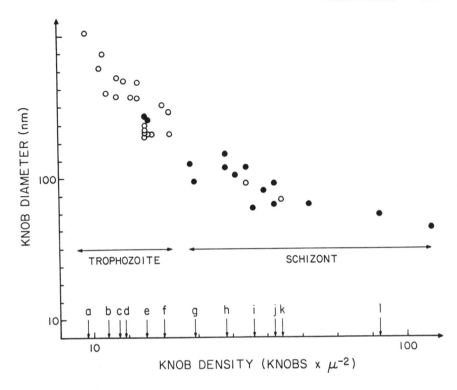

FIGURE 1.   Variation of knob size and density.   Knob diameter (y-axis) and density (x-axis) were determined for a dozen erythrocytes.   (Reproduced by courtesy of the Journal of Cell Biology.)

ranged from 110-160 nm, whereas when the parasites were fully mature schizonts the knobs were more numerous and their diameter was smaller, ranging from 70-100 nm (Figure 1).   Knobs did not appear to be produced continuously during asexual development of the parasite, and there was the implication that knob production increased during the later stages of parasite growth.   Knobs also did not appear to be randomly distributed over the surface of the infected red cell, and frequently knobs were arranged in rows, circles, etc.   Such patterns, more obvious on cells bearing trophozoites suggested that knobs may have been produced in specific domains of the membrane.   Further, the dynamic process of knob formation gave the impression that cytoskeletal components may have been involved in the reorganization-redistribution of membrane constituents.

Changes in the distribution, but not the number, of intramembranous particles (IMP) was found to be associated with parasite maturation (Figure 2). When there was minimal elevation of the red cell membrane a focal IMP cluster was seen; when the membrane was further elevated a central cluster of IMP surrounded by an IMP-free zone and a concentric ring of IMPs was seen; with maximal elevation there was an apparent loss of IMP organization.

The monoclonal antibody 4A3, an IgM, identified a newly exposed antigen on the surface of the live knobby P. falciparum infected red cell (Figure 3). This monoclonal antibody did not react by immunofluorescence with live uninfected red cells or erythrocytes infected with a knobless (K-) line. By immunoelectronmicroscopy the antibody was found to be localized to the elevated portions of the knob itself, and not the intervening regions of the membrane (21).

The monoclonal antibody 4A3 immunoprecipitated an 85 kDa protein from infected red cells that had been previously surface iodinated and extracted with SDS (Figure 4). This antigen was not found in Triton X-100 extracts of surface iodinated infected cells.

Based on our observation that the monoclonal antibody 4A3 recognized band 3 in Triton X-100 extracts made from noninfected erythrocytes and because of the binding of the 85 kD antigen to concanavalin A (Winograd, E. and I. W. Sherman, unpublished observations) the possibility that this antigen might be structurally related to the human red cell anion transporter, band 3, was explored. Comparisons between these two proteins were carried out by means of two-dimensional peptide maps (Figure 5). Examination of the maps revealed a striking similarity between these two proteins despite the reduced number (40%) of spots for the 85 kD protein. All of the spots in the 85 kD map had a correspondent spot in the band 3 map. This result strongly suggested that the 85 kD was either derived from band 3, or that its amino acid sequence was very similar to that of band 3. To gain a better understanding of the structural differences between the 85 kD antigen and band 3, each of the major band 3 fragments--cytoplasmic (TR-41) and the two membrane-associated domains (CH-17 and CH-35)--were isolated, and two-dimensional peptide maps of each were prepared (Figure 5). This information was then used to determine the correspondence of each spot in the band 3 map

(Continued on page 293)

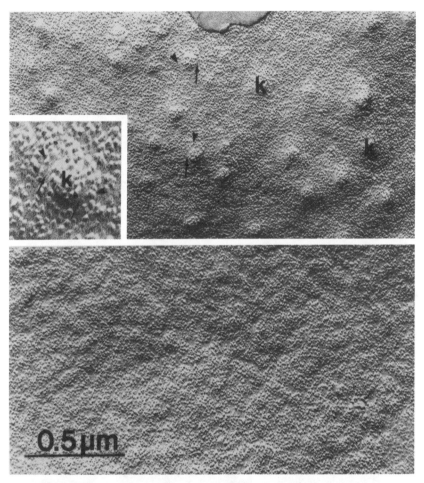

FIGURE 2. Protoplasmic fracture face (PF) of infected
and uninfected red cells; x60,000. Upper--Trophozoite-
infected cell; inset (x200,000) shows the substructure of a
stage (2) knob. Lower--Uninfected erythrocyte. k, knobs;
arrows, IMP-free zone; arrowheads, organized IMP ring.
Platinum-carbon shadowing direction is from the bottom in
all cases. Bar, 0.5 µm. (Reproduced by courtesy of the
Journal of Cell Science.)

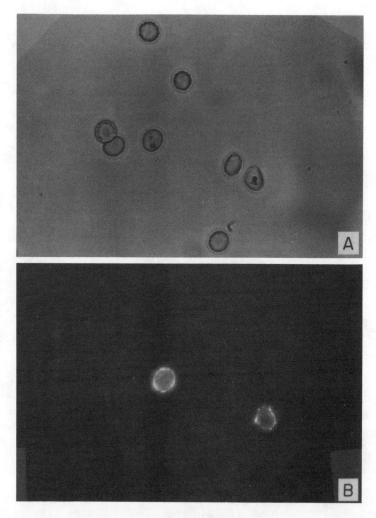

FIGURE 3. Specificity of 4A3 monoclonal antibody. Binding of 4A3 monoclonal antibody to erythrocytes infected with a knobby variant of the FCR-3 strain of P. falciparum by means of an immunofluorescence assay. (A) Phase-contrast microscopy. (B) Same field under fluorescent light. Note that only the two malaria-infected erythrocytes fluoresce. Bars, 8.0 μm. (Reproduced by courtesy of the Journal of Cell Biology.)

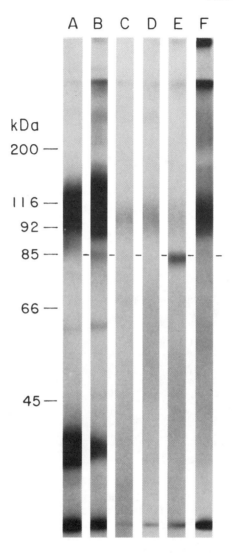

FIGURE 4. Autoradiographic analysis of immunoprecipitates generated by 4A3 monoclonal antibody. The molecular
specificity of 4A3 was studied by incubating the monoclonal
antibody with ^{125}I-labeled membrane proteins extracted with
Triton X-100 or SDS from surface-iodinated red cells.
Isolation of immune complexes was carried out by means of
protein A-Sepharose previously coated with anti-mouse IgM
(see Materials and Methods). Antigens were analyzed by

(Continued on page 292)

292   Sherman and Winograd

running 10-15% linear gradient SDS-acrylamide gels containing mercaptoethanol followed by autoradiography. (Lane
A) triton extract of surface-iodinated infected red cells;
(lane B) SDS extract of surface-iodinated infected red
cells; (landes C and D) immunoprecipitates of the Triton
X-100 extract using 4A3 monoclonal antibody and TEPC 183,
respectively; (lanes E and F) immunoprecipitates of the SDS
extract using 4A3 monoclonal antibody and TEPC 1983,
respectively. Note that only the 4A3 monoclonal antibody
recognized the 85 kD antigen. (Reproduced by courtesy of
the Journal of Cell Biology.)

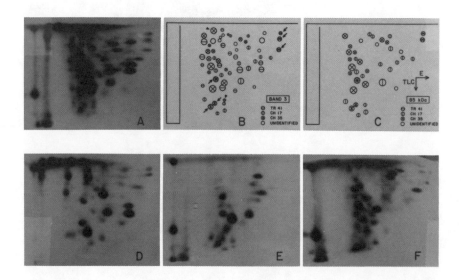

FIGURE 5. Structural analysis of the 85 kD antigen.
(B) Diagrammatic representation showing the assignment of
each proteolytic fragment in the band 3 map (A) to one of
the major band 3 domains; the cytoplasmic domain TR-41 (D),
and the two membrane-associated domains, CH-17 (E) and
CH-35 (F). The origin of some peptide spots could not be
determined unambiguously; arrows indicate peptides with
either dual or triple identity. Analysis of the peptide
map of the 85 kD antigen (C) reveals that most or all of
the TR-41 fragment is absent; a small deletion at the CH-35
domain may have also occurred since two peptide spots were
absent (arrowheads in B). (Reproduced by courtesy of the
Journal of Cell Biology).

to each band 3 fragment; i.e., TR-41, CH-35, or CH-17. With few exceptions, all of the spots could be related to one of the band 3 fragments (Figure 5B). Comparison of the band 3 peptide map with the 85 kD map showed that most or all of the TR-41 cytoplasmic domain was absent from the 85 kD antigen; two spots that corresponded to the CH-35 fragment were also missing; therefore, it appeared that a small deletion at the carboxy-terminal end of band 3 may also have occurred (Figure 5C).

The monoclonal antibody partially blocked (~50%) the adherence of infected cells to formalin-fixed amelanotic melanoma cells (Table 1).

TABLE 1
INHIBITION OF INFECTED RED BLOOD CELL (IRBC, FCR-3 STRAIN) BINDING TO FORMALIN FIXED AMELANOTIC MELANOMA TARGET CELLS BY THE MONOCLONAL ANTIBODY 4A3.

	IRBC/100 target cells	% inhibition
Experiment 1		
PBS	1000	--
4A3	600	40
TEPC 183	1000	0
Experiment 2		
PBS	900	--
4A3	200	78
Experiment 3		
PBS	61	--
4A3 (Lot DM)	37	40
4A3 (Lot 3)	40	33
TEPC 183	65	0

See (21) for description of cytoadherence assay.

DISCUSSION AND CONCLUSIONS

The reports of Leech et al. (27), Howard (15) and Magowan et al. (28) provide evidence for a family of high molecular weight proteins which are present on the surface of the knobby P. falciparum-infected red cell, and are correlated with cytoadherence. The members of this protein family, though they differ in antigenicity and molecular size amongst the various strains studied, did have several features in common including accessibility to surface iodination, solubility in SDS but not Triton X-100, and susceptibility to trypsin concentrations which abolish cytoadherence. In the recent report of Magowan et al. (28) it was not demonstrated that these proteins were metabolically labelled (i.e. encoded by the parasite), however, earlier studies (27,29) did find that proteins of similar molecular size incorporated ^{35}S methionine and ^{14}C isoleucine. By contrast, we have identified an 85 kDa membrane protein that is structurally related to the red cell membrane protein, band 3. We base our conclusions for the structural similarity on: (a) two-dimensional peptide maps, (b) cross-reactivity of naturally occurring anti-band 3 antibodies for the 85 kD antigen (Winograd, E. and I. W. Sherman, manuscript in preparation), (c) concanavalin A binding to the 85 kD antigen (Winograd, E. and I. W. Sherman, unpublished results), and (d) the binding of 4A3 to band 3 in Triton X-100 extracts made from noninfected erythrocytes (Winograd, E. and I. W. Sherman, unpublished results). Importantly, a monoclonal antibody to this 85 kDa antigen partially blocked cytoadherence.

Assuming that the molecular mass of band 3 protein is ~90 kD, then cleavage of the 41 kD cytoplasmic domain from band 3 would be insufficient to explain the formation of an 85 kD protein. It is possible, therefore, that the 85 kD antigen is derived from the covalent nondisulfide bonding between two band 3 monomers, each of which lacks the cytoplasmic domain. Were this the case then our inability to detect reactivity (by immunoprecipitation) of anti-band 3 antisera specific for the cytoplasmic domain of band 3 (30) towards the 85 kD antigen would be explained (Winograd, E. and I. W. Sherman, unpublished observations).

How might the 85 kDa antigen arise? During the intracellular development of the parasite there is a dramatic increase in the levels of Ca^{2+} in the P. falciparum infected red cell; in one report, with a parasitemia of 60%, the Ca^{2+} level was increased 10-fold over that of normal red cells (reviewed in 31). The elevation of intracellular levels of Ca^{2+} in erythrocytes leads to a degradation of the cytoplasmic portion of band 3 and glycophorin due to a calcium-activated protease, called calpain (32). This calcium-dependent proteinase cleaves band 3 at the N-terminal cytoplasmic/membrane interface leaving the intramembranous portion of band 3 intact. Were such an activation to take place in the region of the knob then truncation of band 3 would result. The accumulation of Ca^{2+} by normal human red cells may also result in the formation of high molecular weight membrane proteins.

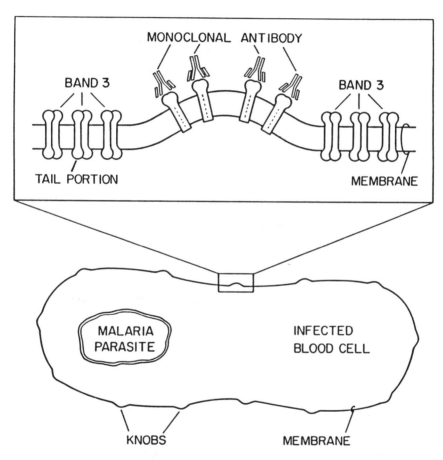

FIGURE 6. Schematic representation of the formation of the 85 kDa antigen in the region of the knob which is recognized by the monoclonal antibody 4A3.

These polymers are heterogeneous in size, and rich in γ-

glutamyl-ε-lysine crosslinks. The formation of such polymers is due to a calcium-activated transglutaminase that
catalyzes the formation of ε-(γ-glutamyl) lysine linkages
between glutaminyl and lysyl residues. Analysis of the
polymers by crossed immunoelectrophoresis indicated that
they were composed of spectrin, band 3 and ankyrin (33).

Thus, we hypothesize that truncation of band 3 is due
to a calcium-activated protease, and when the truncated
band 3 molecules are no longer linked to the cytoskeletal
framework, they are able to redistribute themselves in the
plane of the membrane. And, by a transglutaminase catalyzed linkage of truncated band 3 molecules in the knob
region there is the exposure of a new 85 kDa antigen
(Figure 6) which is in some way involved in cytoadherence.

REFERENCES

1. Bignami A, Bastianelli G (1890). Osservazioni sulle
   febbri malariche estive-autunnali. La Riforma Medica
   223(6):1334-1335.
2. Miller LH (1972). The ultrastructure of red cells
   infected by Plasmodium falciparum in man. Transactions
   of the Royal Society of Tropical Medicine and Hygiene
   66(3):459-462.
3. Aikawa M (1977). Variations in structure and function
   during the life cycle of malarial parasite. Bull WHO
   55:139-156.
4. Aikawa M, Miller L (1983). Structural alteration of
   the erythrocyte membrane during malarial parasite
   invasion and intraerythrocytic development. Ciba
   Foundation Symposium 94:45-63.
5. Aikawa M, Rabbege JR, Udeinya I, Miller LH (1983).
   Electron microscopy of knobs in Plasmodium falciparum-
   infected erythrocytes. J Parasit 69:435-437.
6. Gruenberg J, Allred DR, Sherman IW (1983). Scanning
   electron microscope-analysis of the protrusions
   (knobs) present on the surface of Plasmodium
   falciparum-infected erythrocytes. J Cell Biol
   97:795-802.
7. Langreth SG, Motyl MR, Trager W (1979). Plasmodium
   falciparum: loss of knobs on the infected erythrocyte
   surface after long term cultivation. Exp Parasit
   48:213-219.
8. Schmidt-Ullrich R, et al (1982). Immunogenic antigens
   common to Plasmodium knowlesi and Plasmodium falci-

parum are expressed on the surface of infected erythrocytes. J Parasit 68(2):185-193.

9. Howard RJ, Barnwell JW (1984). Roles of surface antigens on malaria infected red blood cells in evasion of immunity. Contemporary Topics in Immunobiology 12:127-200.
10. Scheibel LW, Ashton SH, Trager W (1979). Plasmodium falciparum: Microaerophilic requirements in human red blood cells. Exptl Parasit 47:410-418.
11. MacPherson GG, Warrell MJ, White NJ, Looareesuwan S, Warrell DA (1985). Human cerebral malaria: a quantitative ultrastructural analysis of parasitized erythrocyte sequestration. Am J Pathol 119:385-401.
12. Pongponratin E, Riganti M, Harinasuta T, Bunnag D (1985). Electron microscopy of the human brain in cerebral malaria. So Asian J Trop Med Pub Health 16(2):219-227.
13. Raventos-Suarez C, Kaul DK, Maculuso F, Nagel RL (1985). Membrane knobs are required for the microcirculatory obstruction induced by Plasmodium flaciparum-infected erythrocytes. Proc Nat Acad Sci USA 82:3829-3833.
14. Smalley ME, Abdalla S, Brown J (1980). The distribution of Plasmodium falciparum in the peripheral blood and bone marrow of Gambian children. Transactions of the Royal Society of Tropical Medicine and Hygiene 75(1):103-105.
15. Howard RJ (1988). Malarial proteins at the membrane of Plasmodium falciparum-infected erythrocytes and their involvement in cytoadherence to endothelial cells. Progr Allergy 41:98-147.
16. Winograd E, Greenan J, Sherman IW (1987). Expression of senescent antigen on erythrocytes infected with a knobby variant of the human malaria parasite Plasmodium falciparum. Proc Nat Acad Sci USA 84:1931-1935.
17. Allred DR, Gruenberg JE, Sherman IW (1986). Dynamic rearrangements of erythrocyte membrane internal architecture induced by infection with Plasmodium falciparum. J Cell Biol 81:1-16.
18. Sherman IW, Greenan JRT (1986). Plasmodium falciparum: Regional differences in lectin and cationized ferritin binding to the surface of the malaria-infected human erythrocyte. Parasit 93:17-32.
19. Sherman IW, Greenan JRT, de la Vega P (1989). Immunofluorescent and immunoelectron microscopic localiza-

tion of protein antigens in red cells infected with the human malaria Plasmodium falciparum. Ann Trop Med Parasit 82:531-545.

20. Trager W, Jensen JB (1976). Human malaria parasites in continuous culture. Science (Washington, DC) 193:673-675.

21. Winograd E, Sherman IW (1989). Characterization of a modified red cell membrane protein expressed on erythrocytes infected with the human malaria parasite Plasmodium falciparum. Possible role as a cyto-adherent mediating protein. J Cell Biol 108:23-30.

22. Drickamer LK (1976). Fragmentation of the 95,000-dalton transmembrane poly-peptide in human erythrocyte membranes. J Biol Chem 251:5115-5123.

23. Appel KC, Low PS (1981). Partial characterization of the cytoplasmic domain of the erythrocyte membrane protein, band 3. J Biol Chem 256:11104-11111.

24. Fukuda M, Eshdat Y, Tarone G, Marchesi VT (1978). Isolation and characterization of peptides derived from the cytoplasmic segment of band 3, the predomi-nant intrinsic membrane protein of the human erythrocyte. J Biol Chem 253:2419-2428.

25. Elder JH, Pickett RA, Hampton J, Lerner RA (1977). Radioiodination of proteins in single polyacrylamide gel slices. J Biol Chem 252:6510-6516.

26. Markowitz S, Marchesi VT (1981). The carboxyl-terminal domain of human erythrocyte band 3. Description, iso-lation and location in the bilayer. J Biol Chem 256:6463-6368.

27. Leech JH, Barnwell JW, Miller LH, Howard RJ (1984). Identification of a strain-specific malarial antigen exposed on the surface of Plasmodium falciparum-infected erythrocytes. J Exp Med 159:1567-1575.

28. Magowan C, Wollish CV, Anderson L, Leech J (1988). Cytoadherence by Plasmodium falciparum-infected erythrocytes is correlated with the expression of a family of variable proteins on infected erythrocytes. J Exp Med 168:1307-1320.

29. Aley AB, Sherwood JA, Howard RJ (1984). Knob-positive and knob-negative Plasmodium falciparum differ in expression of a strain-specific malarial antigen on the surface of infected erythrocytes. J Exp Med 160:1585-1590.

30. Low SP (1986). Structure and function of the cytoplasmic domain of band 3: center of erythrocyte membrane-peripheral protein interactions. Biochim

Biophys Acta 864:145-167.
31. Sherman IW (1985). Membrane structure and function of malaria parasites and the infected erythrocyte. Parasit 91:609-645.
32. Au KS, Hsu L, Morrison M (1988). Ca^{2+}-mediated catabolism of human erythrocyte band 3 protein. Biochim Biophys Acta 946:113-118.
33. Bjerrum O et al (1981). An immunochemical approach for the analysis of membrane protein alterations in Ca^{2+} loaded human erythrocytes. J Supramolec Struc and Cell Biochem 16:289-301.

Cellular and Molecular Biology of Normal
and Abnormal Erythroid Membranes, pages 301–314
© 1990 Alan R. Liss, Inc.

INVASION OF ERYTHROCYTES DEFICIENT IN GLYCOPHORIN C (β,
β_1 AND γ) BY PLASMODIUM FALCIPARUM MALARIA PARASITES.

T.J. Hadley, F.W. Klotz, D.J. Anstee, J.D. Haynes,
L.H. Miller;

Division of Hematology/Oncology, University of
Louisville School of Medicine, Louisville, KY 40292;
Walter Reed Army Institute of Research, Washington, DC;
Southwestern Regional Blood Transfusion Center, Bristol,
UK; National Institutes of Health, Bethesda, MD

ABSTRACT   Previous studies showed that the Camp
strain (Southeast Asia) and the 7G8 strain
(Brazil) of P. falciparum differ in their receptor
requirements. Camp parasites rely heavily on red
cell sialic acid for invasion, whereas 7G8
parasites can invade with 50% or greater efficiency
in the absence of sialic acid. However, invasion
of sialic acid deficient erythrocytes (RBCs) (M^kM^k,
which lack glycophorins A and B, or neuraminidase-
treated RBCs) by 7G8 parasites decreases markedly
after trypsin treatment. Thus, 7G8 parasites use
a sialic acid-independent, trypsin-sensitive
ligand for invasion. This trypsin-sensitive ligand
is not on glycophorin A or B as neuraminidase-
treated M^kM^k cells (which lack sialic acid and
glycophorin A and B) are invaded almost as efficiently as untreated M^kM^k RBCs. However, invasion
of trypsin-treated M^kM^k RBCs by 7G8 is markedly
reduced (JCI 80:1190, 1987). Since glycophorin C
is known to be trypsin-sensitive, we tested
glycophorin C-deficient RBCs from donor PL for
invasion by 7G8 parasites. These cells are
Gerbich negative and lack sialoglycoproteins β, β_1
and γ. The sialic acid-dependent pathway for
invasion on PL RBCs was eliminated by treatment
with neuraminidase. Invasion of neuraminidase-
treated PL RBCs by 7G8 parasites was only minimally reduced compared with untreated PL RBCs.

Invasion of untreated PL RBCs was slightly reduced compared with normal RBCs. Invasion of trypsin-treated PL RBCs was markedly reduced. These data indicate that glycophorin C alone is not the sialic acid-independent, trypsin-sensitive ligand for invasion.

INTRODUCTION

Optimal invasion of erythrocytes by <u>Plasmodium</u> <u>falciparum</u> malaria parasites requires the presence of sialic acid on the erythrocyte membrane. The majority of sialic acid on the erythrocyte membrane is on glycophorin A and this accounts for the importance of glycophorin A in invasion (1,2). The reduction in invasion of En(a-) erythrocytes, which lack glycophorin A, parallels the reduction obtained with neuraminidase-treated erythrocytes (Tables 1 and 2). The suboptimal invasion that does occur with glycophorin A-deficient erythrocytes has been attributed to the presence of a homologous molecule, glycophorin B (3). However, recent data indicate that the presence of glycophorin B cannot totally explain the invasion of En(a-) erythrocytes. These data are derived from experiments using M^kM^k erythrocytes, which lack both glycophorin A and glycophorin B (4). M^kM^k erythrocytes are invaded with efficiencies equal to or greater than En(a-) erythrocytes (Tables 1 and 2).

Studies with En(a-) erythrocytes, M^kM^k erythrocytes, Tn erythrocytes (which lack the O-linked oligosaccharides on the glycophorins) and neuraminidase-treated normal erythrocytes support the conclusion that some strains of <u>P. falciparum</u> are less dependent on erythrocyte sialic acid for invasion than other strains (4,5,6). The original experiments by Mitchell et al. that demonstrated a sialic acid independent pathway for invasion were done with uncloned parasites cultured in Tn erythrocytes (5). Subsequently, a cloned strain (7G8) cultured in normal erythrocytes was also shown to be capable of invading via a sialic acid-independent pathway (4). The 7G8 strain invades neuraminidase-treated M^kM^k erythrocytes with 50% efficiency (or greater) in contrast to the cloned Camp strain that invades neuraminidase-treated M^kM^k erythrocytes with less than 1% efficiency (Table 2). The 50% efficiency of invasion of 7G8 parasites into neuraminidase-treated M^kM^k erythrocytes indicates that this strain utilizes a pathway for invasion that is independent of sialic acid on the erythrocyte membrane and independent of glycophorins A and B. In contrast, the Camp strain relies almost totally on erythrocyte sialic acid for invasion.

The experiments on invasion by 7G8 parasites into M^kM^k erythrocytes also demonstrated that invasion is reduced if the M^kM^k erythrocytes are treated with trypsin (Table 2). This suggests that the non-glycophorin A, non-glycophorin B, sialic acid-independent pathway for invasion involves a ligand on the erythrocyte membrane that is sensitive to degradation by trypsin.

Because glycophorin C is known to be trypsin-sensitive, it was considered as a candidate for the sialic acid-independent, trypsin-sensitive ligand utilized by 7G8 parasites. To test this hypothesis, we studied invasion into erythrocytes of the Leach phenotype. These erythrocytes from donor PL have been well characterized by Anstee et al and lack three sialoglycoproteins β, β_1, γ that make up glycophorin C (7). The sialic acid-dependent pathway for invasion on these PL erythrocytes was eliminated by neuraminidase-treatment prior to testing invasion. If glycophorin C were the sialic acid-independent, trypsin-sensitive ligand for invasion, then invasion of neuraminidase-treated glycophorin C-deficient erythrocytes should be markedly reduced because both pathways for invasion would be absent.

As part of these experiments, we also studied the binding of a putative parasite receptor, designated the 175 kD erythrocyte-binding antigen of P. falciparum, to normal, M^kM^k and glycophorin C-deficient erythrocytes.

METHODS

Schizont-infected erythrocytes from culture were purified by the Percoll-Sorbitol method of Aley et al (8) and incubated with normal uninfected erythrocytes for 12 hours (ratio 1:10) in microtiter wells. At the end of the incubation period, smears were made of the cultured blood and stained with Wright-Giemsa. Newly-invaded erythrocytes were identified as typical ring-forms on light microscopy. Invasion "rates" were determined by counting 1000 RBCs; invasion "rate" is

defined as the percent of RBCs that were invaded (i.e.
parasitized with ring-forms). The term "efficiency of
invasion" is defined as the invasion rate of test cells
expressed as a percentage of the invasion rate obtained
with normal control cells. Glycophorin C-deficient
erythrocytes of the Leach phenotype were obtained from
donor PL. Normal control erythrocytes were obtained in
parallel and handled indentically. PL erythrocytes
have been previously characterized and lack the three
sialoglycoproteins, β, β_1, and γ, that make up glycophorin C (7). PL erythrocytes (1 x 10^8 /ml) and
control erythrocytes were treated with Vibrio cholerae
neuraminidase (GIBCO;50 U/ml) for 1 hour at 37°C and
washed in RPMI 1640 with 10% human serum which had been
preabsorbed with neuraminidase-treated erythrocytes.
Another aliquot of PL erythrocytes was treated with
trypsin-TPCK (Sigma;1 mg/ml for 1 hour at 37°C, washed,
then incubated with soybean trypsin inhibitor (Sigma;1
mg/ml) and washed again in RPMI with 10% serum.
    Experiments with M^kM^k erythrocytes were done in a
similar fashion and the results published elsewhere (4).
Absence of glycophorin A and B on the surface of the
M^kM^k erythrocytes was confirmed by surface-labeling
experiments and by non-reactivity of these erythrocytes
with specific antisera and lectins (4). Experiments
with En(a-) erythrocytes were done with frozen deglycerolized En(a-) erythrocytes from donor GW. Erythrocytes from this donor had been previously studied by
Miller et al. (9) who had obtained a 50% reduction in
invasion (using P. falciparum parasites from
chimpanzees) and by Pasvol et al. (10) who obtained
greater than a 90% reduction in invasion (using
parasites of a different strain which were maintained
in culture). Frozen deglycerolized En(a-) erythrocytes
were used because we were unable to obtain fresh En(a-)
erythrocytes. The normal control erythrocytes in
En(a-) experiments were freshly obtained.
    Experiments to determine whether the 175 kD
erythrocyte-binding antigen of P. falciparum binds to
M^kM^k erythrocytes and glycophorin C-deficient erythrocytes were done using the method described by Haynes et
al. (11). Briefly, culture supernatants of biosynthe-
tically radio-labeled parasites, containing radio-
labeled proteins, were incubated with erythrocytes.
Under these conditions the 175 kD erythrocyte-binding
antigen binds to normal erythrocytes but not to

neuraminidase-treated erythrocytes, trypsin-treated erythrocytes or Tn erythrocytes (11,12, and JD Haynes, unpublished). Unbound proteins are removed by centrifuging the erythrocytes through silicone oil (GE Versilube F50). Proteins that are bound to erythrocytes are eluted by 1.5 M NaCl and analyzed by SDS-polyacrylamide gel electopheresis.

RESULTS

Invasion of En(a-) Erythrocytes

Reduction in invasion of En(a-) erythrocytes by two different parasite strains parallels the reduction obtained with neuraminidase-treated erythrocytes.
Table 1 shows the percent invasion compared with control normal erythrocytes obtained with En(a-) and neuraminidase-treated En(a-) erythrocytes.

TABLE 1
INVASION OF UNTREATED AND ENZYME-TREATED NORMAL AND En(a-) ERYTHROCYTES BY TWO CLONED STRAINS OF PLASMODIUM FALCIPARUM (Camp and 7G8)*

Cell	Enzyme-Treatment	7G8	Camp	Ratio
Control	None	100	100	
Control	NANase	70	17	4.1:1
En(a-)	None	36	8	4.5:1
En(a-)	NANase	32	8	4 :1
En(a-)	Trypsin	1	1	

* Abbreviations: NANase, neuraminidase. Invasion is expressed as a percentage of the invasion rates into normal control erythrocytes. Invasion rate is the percentage of erythrocytes in culture that were invaded.

The En(a-) erythrocytes were thawed from cryopreservation; the absolute invasion rates obtained with these cells may be lower than those obtained with freshly obtained En(a-) cells because of the undefined effects of cryopreservation and thawing. Freshly obtained

En(a-) erythrocytes were not available for testing. However, the major finding of this experiment is that there is a difference in the efficiencies of invasion of the two stains (Camp and 7G8) tested and that this difference parallels the difference in the capabilities of these strains to invade neuraminidase-treated erythrocytes. The Camp strain, which invades neuraminidase- treated erythrocytes poorly, also invades En(a-) erythrocytes poorly; the 7G8 strain, which invades neuraminidase-treated erythrocytes with higher efficiency than the Camp strain (Table 2), also invades En(a-) erythrocytes with higher efficiency than the Camp strain. These findings suggest that glycophorin A is important for invasion because of its sialic acid residues. Also, the data indicate that there is a trypsin-sensitive ligand on En(a-) erythrocytes which is important for invasion.

Invasion of M^kM^k Erythrocytes

TABLE 2

INVASION OF UNTREATED AND ENZYME-TREATED
M^kM^k ERYTHROCYTES BY TWO CLONES OF
PLASMODIUM FALCIPARUM (Camp and 7G8)*

Cell	Enzyme-Treatment	Camp	7G8
M^kM^k	None	20	86
M^kM^k	NANase	0.8	55
M^kM^k	Trypsin	27	14
Control	None	100(6)	100 (17.0)
Control	NANase	1.6	70
Control	Trypsin	8.5	0.6

* Abbreviations: NANase, neuraminidase. The data are expressed as the percentage of the maximum invasion rate obtained with untreated normal control erythrocytes. The maximum invasion rate is in parenthesis and represents the percentage of erythrocytes in the culture that were invaded.

Glycophorins A and B are not required for invasion. The residual invasion of En(a-) erythrocytes by Plasmodium falciparum parasites has been attributed to glycophorin B which is homologous to glycophorin A for the first 26 N-terminal amino acids (10). In order to test this hypothesis, we tested invasion of P. falciparum parasites into M^kM^k erythrocytes which lack both glycophorin A and glycophorin B. The results of these experiments have been reported in full elsewhere (4); Table 2 shows the result of a representative experiment.

The data shown in Table 2 indicate that M^kM^k erythrocytes can be invaded by P. falciparum parasites. Also, a difference in the efficiencies of invasion is again noted between the two strains of parasites (Camp and 7G8) tested. The Camp strain, which is more dependent on erythrocyte sialic acid for invasion, invades M^kM^k erythrocytes less efficiently than the 7G8 strain which is less dependent on erythrocyte sialic acid for invasion. These results are similar to those obtained with En(a-) erythrocytes, and again suggest that the glycophorins are important for optimal invasion because of their sialic acid residues. These data also indicate that glycophorin A and glycophorin B, are not required for invasion by the parasite. However, the presence of at least glycophorin A appears to be necessary for optimal invasion.

There is a striking difference between the Camp strain and the 7G8 strain in terms of their abilities to invade neuraminidase-treated M^kM^k erythrocytes. Invasion of neuraminidase-treated M^kM^k erythrocytes by Camp parasites falls almost to zero, whereas invasion by 7G8 parasites occurs with about 50% efficiency. Thus, 7G8 parasites appear to be capable of invading by a pathway that is independent of sialic acid on the erythrocyte membrane. In contrast, when M^kM^k erythrocytes are first treated with trypsin, invasion by 7G8 parasites decreases significantly. This finding suggests that the sialic acid-independent ligand (or ligands) is sensitive to degradation by trypsin. It is interesting that in these experiments, trypsin-treatment of normal cells had a more profound effect on invasion than trypsin-treatment of M^kM^k cells. M^kM^k cells may have other undefined abnormalities, such as alternate glycosylation, which render the sialic acid-independent pathway less susceptible to trypsin.

Invasion of Glycophorin C-Deficient Erythrocytes

Glycophorin C alone is not the sialic acid-independent ligand. Glycophorin C is known to be sensitive to degradation by trypsin when intact erythrocytes are treated with the enzyme (1). Therefore, glycophorin C was considered to be a candidate for the sialic acid-independent, trypsin-sensitive ligand. The approach taken to test this possibility was to test invasion of 7G8 parasites into glycophorin C-deficient erythrocytes that had been treated with neuraminidase to remove the sialic acid-dependent pathway for invasion. Based on the 14 percent efficiency of invasion of trypsin-treated M^kM^k erythrocytes, the efficiency of invasion of neuraminidase-treated PL erythrocytes by 7G8 parasites, should also be 14 percent or less if glycophorin C constitutes the sialic acid-independent, trypsin-sensitive ligand. The results of the experiment are shown in Tables III and IV.

TABLE 3

INVASION OF UNTREATED AND ENZYME-TREATED GLYCOPHORIN C-DEFICIENT ERYTHROCYTES OF THE LEACH PHENOTYPE (PL) BY TWO CLONES OF PLASMODIUM FALCIPARUM*

Cell	Enzyme- Treatment	Camp	7G8
Control	None	100 (16.0)	100 (14.1)
Control	Trypsin	7.5	0.2
Control	NANase	0.6	39.7
PL	None	85.6	91.5
PL	Trypsin	3.8	0.6
PL	NANase	2.5	83.0

* Abbreviations: NANase, neuraminidase; PL, glycophorin C-deficient erythrocytes of the Leach phenotype. The data are expressed as the percentage of the maximum invasion rate obtained with untreated normal control erythrocytes. The maximum invasion rate is given in parenthesis and is the percentage of erythrocytes in the culture that were invaded.

TABLE 4

INVASION OF UNTREATED AND ENZYME-TREATED
GLYCOPHORIN C-DEFICIENT ERYTHROCYTES (PL)
OF THE LEACH PHENOTYPE (PL) BY TWO CLONES
OF <u>PLASMODIUM FALCIPARUM</u>*

Cell	Enzyme-Treatment	Camp	7G8
Control	None	100 (17.5)	100 (22.8)
PL	None	45.1	50
PL	NANase	12.0	32

* The erythrocytes in this experiment were thawed from cryopreservation; however, the invasion rate obtained with thawed cryopreserved control erythrocytes (17.5% and 22.8%) were essentially the same as those obtained with freshly obtained erythrocytes (data not shown). The data are expressed as the percentage of the maximum invasion rate obtained with untreated normal control erythrocytes.

The data in Tables 3 and 4 indicate that invasion of neuraminidase-treated PL erythrocytes did not fall to the low level expected if glycophorin C were the trypsin-sensitive ligand. Furthermore, invasion of PL erythrocytes <u>did</u> fall dramatically after trypsin-treatment. These data indicate that glycophorin C alone is not the sialic acid independent, trypsin-sensitive ligand. The data does not exclude the N-linked oligosaccaride as a receptor; this oligosaccharide is found on both glycophorin A and glycophorin C.

In the experiment shown in Table 3 using freshly obtained erythrocytes, the invasion of PL erythrocytes was only slightly reduced compared with controls. This result is somewhat different from the result reported by Pasvol et al. who found nearly a 50% reduction in invasion into freshly obtained PL erythrocytes (13). In the experiment shown in Table 4, in which PL and control erythrocytes had been thawed from cryopreservation, we obtained a reduction in invasion similar to that observed by Pasvol et al (13).

Binding of the 175kD Erythrocyte-Binding Antigen

The 175kD protein binds to glycophorin C-deficient erythrocytes but binding is reduced or absent with M^kM^k erythrocytes. Previous studies have identified a 175 kD protein of P. falciparum that binds in a receptor-specific fashion to human erythrocytes with a normal sialic acid content (12). The 175 kD antigens does not bind to neuraminidase-treated erythrocytes or to Tn erythrocytes, both of which show markedly reduced invasion with Camp parasites (12). An experiment was therefore done to determine whether the 175 kD protein binds to M^kM^k erythrocytes and to PL erythrocytes. The results indicate that the 175 kD protein of Camp parasites shows reduced or absent binding with M^kM^k erythrocytes and binds normally to PL erythrocytes. (Data not shown). Similar experiments have not yet been done with the 175 kD protein of 7G8 parasites.

DISCUSSION

The goal of identifying erythrocyte ligands for malaria parasites is important because information about erythrocyte ligands can be used to identify parasite receptors. It is hoped that parasite receptor molecules can be used as immunogens to induce anti-receptor antibodies that block invasion (2). Identification of sialic acid on the erythrocyte membrane as important for invasion contributed to the identification of a 175 kD protein of P. falciparum that binds to erythrocytes in a sialic acid-dependent fashion (12). The 175 kD protein is currently considered as a candidate for a parasite receptor and the protein is being purified for further studies.

A protein analogous to the 175kD protein of P. falciparum has been identified from the monkey malaria parasite, P. knowlesi. (11) This protein, which is 135 kD, binds to human erythrocytes that contain the Duffy blood group antigens but not to erythrocytes which lack the Duffy blood group antigens. This specificity of binding is what would be expected of a P. knowlesi receptor because P. knowlesi can invade only human erythrocytes that contain the Duffy blood group antigens and cannot invade human erythrocytes that lack these antigens (9, 14). The 135 kD protein is also considered to be a potential parasite receptor of P. knowlesi and is being purified for further studies.

Previous work on erythrocyte ligands for P. falciparum parasites focused on glycophorins A and B. However, the studies presented and reviewed here indicate that some strains of P. falciparum can invade erythrocytes in the absence of glycophorins A and B. Furthermore, the studies suggest that some strains of P. falciparum have more than a single receptor for invasion and utilize more than a single ligand on the erythrocyte membrane.

A two receptor model for invasion was first proposed for P. knowlesi by Miller et al (14). This model was based on the finding that P. knowlesi parasites bind to both Duffy-positive and Duffy-negative erythrocytes (14), but can invade only Duffy-positive erythrocytes. Electron microscopic studies showed that the attachment of P. knowlesi parasites to Duffy-negative erythrocytes is characterized by fine fibrillar material extending between the surface of the parasite and the surface of the erythrocyte, whereas attachment of P. knowlesi parasites to Duffy-positive erythrocytes is characterized by a tight junction between the parasite and the erythrocyte (14). Thus, at least two erythrocyte ligands (and presumably parasite receptors) appear to be operative: one is required for attachment and is found on Duffy-positive and Duffy-negative erythrocytes; the other is required for junction-formation (and subsequent invasion) and is found only on Duffy-positive erythrocytes.

Based on the work presented and reviewed here, we propose a two receptor model for some strains of P. falciparum. One receptor (the 175 kD erythrocyte-binding protein) binds to a sialic acid-dependent site predominantly on glycophorin A; the other receptor (not yet identified) binds in a sialic acid-independent fashion to a ligand (also not yet identified) other than glycophorin A or B.

Because the non-glycophorin A, non-glycophorin B ligand appears to be sensitive to degradation by trypsin, the possibility arose that it may be glycophorin C. Also, glycophorin C-deficient erythrocytes had previously been shown to be somewhat resistant to invasion by P. falciparum (13). However, the studies reported here indicate that glycophorin C alone is not the sialic acid-independent, trypsin-sensitive ligand for invasion. This conclusion is based on the finding that neuraminidase treatment of glycophorin C-deficient erythrocytes (which eradicates the sialic acid-dependency pathway for invasion) caused only a slight reduction in invasion by 7G8 parasites.

The slight reduction in invasion obtained with untreated glycophorin C-deficient erythrocytes may be due to the fact that these erythrocytes are ellipto-cytic; other elliptocytic erythrocytes such as those deficient in band 4.1, with a partial deficiency of glycophorin C, are somewhat refractory to invasion by both P. falciparum and P. knowlesi (15). (As these parasites utilize different erythrocyte ligands for invasion, the refractoriness observed is probably due a disruption of the invasion process at a step following reception). Mohandas et al. have shown that erythro-cytes with increased membrane rigidity, such as Melanesian ovalocytes, are resistant to invasion, presumably by a mechanism independent of receptor-ligand interactions (16). Such mechanisms of resistance to invasion must be considered when using erythrocyte variants or anti-erythrocyte antibodies that cause reduced invasion (15).

The studies reviewed here indicate that the peptide portions of glycophorins A, B and C are not required for invasion. The glycophorins, especially glycophorin A, appear to supply the sialic acid-dependent site required for optimal invasion. Binding may require N-acetylneuraminic acid plus adjacent sugars on the O-linked oligosaccarides (17). However, the biologic evidence points to the existence of another important ligand-site for invasion which is independent of sialic acid. The N-linked oligosaccha-ride on glycophorins A and C should be considered. Also, molecules other than glycophorin A, B and C should be considered. Identification of a second ligand and second receptor may be important for development of a vaccine; both receptors may be required to induce antibodies that block invasion.

ACKNOWLEDGMENTS

We gratefully acknowledge Dr. Yasuto Okubo at the Osaka Red Cross Blood Center, Osaka, Japan for providing M^kM^k erythrocytes and Rachel Moore at the American Red Cross Medical Operations Laboratory in Bethesda, Maryland for providing En(a-) erythrocytes.

REFERENCES

1. Anstee DJ (1981). The blood group MN
    Ss-active sialoglycoproteins. Semin Hematol
    18:13.

2. Hadley TJ, Miller LH (1989) Invasion of
    erythrocytes by malaria parasites: erythrocyte
    ligands and parasite receptors. Prog Allery
    41:49.

3. Pasvol G, Jungery M, Weatherall DJ, Parsons
    SF, Anstee DJ, Tanner MJA (1982) Glycophorin
    as a possible receptor for Plasmodium
    falciparum. Lancet ii:937.

4. Hadley TJ, Klotz FW, Pasvol G, Haynes JD,
    McGinniss MH, Okubo Y, Miller LH (1987).
    Falciparum malaria parasites invade erythrocytes
    that lack glycophorin A and B ($M^k M^k$). Strain
    differences indicate receptor heterogeneity and
    two pathways for invasion. J Clin Invest 80:1190.

5. Mitchell GH, Hadley TJ, Klotz FW, McGinniss
    MH, Miller LH (1986) Invasion of erythrocytes
    by Plasmodium falciparum malaria parasites:
    evidence for receptor heterogeneity and two
    receptors. Blood 67:1519.

6. Perkins ME, Holt EH (1988) Erythrocyte receptor
    recognition varies in Plasmodium falciparum
    isolates. Mol Biochem Parasit 27:23

7. Anstee DJ, Parsons SF, Ridgewell K, Tanner
    MJA, Merry AH, Thomson EE, Judson PA, Johnson
    P, Bates S, Fraser ID (1983). Two individuals
    with elliptocytic red cells apparently lack minor
    erythrocyte membrane sialoglycoproteins. Biochem
    J 218:615.

8. Aley SB, Sherwood JA, Howard RJ (1984).
    Knob-positive and knob-negative Plasmodium
    falciparum differ in expression of a strain-
    specific malarial antigen on the surface of
    infected erythrocytes. J Exp Med 160:1585

9. Miller LH, Haynes JD, McAuliffe FM, Shiroishi T,
    Durocher JR, McGinniss MH (1977). Evidence for
    differences in erythrocyte surface receptors for
    the malarial parasites, Plasmodium falciparum
    and Plasmodium knowlesi. J Exp Med 146:277.

10. Pasvol G, Wainscot JS, Weatherall DJ (1982).
     Erythrocytes deficient in glycophorin resist
     invasion by the malarial parasite, Plasmodium
     falciparum. Nature 297: 64.
11. Haynes JD, Dalton JP, Klotz FW, McGinniss MH,
     Hadley TJ, Hudson DE, Miller LH (1988).
     Receptor-like specificity of a Plasmodium knowlesi
     malarial protein that binds to Duffy antigen
     ligands on erythrocytes. J Exp Med 167:1873.
12   Camus D, Hadley TJ (1985). A Plasmodium
     falciparum antigen that binds to host
     erythrocytes and merozoites. Science 230,
     553.
13. Pasvol G, Anstee D, Tanner MJA (1984).
     Glycophorin C and the invasion of red cells by
     Plasmodium falciparum Lancet. i:907.
14. Miller LH, Aikawa M, Johnson JG, Shiroishi T
     (1979) Interaction between cytochalasin B-treated
     malarial parasites and erythrocytes. Attachment
     and junction formation. J Exp Med 149:172.
15. Hadley TJ, Erkman Z, Kaufman BM, Futrovsky S,
     McGinniss M (1986) Factors influencing invasion of
     erythrocytes by Plasmodium falciparum parasites:
     The effects of an N-acetylglucosamine neoglyco-
     protein and an anti-glycophorin A antibody.
     Am J Trop Med Hyg 35:898.
16. Mohandas N, Lie-Imjo LE, Friedman M, Mak JW (1984)
     Rigid membranes of Malayan ovalocytes: a likely
     genetic barrier against malaria. Blood 63: 1385.
17. Hermentin P, Enders B. (1984) Erythrocyte invasion
     by malaria (Plasmodium falciparum) merozoites:
     Recent advances in the evaluation of receptor
     sites. Behring Inst Mitt 76: 121.

Cellular and Molecular Biology of Normal
and Abnormal Erythroid Membranes, pages 315–332

A MALARIA PHOSPHATIDYLINOSITOL-SPECIFIC PHOSPHOLIPASE C: A POSSIBLE ROLE IN MEROZOITE MATURATION AND ERYTHROCYTE INVASION

Catherine Braun Breton, Gordon Langsley, Jean-Christophe Barale and Luis H. Pereira da Silva

Unit of Experiment Parasitology, URA CNRS 146, Department of Immunology, Institut Pasteur, 25, rue du Docteur Roux, 75624 PARIS Cedex 15, FRANCE

ABSTRACT   The signal induced turnover of inositol phospholipids involves specific phospholipase C in different tissues. Here, we described a developmentally regulated phosphatidylinositol-specific phospholipase C of malaria parasites. The enzyme is a membrane bound, calcium independent phospholipase C and as such resembles the glycosyl-phosphatidylinositol-specific phospholipases C purified from rat liver plasma membranes and *Trypanosoma brucei* parasites. We also described the regulation by the malaria phospholipase C of a second parasite enzyme, a membrane bound serine protease. Finally, we discuss the possible role of phospholipase C in the generation of second messengers and how these might be involved in the invasion of erythrocytes by malaria merozoites.

This investigation received financial support from the UNDP/World Bank/WHO Special Programme for Research and Training in Tropical Diseases and grants from the Ministère de la Recherche et l'Enseignement Supérieur (Aide no. 87W0043-Eureka).

INTRODUCTION

Phosphatidylinositol and phosphatidylinositol phosphates have become a subject of great interest in the last few years because of their role in cellular transmembrane signalling (1). The hydrolysis of inositol lipids which can result from external stimuli (hormones, growth factors, neurotransmitters) gives rise to diacylglycerol and inositol trisphosphate which both act a second messengers (1). Diacylglycerol remains within the plane of the plasma membrane and activates protein kinases C, resulting in the phosphorylation of specific cellular proteins. Activation of protein kinase C has been correlated with the mobilisation of the enzyme from the cytoplasm and its binding to the plasma membrane (2-4). This translocation is probably also mediated by calcium (5). Inositol trisphosphate is released into the cytosol and causes a flux of calcium from the endoplasmic reticulum (6). Much of the calcium released from the internal reservoir is rapidly pumped out of the cell, but calcium entry across the plasma membrane is also enhanced (1).

Recently a novel inositol phosphate glycan has been implicated as a second messenger which regulates cyclic AMP phosphodiesterase in response to insulin (7). This substance is produced by the hydrolysis of a glycosyl phosphatidylinositol precursor, similar to the glycosyl phosphatidylinositol (GPI) anchor domain of various eukaryotic membrane proteins (8,9). The hydrolysis is catalyzed by a GPI specific phospholipase C (PLC) which has been recently purified from a liver plasma membrane fraction (10).

The possibility of calcium acting as a second messenger in the invasion of human erythrocytes by malaria parasites has been investigated (11). Although EGTA has been shown to reversibly inhibit invasion, it has no effect on the attachment of the merozoite to the red blood cell (11, 12). Moreover, EGTA trapped within erythrocyte ghosts fails to inhibit invasion (13). In agreement with this latter observation is that the level of intraerythrocytic calcium does not seem to be important for the invasion process (pers. comm.,14). Therefore, intraparasitic rather than intraerythrocytic calcium might be important during invasion. Mendoza and Wasserman have proposed that calcium might be liberated with the rhoptry contents, producing a transient and local higher concentration of calcium at the junction between the parasite and the red blood cell (14). The effect of calmodulin inhibitors in arresting invasion (15), suggests that calcium might be acting as a second messenger to induce changes in the erythrocyte cytoskeleton, necessary for the penetration of the parasite.

We have recently reported the characterization of a developmentally regulated phosphatidylinositol-specific phospholipase C (PI-PLC) in malaria merozoites (16). The properties of this enzyme are consistent with it playing a role in merozoite maturation and red blood cell invasion and here we describe these properties and discuss some of the possible regulatory roles for PI-PLC.

RESULTS

Time of synthesis of phospholipase C

If a phospholipase has a role in invasion, one would expect this enzyme to be synthesized, or to become active, at the time or about the time of erythrocyte invasion. The time course of synthesis has been investigated by exploiting the observation that PI-PLC can cleave the membrane form of a GPI anchored protein, to yield a soluble form of the protein and diacylglycerol (17). Our enzyme assay estimated the ability of 1% NP40 extracts of *Plasmodium falciparum* and *Plasmodium chabaudi* to liberate ^{3}H-myristate labelled dimyristoyglycerol from membrane form variant surface glycoprotein (mfVSG) of *Trypanosoma equiperdum* (18). In this way, a GPI anchor degrading activity can be detected at the end of the intraerythrocytic cycle, increasing as young schizonts (less than 4 nuclei) matured into merozoites (Table 1). The PI-PLC enzyme is 3 times more active in merozoites than in mature schizonts.

		relative PI-PLC activity	
		P. falciparum	*P. chabaudi*
mature trophozoites		<0.05	<0.05
schizonts	<4 nuclei	0.3	0.2
	4 to 8 nuclei	1	1
	>8 nuclei	1.5	2
merozoites		3	3
merozoites+pCMPS		<0.05	n t

Table 1: time-course of PI-PLC activity in *P. falciparum* and *P. chabaudi* parasites: 2 ug of ^{3}H myristate labelled membrane form VSG from *T.equiperdum* were incubated for 30 mn at 37°C in 50 mM Tris HCl, 5mM EDTA, 1% NP 40, pH 8,0 with 1% NP 40 extracts of *P. falciparum* and *P. chabaudi* proteins; the 3H di-acylglycerol released from VSG by phospholipase was recovered and measured in the organic phase after butanol extraction; the parasite extracts were prepared from synchronous cultures of parasites harvested at different stages of the intraerythrocytic cycle.

Type of phospholipase C

Using the same enzyme assay, we have compared the effects of various reagents on different GPI-anchor degrading activities : the plasmodial lipases, the *Trypanosoma brucei* VSG lipase and the *Bacillus cereus* PI-PLC. As shown in Table 2, the plasmodial phospholipases have a number of characteristics. They are unaltered by the presence of protease inhibitors. They exhibit an acute sensitivity to thiol reagents like DTT, $ZnCl_2$ and pCMPS, characteristics consistent with the involvement of a thiol group in the conformation of the active enzyme and finally, calcium and EDTA have no effect on these activities, indicating that they are calcium-independent PI-PLC. The fact that malaria PI-PLC are calcium independent enzymes makes them much more similar to bacterial and typanosome phospholipases C, that to mammalian PI-PLC.

| | PI-PLC | | | |
	P. falciparum 60kDa	P. chabaudi 50kDa	T.brucei 40kDa	B.cereus 30kDa
none	100	100	100	100
CaCl2 2mM	100	100	100	nt
10mM	80	90	95	90
EDTA 2mM	80	nt	85	nt
10mM	100	100	95	100
pCMPS 5mM	1	10	20	100
ZnCl2 2mM	50	nt	90	100
10mM	30	2	0	2
DTT 2mM	140	130	170	100
10mM	200	150	205	100
Triton 0.2%	100	nt	95	100
1%	66	40	70	70
Nacholate 0.2%	15	25	15	85
1%	2	2	2	70
leupeptine pepstatine 50ug/ml	100	100	100	100

Table 2: effects of various reagents on the glycosyl phosphatidylinositol anchor degrading activities

Localisation of the PI-PLC enzyme

A marked difference between the *T.brucei* PI-PLC and bacterial PI-PLC is the membrane association of the former enzyme, whereas the bacterial enzymes are soluble (19, 20). The *P.*

falciparum and *P. chabaudi* GPI-specific lipases behave as membrane associated proteins, since detergent was required for the solubilisation of the activities (Table 3). Moreover, greater than 80% of the PI-PLC activity was recovered in the detergent phase, in phase-partition experiments with Triton X114 (Table 3 and ref. 16). In conclusion, due to their association with membranes and their insensitivity to calcium, the malarial enzymes appear to be very similar to the trypanosome VSG lipase.

	fraction	relative activity
P. falciparum	osmotic lysis	
	soluble fraction	<0.05
	membrane pellet	0.4-0.5
P. chabaudi	TritonX114 partition	
	aqueous phase	<0.05
	detergent phase	0.8-0.9

Table 3: relative PI-PLC activity in soluble and membrane fractions. a relative activity of 1 corresponds to a 1% NP 40 extract of parasite proteins.

Partial purification of the PI-PLC activity

The malaria PI-PLC were partially purified on a phenylboronate column. As shown in Figure 2, the *P.falciparum* and *P.chabaudi* PI-PLC activities were concentrated in the 100 mM sorbitol eluate. These results suggest that the PI-PLC might be glycosylated and the purification should enable the enzyme kinetics to be studied.

Identification of the enzyme

Identification of the parasite proteins with GPI-PLC activities exploited the similarity between the malarial and trypanosomal enzymes. This similarity enable us to use a monoclonal antibody, mAT3, raised to *T. brucei* VSG lipase (21). In immunoblotting experiments, mAT3 reacted with a 60 kDa polypeptide in *P.falciparum* schizonts (Figure 1) and merozoites and a 50 kDa polypeptide in *P.chabaudi*.

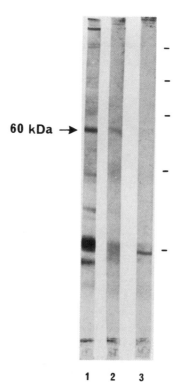

60 kDa →

1   2   3

Figure 1: Western-blot analysis of *P. falciparum* schizont extracts with monoclonal antibody mAT3 (lane 1) and polyclonal serum (lane 2) raised to VSG lipase and a non-immune serum (lane 3).

These mAT3 reactive polypeptides were also essentially recovered in the 100 mM sorbitol eluate of the phenylboronate column (Figure 2). This was the fraction which contained the PI-PLC activity. Finally, mAT3 immunoprecipitated the PI-PLC activities detected in the enzyme assay (Table 4). Taken together, these results are consistent with the idea that the 60 kDa *P.falciparum* and 50 kDa *P.chabaudi* proteins correspond to the PI-PLC enzymes.

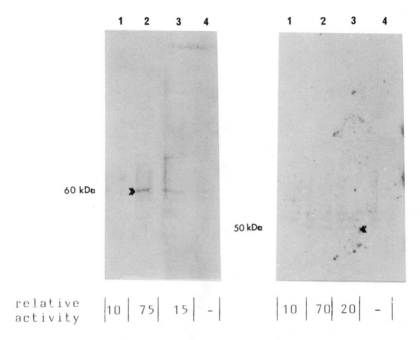

relative activity |10 | 75| 15| - | |10 | 70| 20| - |

Figure 2: mAT3 reactive polypeptides by Western blot and PI-PLC activity of different parasite protein fractions purified by phenylboronate chromato-graphy. lane 1: 10mM sorbitol eluate, lane 2: 100mM sorbitol eluate, lane 3: 1M guanidine eluate and lane 4: 3M guanidine eluate. The relative activity of the parasite extract loaded on the column was 100; that of unbound material was less than 1; - means less than 1.

relative GPI anchor degrading activity

	P. falciparum 1% NP 40	P. chabaudi 1% NP 40	T.brucei pure
NI serum	100	100	100
mAT3	60	60	50

Table 4: residual activity after immunoprecipitation with non immune serum (NI) and monoclonal antibody mAT3 purified immunoglobulins (mAT3).

Malaria proteins that are substrates for PI-PLC

Information on the possible physiological role of these enzymes can be expected from studies on solubilisation of GPI anchored membrane proteins from malaria merozoites, since the PI-PLC activity seems to be specific for this particular stage of the parasite cycle (see above). We have recently reported the identification of 7 membrane proteins of *P.falciparum* schizonts which fulfill the criteria of being GPI anchored proteins (17). They contain myristic acid and ethanolamine, they are solubilized by exogenous PI-PLC and after PI-PLC cleavage, they exhibit a cross-reactive determinant (CRD) epitope (22). Four of these proteins (the 45 kDa, 40 kDa, p76 polypeptides and a 80 kDa processing product of the p190 protein) were detected in merozoites (22, 23). Although it remains to be demonstrated that all of these antigens are substrates for the endogenous enzyme, we have clearly shown that the p76 protein is a substrate for the malaria PI-PLC.

A regulatory role for PI-PLC

In osmotically lysed schizonts, the p76 protein can be essentially recovered in the membrane fraction (Figure 3). In contrast, two forms of p76 are detected in osmotically lysed merozoites : a GPI anchored membrane form and a soluble form (Figure 3). In addition, this naturally occuring soluble form of p76 has been shown to exhibit a CRD epitope (22). Therefore, solubilisation of p76 is due to a PI-PLC activity, and when the osmotic lysis of merozoites was performed in the presence of 5 mM pCMPS, p76 was detected only as a membrane bound protein.

Interestingly, solubilisation of the membrane form of p76 by PI-PLC reveals a proteolytic activity (Figure 4, ref. 24). The solubilisation by PI-PLC is not true activation of the enzyme, since the membrane form of p76 binds DFP, indicating that the conformational change of the protein giving the active site of the enzyme has already taken place (23). Although the membrane form of p76 possesses an active site we were unable to detect a proteolytic activity associated with the membrane form, event after detergent extraction of the protein. In contrast, the soluble form of p76, released from schizont membranes, either by exogenous PI-PLC or by endogenous PI-PLC in merozoites, exhibits a gelatin gel sensitive protease activity (Figure 4). Both inhibitor studies and reaction with anti-chymotrypsin antibodies indicates that p76 is a chymotrypsin-like serine protease (23-24).

324   Breton et al.

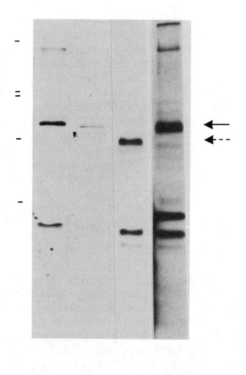

Figure 3: soluble and membrane associated forms of 35S methionine labelled p76 immunodetected with mAb Hb31cl3: schizont membranes (lane 1), schizont soluble fraction (lane 2), merozoite membranes (lane 3) and merozoite soluble fraction (lane 4).

Localisation of p76

IFA studies using monoclonal antibodies reacting with p76 suggested that p76 is associated with the rhoptries (25, 26). It is noteworthy that the rhoptry contents have been reported to play an important role in the invasion process and that a parasite serine protease is implicated in the red blood cell invasion by malaria merozoites (27-29). Even though the rhoptries are internal organs of merozoites, p76 must be in contact with the exterior, because the exogenous addition to intact merozoites of PI-PLC leads to release of the protein (24). The possible interaction between a membrane associated endogenous PI-PLC and the membrane form of p76 and the implications of this interaction for the invasion process are discussed.

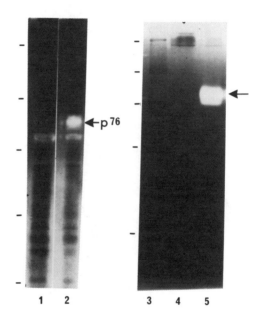

Figure 4:   exogenous activation of p76 serine protease: p76 protease was detected in schizont membrane extracts on gelatin-substrate polyacrylamide gels in schizont membranes (lane 1), schizont membranes treated with *S.aureus* PI-PLC (lane 2); p76 was identified by immunoprecipitation with mAb Hb31cl3 followed by gelatin-substrate PAGE using schizont membranes non treated (lane 4) and treated with PI-PLC (lane 5). lane 3 corresponds to molecular weight markers: 200, 97.4, 68, 43 and 30 kDa.

A regulatory role for PI-PLC in other Plasmodia

If such a mechanism of enzyme regulation is associated with red blood cell invasion, then it might be a common feature of all cell invading parasites, especially those having rhoptry organelles and therefore, present in other Plasmodia species. consistent with this hypothesis, we have identified in the rodent malaria parasite *P.chabaudi* a similar serine protease activity (65 kDa protein), which also depends on cleavage by PI-PLC (Figure 5 ref. 30). As for *P. falciparum*, *in vivo* induction of the 65 kDa proteolytic activity was detected in osmotically lysed merozoites (Figure 5).

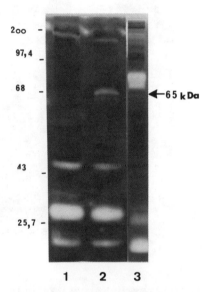

Figure 5: gelatin-substrate PAGE of *P. chabaudi* schizonts without PI-PLC treatment (lane 1) or treated with *S.aureus* PI-PLC (lane 2) and *P. chabaudi* merozoites without PI-PLC treatment (lane 3).

DISCUSSION

We have identified in two different *Plasmodium* species a developmentally regulated PI-PLC. The *P. falciparum* and *P. chabaudi* PI-PLC activities increased during the last step of the parasite maturation being maximal in merozoites, the form invasive for erythrocytes. What is inducing the PI-PLC activity remains to be determined, though several attractive possibilities exist. One form of regulation could involve the level of mRNA synthesis and the recent cloning of the *P. falciparum* PI-PLC gene should help elucidate this point (16). A second possibility might be that the PI-PLC activity is induced by some specific activator, in a way analogous to that by which insulin stimulates rat liver plasma membrane PI-PLC (31).

The Triton X114 partition experiments have shown that the plasmodial PI-PLC enzymes are membrane bound. Although preliminary IFA studies with mAT3 gave a faint fluorescence with the merozoite (not shown), the precise location within the merozoite is for the moment unknown. Expression of a large portion of the cloned gene and immunisation with the recombinant protein should yield a serum of sufficient quality to perform immunoelectron microscopy. This should define the localisation of PI-PLC within the parasite. Due to the similarity between the plasmodial PI-PLC and the *T. brucei* VSG lipase, our current working hypothesis however, is that the malaria enzyme is located in sub-membrane vesicles.

A precise cellular localisation for PI-PLC is important as the localisation could influence the substrate specificity. We have shown that several malaria GPI- anchored proteins are potential substrates for this enzyme. They contain ethanolamine and myristic acid and following solubilisation by exogenous PI-PLC display the CRD epitope. For one of these polypeptides, namely the p76, we have clearly demonstrated that it is a substrate for the endogenous enzyme. PI-PLC cleavage of the membrane form of p76 is only seen however, when the merozoites are lysed by osmotic shock. We interpret this as being a reflection of the compartmentalisation of the vesicular PI-PLC and the rhoptry membrane bound p76. The osmotic shock substituting for the signal necessary to induce fusion between the PI-PLC containing vesicles and the rhoptry membrane.

The question arises as to whether function of the malaria PI-PLC is simply to solubilize certain membrane bound proteins, or whether its role in the generation of the secondary messengers diacylglycerol and inositoltrisphosphate is also important. The malaria PI-PLC activity that we have identified appears to be a GPI-PLC activity. Cleavage of GPI produces diacylglycerol and an inositolphosphate glycan (9). Diacylglycerol is a well characterized activator of protein kinase C and in plasmodia, this could be responsible for the phosphorylation of the erythrocyte cytoskeleton during invasion (pers. comm., 32). Inositolphosphate glycan appears to be a promising candidate as a second messenger of insulin action (31) and if it results in an alteration of the calcium flux in way analogous to inositoltrisphosphate, then the PI-PLC described here, could also mediate the changes in calcium concentration which are associated with merozoite invasion of red blood cells (14).

Finally, regarding the regulation of the p76 serine protease by PI-PLC and its possible role in invasion, the following model appears attractive. The serine protease is first synthesised as an inactive zymogen, which is rapidly processed at the C-terminal end, resulting in the addition of the GPI anchor. A subsequent N-terminal processing event occurs leading to the conformational change which gives the active site. The membrane bound p76 binds DFP consistent with this model. Although possessing the active site the membrane bound form of p76 is catalytically inert. The merozoite stockpiles pre-activated, but inert p76 on the rhoptry membrane. At the moment of invasion a signal is received which causes the PI-PLC containing vesicles to fuse with the rhoptry membrane, such that when the rhoptry contents are released, the PI-PLC has solubilised the activated p76 resulting in a local high concentration of this chymotrypsin like serine protease. The activity of which appears to be necessary for invasion of erythrocytes to take place.

REFERENCES

1.   Berridge M.J. (1987). Inositol trisphosphate and diacylglycerol : two interacting second messengers. Ann. Rev. Biochem. 56: 159-193.

2.   Kraft AS and Anderson WA (1983). Phorbol esters increase the amount of Ca^{++}, phospholipid-dependent protein kinase associated with plasma membrane. Nature 301 : 621-623.

3.   Nishizuka Y. (1984). The role of protein kinase C in cell surface signal transduction and tumour promotion. Nature 308: 693-698.

4.   Wolf M, Le Vine Harry III, May WS Jr, Cuatrecasas P and Sahyoun N (1985). A model for intracellular translocation of protein kinase C involving synergism between Ca^{++} and phorbol esters. Nature 317: 546-549.

5.   May WS Jr, Sahyoun N, Wolf M and Cuatrecasas P (1985). Role of intracellular calcium mobilization in the regulation of protein kinase C-mediated membrane processes. Nature 317: 549-551.

6.   Berridge MJ and Irvine RF (1984). Inositol trisphophate, a novel second messenger in cellular signal transduction. Nature 312: 315-321.

7.   Saltiel AR, Fox JA, Sherline P & Cuatrecasas P (1986). Insulin-stimulated hydrolysis of a novel glycolipid generates modulators of cAMP phosphodiesterase. Science 233: 967-972.

8.   Saltiel AR & Cuatrecasas P (1986). Insulin stimulates the generation from hepatic plasma membranes of modulators derived from an inositol glycolipid. Proc. Nat. Acad. Sci. USA 83 : 5793-5797.

9.   Saltiel AR, Sherline P & Fox JA (1987). Insulin-stimulated diacylglycerol production results from the hydrolysis of a novel phosphatidylinositol glycan. J. Biol. Chem. 262: 1116-1121.

10.   Fox JA, Soliz NM & Saltiel AR (1987). Purification of a phosphatidylinositol-glycan specific phospholipase C from liver plasma membranes : a possible target of insulin action. Prot. Nat. Acad. Sci. U.S.A. 84: 2663-2667.

11.   Wasserman M, Alarcon C & Mendoza PM (1982). Effects of Ca^{++} depletion on the asexual cell cycle of *P.falciparum*. Am. J. Trop. Med. Hyg. 31: 711-717.

12.   Johnson JG, Epstein N, Shiroishi T & Miller LH (1980). Factors affecting the ability of isolated *P. knowlesi* merozoites to attach to and invade erythrocytes.

Parasitology 80: 539-550.

13.   Dluzewski AR, Rangachari K, Wilson RJM and Gratzer WB (1983). A cytoplasmic requirement of red cell for invasion by malaria parasites. Mol. Biochem. Parasitol. 9: 145-160.

14.   Mendoza PM and Wasserman M . The role of Ca^{++} in the invasion of human erythrocytes by *P. falciparum*. Manuscript in preparation.

15.   Matzumoto Y, Perry G, Scheibel LW and Aikawa M (1987). Role of calmodulin in *P. falciparum*. Implications for erythrocyte invasion by the merozoite. Eur. J. cell. Biol. 45: 36-43.

16.   Braun Breton C, Blisnick T, Barbot P, Bülow R, Pereira da Silva L & Langsley G. Characterization of a glycosyl phosphatidylinositol-specific phospholipase C from malaria parasites. J. Biol. Chem. (Submitted).

17.   Low MG & Saltiel AR (1988). Structural and functional roles of glycosyl-phosphatidylinositol in membranes. Science 239 : 268-275.

18.   Cardoso de Almeida ML & Turner MJ (1983). The membrane form of variant surface glycoprotein of *T. brucei*. Nature 302 : 349-352.

19.   Ikezawa H and Taguchi R (1981). Phosphatidylinositol-Specific Phospholipase C from *Bacillus cereus* and *Bacillus thuringiensis*. Methods Enzymol. 71: 731

20.   Low   MG   (1981).   Phosphatidylinositol-Specific Phospholipase C from *Staphylococcus aureus*. Methods Enzymol. 71: 741

21.   Bülow R and Overath P (1986). Purification and characterization of the membrane form variant surface glycoprotein hydrolase of *T. brucei*. J. Biol. Chem. 261 : 11918-11923.

22.   Braun-Breton C, Rosenberry TL & Pereira da Silva LH Glycolipid anchorage of *P. falciparum* membrane

proteins. Proc. Natl. Acad. Sci. USA (Submitted).

23.   Braun-Breton C & Pereira da Silva LH (1988). Activation of a *P. falciparum* protease correlated with merozoite maturation and erythrocyte invasion. Biol. of the Cell 64: 223-231.

24.   Braun-Breton C, Rosenberry TL & Pereira da Silva LH (1988). Induction of the proteolytic activity of a membrane protein in *P. falciparum* by phosphatidylinositol-specific phospholipase C. Nature 332 : 457-459.

25.   Clark JT, Anand R, Akoglu T & MacBride JS (1987). Identification and characterization of proteins associated with the rhoptry organelles of *P. falciparum* merozoites. Parasitol. Res. 73 : 425-434.

26.   Schofield L, Bushell GR, Cooper JA, Saul AJ, Upcroft JA & Kidson C (1986). A rhoptry antigen of *P. falciparum* contain conserved and variable epitopes recognized by inhibitory monoclonal antibodies. Mol. Biochem. Parasitol. 18 : 183-195.

27.   Aikawa M, Miler LH, Johnson J and Rabbege J (1978). Erythrocyte entry by malarial parasites : a moving junction between erythrocyte and parasite . J. Cell. Biol. 77 : 72-82.

28.   Hadley T, Aikawa M & Miller LH (1983). *P. knowlesi* : studies on invasion of rhesus erythrocytes by merozoites in the presence of protease inhibitors. Exp. Parasitol. 55: 306-311.

29.   Dluzewski AR, Rangachari K, Wilson RJM & Gratzer WB (1986). *P. falciparum* : protease inhibitors and inhibition of erythrocyte invasion. Exp. Parasitol. 62: 416-422.

30.   Braun-Breton C, Blisnick T, Barale JC, & Pereira da Silva LH. *P. chabaudi* : Phospholipase C cleavage of a protein results in ints activation as a serine protease. Submitted.

31.   Saltiel AR, Osterman DG, Darnell JC, Sorbara Cazan LR, Chan BL, Low MG & Cuatrecasas P (1988). The function of glycososyl phosphoinositides in hormone action. Phil. Trans. R. Soc. Lond. B 320: 345-358.

32.   Vernot JP, & Wasserman M. Changes in the phosphorylation of the erythrocyte cytoskeleton during invasion of *P. falciparum*. Manuscript in preparation.

Index

Acanthocytosis, 29
Actin, 27
    protein 4.1 and, 66
Alpha spectrin
    brain and, 6–7
    exon/intron organization of,
        202–205
    hereditary elliptocytosis and,
        211–221
    kinase activity and, 119–120
    mammalian cells and, 147
Alpha1 variants of spectrin, 235–248
Alternative RNA splicing, 62–63
    protein 4.1 and, 67–69
Aminophospholipid, 162
Anemia, hemolytic; *see* Hereditary
        elliptocytosis; Hereditary pyropoi-
        kilocytosis
Ankyrin
    brain membrane and, 1
    mammalian cells and, 149–151
    phosphorylation and, 98–99
Ankyrin binding site, 27–41
    cdb3 binding assays and, 30
    non-denaturing gel shift electrophor-
        esis and, 30–31
    N-terminal band 3 peptides and, 31,
        34
    in vitro translated band 3 fragments
        and, 35
Ankyrin/cdb3 binding assay, 30
Ankyrin-independent site
    brain membrane and, 7–8
    discussion of, 16–19
    erythrocyte membranes and, 8–9
    stripped brain membranes and, 3–4
Antigen 85 kD, 292, 294–295

Aotus monkey erythrocytes, 249–265;
        see also Plasmodium falciparum-
        infected erythrocytes
Aspiration pressure, 195, 196
Autophosphorylation, spectrin,
        118–120
Avian erythroid cell, 146
    spectrin and, 147–149

Band 3
    ankyrin binding site on, 27–41
    mammalian cells and, 151–152
Band 7, 165
Band 4.9 phosphorylation, 99–100
Band 3 protein, modified, 283–299
Binding, 187, 188, 195
Beta spectrin
    brain and, 6–7
    kinase activity and, 119–120
    mammalian cells and, 147
    phosphorylated, 121–122
    structural characteristics of, 114
BFU-E; *see* Burst-forming uniterythroid
Brain membrane proteins, spectrin with,
        1–26; *see also* Spectrin, brain
        membrane proteins and
B6SUtA cells, 139
Burst-forming uniterythroid, 145

Calcium, 12–13
Calcium-calmodulin dependent kinase,
        103–104, 126
Calmodulin, spectrin and, 9–12
    inhibition and, 12–13
    membrane protein interactions and,
        19
Calpain, 295–296

cAMP dependent kinase, 126
Casein kinase, 115, 119
cDNA clone
    band 3 and, 33
    protein 4.1 and, 45, 46, 63–64
CFU-E; *see* Colony-forming unit-er-
        ythroid
Clone, cDNA
    band 3 and, 33
    protein 4.1 and, 45, 46, 63–64
Colony-forming unit-erythroid, 145
Cycloheximide in *Plasmodium falci-
        parum*-infected erythrocytes, 275
Cytoadherence, 283–299
Cytoplasmic aggregates, 19–20
Cytoplasmic domain of band 3, 27–41
Cytoskeleton, phospholipid and,
    163–164

Deformability, 185–199
Deformation
    phosphorylation and, 93–95
    ultrastructural basis of, 175–176
Detergent-solubilized stripped brain
        membrane, 14–16
Dimer, rigidity and, 197
Dimethylsulfoxide, 133
DMSO; *see* Dimethylsulfoxide

Echinocytic red cell ghost, 179
EDTA, 319
EGTA, 316, 317
85 kD antigen, 292, 294–295
Electrophoresis, sodium dodecyl sulfate
        polyacrylamide gel, 115–116,
        117
Elliptocytosis, hereditary
    alpha spectrin abnormalities and,
        213–214
    alpha spectrin and, 211–221
    function and structure of mutant
        spectrin and, 215–216
    North Africa and, 223–234
    polymerase chain reaction and,
        201–210
    primary defect and, 216–217

spectrin A1 variants and, 235–248
spectrin deficiency and, 189, 191
En(a-) erythrocytes, 302, 305–306
Endothelium, malarial parasite and, 284
Epinephrine, skeletal protein phosphor-
        ylation and, 103
Erythroblast, development of, 146–147
Erythroid-specific motif, 56–57
Erythroleukemia cell, murine, 18
    erythropoietin and, 133
Erythropoietin receptor expression,
        131–144
    cell culture and, 133
    discussion of, 138–140
    growth factors and, 135–138
    quantitation of receptors and,
        133–134
    time course of binding, 134–135
Excrescences, malarial parasite and, 284
Exon/intron organization of A spectrin
        gene, 202–205

Fibonectin matrix, 18
Fragmentation, 93–95

G-CSF; *see* Human granulocyte colony-
        stimulating factor
Ghost, red cell, 179
Glycophorin C, *Plasmodium falciparum*
        and, 301–314
    deficiency and, 308–309
    En(a-) erythrocytes and, 305–306
    175kD erythrocyte-binding antigen
        and, 310
    M^kM^k erythrocytes and, 306–307
Glycosyl phosphatidylinositol, 316,
        317, 318, 323
Granulocyte-macrophage colony-stimu-
        lating factor, 135–136
Growth factors, erythropoietin and,
        135–138

HE; *see* Hereditary elliptocytosis
Hemolytic anemia; *see* Hereditary ellip-
        tocytosis; Hereditary Pyropoikilo-
        cytosis

Hereditary defect of band 3, 29
Hereditary elliptocytosis
    alpha spectrin abnormalities and,
        213–214
    alpha spectrin and, 211–221
    function and structure of mutant
        spectrin and, 215–216
    North Africa and, 223–234
    polymerase chain reaction and,
        201–210
    primary defect and, 216–217
    spectrin A1 variants and, 235–248
    spectrin deficiency and, 189, 191
Hereditary pyropoikilocytosis, 153–155
    alpha spectrin and, 211–221
    ultrastructural alterations in,
        176–177
Hereditary spherocytosis, 152–153
    membrane lipid loss and, 178
    spectrin deficiency and, 189
    ultrastructural alterations in,
        176–177
Heterodimer, spectrin, 212–213
Hormone, skeletal protein phosphoryla-
    tion and, 103
HPP; see Hereditary pyropoikilocytosis
HS; see Hereditary spherocytosis
Human granulocyte colony-stimulating
    factor, 136

αI/50a kD abnormality, 206
αI/50b kD abnormality, 207
αI/68 kD abnormality, 205–206
Inner leaflet, phospholipid and, 162,
    163–164
Inositol phosphate glycan, 316
Inside out vesicle, 215
Intramembranous particles in malarial
    parasite, 288
In vitro spectrin phosphorylation, 114,
    121, 122, 124–127
    beta, 123
In vivo spectrin phosphorylation, 114,
    124–125
Isoforms, spectrin and, 20

Isotropic deformation, 187, 188
ITC-phlorizin, 276

Kinase phosphorylation, 89–112
    discussion of, 103–106
    multiple, 113–130
        autophosphorylation and,
            118–120
        discussion of, 125–127
        quantitation of, 121–124
        spectrin and, 116–118
    possible functions of, 91–95
    specific effects of, 95–102
Knobby line of *Plasmodium falciparum*,
    283–299

Lipid bilayer deformability, 187–188
Lipid bilayer-skeleton uncoupling,
    178–180
Lymphoid protein 4.1 isoforms, 55

Malaria parasite
    glycophorin C and, 301–314
        deficiency and, 308–309
        En (a-) erythrocytes and,
            305–306
        175kD erythrocyte-binding anti-
            gen and, 310
        M^kM^k erythrocytes and, 306–307
    knobby line of *Plasmodium falci-
        parum* and, 283–299
    permeation sites and, 267–281
    phosphatidylinositol-specific phos-
        pholipase C, 315–332
        enzyme identification and,
            320–322
        localization of p76 and, 324–326
        location of enzyme and, 319–320
        in other *Plasmodia*, 326
        partial purification and, 320
        regulatory role of, 323
        substrates and, 323
        synthesis and, 317
        type of, 318
    phosphorylation and, 94–95
    rosetting and, 249–265

Mammalian erythrocyte, 145–160
  ankyrin and protein 4.1 and,
    149–151
  band 3 and, 151–152
  hereditary pyropoikilocytosis and,
    153–155
  hereditary spherocytosis and,
    152–153
  spectrin synthesis and, 147–149
Matrix, fibonectin, 18
Mechanical properties of membrane,
  185–199
Membrane skeletal protein
  ankyrin-binding site on, 27–41
  brain and, 1–26; see also Spectrin,
    brain membrane proteins and
  protein 4.1 and, 43–60
Membrane skeleton
  mammalian, 145–160
  mechanical properties and, 185–199
  molecular anatomy of, 171–183
  phosphatidylserine transport and,
    161–170
  phospholipid and, 163–164
  phosphorylation and; see Phosphory-
    lation, kinase
  phosphorylation mediated associa-
    tions of, 89–112
  protein 4.1 mRNA and, 61–74
  Rh polypeptides and, 75–87
Merozoite maturation, 315–332
M^kM^k erythrocytes, 301–303, 306–307
Monoclonal antibody 4A3, 288, 290,
  291, 293
Motifs I-V, 47–48
mRNA
  protein 4.1, 63
    detection of, 49, 52, 53
  protein 4.1 and, 61–74
mRNA splicing events, 43, 44
Murine erythroleukemia cell, 18
  erythropoietin and, 133
Murine GM979 cells, 131, 136
Mutation, protein 4.1 and, 69–70

Neural spectrin-based membrane skeleton, 2–3

Non-denaturing gel shift electrophoresis,
  30–31
Nonerythroid cell, 54–56
Nonerythroid protein 4.1, 70–71
Non-rosetting parasites, 253
N terminal band 3 peptide, 31, 34
N terminal :ga I domain, 212–213

OCIM1 cell line, 131, 134–138
Open reading frames, protein 4.1 and,
  67–67
Outer leaflet, phospholipid and, 162,
  163–164, 165–166

Parasite, malaria; see Malaria parasite
Peptide, N-terminal band 3, 31, 34
Permeation sites, Plasmodium falciparum-infected erythrocytes and,
  267–281
pHB3-45, 33, 34
Phlorizin analog, 276–279
Phosphatase, role of, 105
Phosphatidylinositol-specific phospholipase C, 315–332
  enzyme identification and, 320–322
  location of enzyme and, 319–320
  in other Plasmodia, 326
  partial purification and, 320
  substrates and, 323
  type of, 318
Phosphatidylserine, 161–170
Phospholipid asymmetry, 162–165
Phosphorylation, kinase
  mechanical stress and, 93–95
  multiple, 113–130
    autophosphorylation and,
      118–120
    discussion of, 125–127
    quantitation of, 121–124
    spectrin and, 116–118
  possible functions of, 91–95
  specific effects of, 95–102
Phosphorylation mediated associations
  of membrane skeleton, 89–112
PI-PLC; see Phosphatidylinositol-specific phospholipase C
Plasma membrane, 3

Plasmodium berghei, 94–95
Plasmodium chabaudi, 317, 320, 321, 322, 326, 327
Plasmodium cynomolgi, 251, 260
Plasmodium falciparum
    glycophorin C and, 301–314
        En(a-) erythrocytes and, 305–306
        175kD erythrocyte-binding antigen and, 310
        M^{k}M^k erythrocytes and, 306–307
    phosphatidylinositol-specific phospholipase C and, 315–332
        enzyme identification and, 320–322
        location of enzyme and, 319–320
        partial purification and, 320
        substrates and, 323
        type of, 318
Plasmodium falciparum-infected erythrocytes, 249–265
    assay for rosetting and, 251
    discussion of, 260–263
    identification of rosettes and, 253–260
    modified band 3 protein and, 283–299
    parasites and, 252–253
    permeation sites in, 267–281
        biophysical properties and, 272–274
        measurement and evaluation of transport and, 270–272
        pores and, 275–280
Plasmodium fragile, 251, 260, 261
Plasmodium vivax, 251, 260
PL erythrocyte, 304, 309
Polymerase chain reaction, 201–210
    protein 4.1 and, 63
Polypeptides, Rh, 75–87
    comparison of, 80–81
    fatty acid acylation of, 83–84
    identification of, 76–78
    isolation of, 78–79
    nonhuman analogs of, 81
Pore in *Plasmodium falciparum*-infected erythrocytes, 273–280
Pre-mRNA, 62–63

Pressure, aspiration, 195, 196
Prostaglandin, skeletal protein phosphorylation and, 103
Protein
    ankyrin-binding site on, 27–41
    brain membrane, 1–26; *see also* Spectrin, brain membrane proteins and
    Plasmodium falciparum-infected erythrocytes, 283–299
    spectrin-membrane interactions and, 13
Protein 4.1
    abnormal, 192, 197–198
    isoforms of, 43–60
        erythroid and non-erythroid cells and, 49, 52–56
        sequence blocks of, 47–48
    mammalian cells and, 149–151
    mRNA structure and, 61–74
    phosphorylation and, 98
    spectrin and actin and, 27
PS; *see* Phosphatidylserine
Pyropoikilocytosis, 153–155
    alpha spectrin and, 211–221
    function and structure of mutant spectrin and, 215–216
    primary defect and, 216–217
    ultrastructural alterations in, 176–177

Reverse transcriptase/polymerase chain reaction, 65–67
Rh polypeptides, 75–87
    comparison of, 80–81
    fatty acid acylation of, 83–84
    identification of, 76–78
    isolation of, 78–79
    nonhuman analogs of, 81
Rigidity of membrane, 193–197
RNA spicing, alternative, 62–63
Rosetting, *Plasmodium falciparum*-infected erythrocytes and
    assay for, 251
    identification of, 253–260
    purification of, 259

Schizont, 284, 303
SDS PAGE, 115–116, 117
Self-association, Sp, 215
Self-association, SpD, 212–213
Sequestration, malarial parasite and, 284–285
Shear stress, 187, 188
  phosphorylation and, 93–95
Sodium dodecyl sulfate polyacrylamide gel electrophoresis, 115–116
SpD self-association, 212–213
Spectrin
  abnormalities in, 197–198
  alpha
    exon/intron organization of, 202–205
    hereditary elliptocytosis and, 211–221
    kinase activity and, 119–120
  A1 variants of, 235–248
  ankyrin binding and, 98–99
  ankyrin-independent sites and, 7–8
  autophosphorylation and, 118–120
  brain membrane proteins and, 1–26
    alpha and beta subunits and, 6–7
    ankyrin-independent protein sites and, 3–9
    calmodulin and, 9–12
    calmodulin inhibition and, 13
    detergent-solubilized stripped brain membranes and, 14, 16
    differential regulation and, 13
    discussion of, 16–20
    stripped synaptosomal membranes and, 12–13
  deformation and, 189
  elliptocytosis and, 201–210
  kinase phosphorylation and, 113–130; see also Kinase phosphorylation
  mammalian cells and, 147–149
  phosphorylation, 121–124
  skeletal mass and, 172
  Spα$^{I/65}$ abnormality and, 228–229
  variants of, 192–196

Spectrin-actin-band 4.1 complex formation, 95, 98
Spectrin/actin binding domain, 66
Spectrin heterodimer, 212–213
Spectrin-membrane protein interaction, 13
Spectrin Tunis, 230–231
Spherocytosis, hereditary, 152–153
  membrane lipid loss and, 178
  spectrin deficiency and, 189
  ultrastructural alterations in, 176–177
Spα$^{I/65}$ abnormality, 228–229
Spicule, membrane, 178–180
Splicing, alternative RNA, 62–63
  protein 4.1 and, 67–69
Splicing events, mRNA, 43, 44
Sp self-association, 215
Stability, membrane skeletal, 100–102
Stiffness, 195
Stress, mechanical, 187, 188
  phosphorylation and, 93–95
Stretch, phosphorylation and, 94
Stripped brain membrane, 14–16
Stripped synaptosomal membrane, 12–13
Synaptosomal membrane, stripped, 12–13

12-o-Tetradecanoyl phorbol 13-acetate, 100–102
TPA; see 12-o-Tetradecanoyl phorbol 13-acetate
Transbilayer movement of phospholipid, 164
Transcriptase, 65–67
Transport
  phosphatidylserine, 161–170
  Plasmodium falciparum-infected erythrocytes and, 267–281; *see also Plasmodium falciparum*-infected erythrocytes
Trifluoperazine, 11
Trophozoite, 284
  knobs and, 286–287
Trypanosoma brucei, 318

Trypanosoma equiperdum, 317
Tyrosine kinase, 104–105

Uncoupling, lipid bilayer-skeleton,
    178–180

Venular endothelium, malarial parasite
    and, 284
Vesicle, inside out, 215